Progress in Polio Eradication: Vaccine Strategies for the End Game

Developments in Biologicals

Vol. 105

This series «Developments in Biologicals» begins with Vol. 102 and is the continuation of IABs symposia series «Progress in Immunobiological Standardization», Vols 1-5, «Immunobiological Standardization», Vols 1-22 and «Developments in Biological Standardization», Vols 23-101.

KARGER

Basel · Freiburg · Paris · London · New York ·
New Delhi · Bangkok · Singapore · Tokyo · Sydney

Progress in Polio Eradication: Vaccine Strategies for the End Game

Institut Pasteur, Paris
June 28-30, 2000

Volume Editor *F. Brown*
Plum Island Disease Center, Greenport, New York, USA

Meeting Organisers *† Florian Horaud*
Institut Pasteur, Paris, France

Geoffrey Schild
N.I.B.S.C., Potters Bar, UK

David Wood
World Health Organization, Geneva, Switzerland

Proceedings of a symposium organized by
International Association for Biologicals, Geneva
with the co-operation of World Health Organization, Geneva
Pan American Health Organization, Washington
Institut Pasteur, Paris

43 figures and 26 tables, 2001

KARGER

Basel · Freiburg · Paris · London · New York ·
New Delhi · Bangkok · Singapore · Tokyo · Sydney

Developments in Biologicals

Bibliographic Indices. This publication is listed in bibliographic services, including Current Contents® and Index Medicus.

Drug dosage. The authors and the publisher have exerted every effort to ensure that drug selection and dosage set forth in this text are in accord with current recommendations and practice at the time of publication. However, in view of ongoing research, changes in government regulations, and the constant flow of information relating to drug therapy and drug reactions, the reader is urged to check the package insert for each drug for any change in indications and dosage and for added warnings and precautions. This is particularly important when the recommended agent is a new and/or infrequently employed drug.

Printed in Switzerland by Médecine et Hygiène, Genève.
ISBN 3-8055-7285-9

Organization of the Symposium

Session I	Status of Polio Eradication Chairperson: *Walt Orenstein*
Session II	The Biology and Molecular Biology of Polioviruses Chairperson: *Jeff Almond*
Session III	Current Poliovirus Vaccines Chairperson: *David Wood*
Session IV	When and How Can we Stop Vaccination? Chairperson: *John Furesz*
Session V	Risks of Reintroduction of Polio Post Eradication Chairperson: *Tapani Hovi*
Poster Session I	
Session VI	Post Eradication Issues Chairperson: *Barry Schoub*
Session VII	Possible Strategies for Stopping Immunisation Chairperson: *Sir Joe Smith*
Session VIII	What Vaccines Could be Used Post Eradication if They Were Needed? Chairperson: *John Petricciani*
Poster Session II	
Poster Session III	

Programme Committee

R. Crainic	Institut Pasteur
C. de Quadros	PAHO
M. Greco	IFPMA
† F. Horaud	IABs
H. Hull	WHO
R. Perez Bercoff	University of Rome
D. Salisbury	UK Department of Health
G. Schild	NIBSC, Coordinator
R. Sutter	CDC
D. Wood	NIBSC, Rapporteur
K. Zoon	CBER

The International Symposium on Progress in Polio Eradication: Vaccine Strategies for the End Game are grateful to the following companies for their financial support.

- Aventis Pasteur, France
- Chiron Behring GmbH, Germany
- Fondation Mérieux, France
- SmighKline Biologicals SA, Belgium

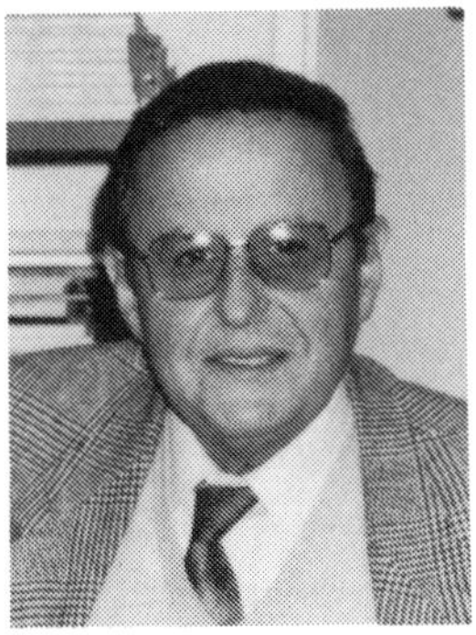

Professor Florian Horaud (1925-2000)

An Appreciation

Professor Florian Horaud, to whose memory this special volume of Developments in Biologicals is dedicated, passed away on 28 July 2000, in Paris at the age of 75. He had been fully active professionally and scientifically right up to the end of his life and was a wonderful friend and colleague of the many who were privileged to know and work with him.

Florian was a virologist par excellence who spent much of his career working on poliovirus and polio vaccine, both in his native Romania and at the Institut Pasteur in Paris. He had an enquiring mind and made an important contribution to polio research. His scientific memory was legendary and his knowledge of the history of vaccines and vaccination was second to none. His long career had brought him in touch with the great and he had been a friend and confidant of both Jonas Salk and Albert Sabin and many other famous figures of virology and medical science.

From 1992-2000 Florian served with great distinction as President of the International Association for Biological Standardization and took a great personal interest in the Symposia it organized. He worked tirelessly for the success of the Association. As President of the IABs, he was a great advocate for scientific research underpinning the quality, safety and standardization of biologicals.

Florian was born in Romania and graduated in medicine in 1951. He worked for several years (1953-1971) on poliovaccine development at the Cantacuzino Institute in Bucharest. In 1971 an opportunity arose to take up a Research Fellowship at the Institut Pasteur in Paris. There his talents were quickly recognised and shortly afterwards he was appointed Chief of the Laboratory of Medical Virology and eventually to a full Professorship and Headship of the Department of Virology. His work on poliovirus continued to flourish at the Pasteur and he was a major contributor to the work of a group at Pasteur who made important contributions to poliovirus research combining biological studies with modern molecular approaches.

Florian's long and wide experience of vaccines and vaccination and public health issues made him a most valuable participant in any forum on vaccines and other biologicals and their regulation. His advice was much sought after internationally. He was a frequent and active participant in many WHO committees. I well recall his important contributions to the work of the WHO Steering Committee on Poliovaccines in the 1980s. He was also a very prominent and active member of the Biotechnology Working Party - a scientific working party advising the Committee on Proprietory Medical Products of the EU - and took an active role from 1986 onwards in the drafting of the key European guidelines in relation to the production, quality control and standardization for biological and biotechnology products, a field in which his long and wide experience and scientific understanding were of great value. He remained an active and effective member of the Biotechnology Working Party right up to his death. In France he made a major contribution to the safety of biologicals. He was a special adviser to the Agence Française de Sécurité Sanitaire des Produits and the Chairman of its Advisory Committee on Viral Safety from 1993-2000. It should not be assumed that Florian was a 'yes' man in committee. He was indeed a vigorous, highly articulate defender of his views which almost always were strongly based on science, practical experience and common sense.

Florian had a successful entrepreneurial bent to his character. He was much involved in establishing a Biotechnology Service Unit (Texcell) at the Institut Pasteur and was its Scientific Director from 1987-1993.

One of Florian's last achievements was the organization of the Symposium on Progress in Polio Eradication; its great success reflected his wisdom and eminence in the field. This volume will be a fitting and lasting tribute to Florian and his work and I am sure it will remain a standard reference work on polio and poliovaccines for many years to come.

Florian was a scientist of great personal charm and generosity of spirit. He had an extraordinarily infectious enthusiasm for science and international co-operation. He will be much missed by all his very many colleagues and friends around the world. Florian is survived by his wife Thea, an eminent microbiologist, and their two sons.

G. C. Schild
NIBSC, Potters Bar

Contents

Brown F (ed): Progress in Polio Eradication: Vaccine Strategies for the End Game.
Dev Biol. Basel, Karger, 2001, vol 105, p 1

SESSION I

Status of Polio Eradication

Chairperson: *Walt Orenstein*

Brown F (ed): Progress in Polio Eradication: Vaccine Strategies for the End Game.
Dev Biol. Basel, Karger, 2001, vol 105, pp 3-7

Progress Towards Global Polio Eradication

H.F. Hull

Department of Vaccines and Biologicals, World Health Organization, Geneva, Switzerland

Abstract: In the 12 years since the global polio eradication goal was set in 1988, the eradication initiative has reached every polio-endemic country. Mass immunization campaigns have reached as many as 450 million children per year and 134 million children in a single day. The number of reported cases has declined from 35,251 to 7088 cases during that time span. Because surveillance has improved the decline in cases occurring is significantly greater. Wild poliovirus transmission is now confined to South Asia and West and Central Africa and the Horn of Africa. Although significant obstacles remain, it appears likely that polio will be eradicated world-wide by the end of the year 2002.

Introduction

In 1988, the World Health Assembly set a target for WHO to eradicate polio world-wide by the year 2000. Twelve years later, the polio eradication initiative has reached every polio-endemic country. As a result, the burden of disease has been dramatically reduced and wild poliovirus transmission contained to a limited number of countries. The progress achieved makes it likely that polio will be eradicated world-wide in the near future. This report provides an update on the status of the initiative and lays out the pathways being taken to ensure that the challenges of the post eradication era are met.

Strategies for Eradication

Because the vast majority of poliovirus infections are subclinical, eradication of polio implies that there be no new cases of the disease and that all wild poliovirus transmission ceases. To achieve this, WHO has elaborated four basic strategies: Routine immunization, National Immunization Days (NIDs), Acute Flaccid Paralysis (AFP) Surveillance and Mopping-up Immunization [1].

Routine immunization provides the foundation for polio eradication. WHO recommends that all children receive a minimum of three doses of oral polio vaccine in the first year of life. A fourth dose of OPV is recommended in polio-endemic countries, either at birth or with measles vaccine at the nine-month visit. In practice, though, few countries are providing this fourth dose. Because the vaccine efficacy of three doses of OPV is only 70%-80% in tropical developing countries [2,3], polio cannot be eradicated with routine immunization alone.

National Immunization Days are mass campaigns delivering OPV to all children aged less than five years. NIDs act by rapidly raising population immunity, particularly intestinal secretory immunity, thereby interrupting circulation of wild polioviruses [4]. Generally two doses are given approximately one month apart. Children are immunized regardless of previous immunization status. To be successful, NIDs must reach all children. Emphasis must be placed on reaching zero-dose children, those who have never been vaccinated before. Distribution to minorities and migratory populations is essential. NIDs are required for a number of years to achieve eradication, the number being dependent on the ability to identify and vaccinate high risk, under-immunized populations.

Effective disease surveillance is essential to any eradication effort. Because there is no pathognomonic clinical syndrome for poliomyelitis, final diagnosis must be confirmed in the laboratory. For the purposes of polio eradication, a system was developed in which all cases of acute onset, flaccid paralysis occurring in persons less than 15 years of age are reported. These cases are then investigated with a clinical examination, epidemiological history and two stool specimens collected for laboratory examination. Surveillance data are then used to monitor trends and to identify high risk populations where virus transmission persists. To ensure that every polio-endemic country has access to a laboratory with the necessary proficiency to detect wild poliovirus in stool samples reliably, WHO has created a global network of 148 laboratories. More than 90% of these laboratories are fully accredited. Active efforts are underway to bring the remainder fully up to standard.

When poliovirus circulation is reduced to low levels, high-risk populations are targeted for additional localised immunization campaigns known as mopping-up campaigns. An important difference between NIDs and mopping-up is that vaccine is taken from house to house rather than expecting parents to bring children to a central immunization clinic. Door-to-door immunization may reach as many as 50% more children compared with clinic based campaigns [5]. Mopping-up is an end-game strategy aimed at interrupting the final chains of poliovirus transmission in a country.

Trivalent, oral polio vaccine is the only vaccine recommended by WHO for the purposes of eradication. It is preferred because of its superior ability to induce secretory immunity in the intestines, the primary site for poliovirus replication [6]. OPV has the additional advantages of ease of administration and lower cost. All OPV vials purchased through UNICEF now carry individual theromosensitive vaccine vial monitors to detect heat exposure during storage and transport, permitting OPV to be used outside the cold chain for limited periods while eliminating the risk of administering vaccine that has lost its potency.

Progress Towards Global Eradication

By the end of 1999, at least one set of NIDs had been conducted in every polio-endemic country in the world. The last two countries to conduct NIDs were the Democratic Republic of the Congo and Sierra Leone in the third and fourth quarters of 1999 respectively. As many as 470 million children have been immunized world-wide during NIDs in a single year. China was able to immunize 84 million children in two days. India has immunized up to 134 million children in one day and 147 million children in one week. To enhance the impact of NIDs in suppressing poliovirus transmission at the regional level, multi-country NIDs have been co-ordinated in 18 Countries in the Middle East, Caucasus and Central Asia, nine countries in Asia and 35 countries in Africa. Currently, only 80% of infants born world-wide receive three doses of OPV through routine immunization. Performance of immunization systems is lowest in Africa where less than half of all children receive three routine doses of OPV during the first year of life.

The result of these immunization efforts is a decline in the number of polio cases from a total of 35,251 cases reported world-wide in 1988 to 7086 reported in 1999. Because improved surveillance systems are now detecting a greater percentage of cases, the percentage decline is probably greater. WHO estimates that 350,000 cases occurred world-wide in 1988, but no more than 20,000 in 1999 – a 94% decline. The geographical distribution of cases has also undergone a remarkable alteration. At the start of the initiative, 125 countries on five continents were polio-infected, while, by the end of 1999, 30 countries on two continents were infected. Poliovirus transmission is now concentrated in South Asia and West and Central Africa. The last case reported in WHO's American Region was in Peru in 1991. At the time of writing, it has been three years since the last case in WHO's Western Pacific Region in Cambodia (March 1997) and 18 months since the last case in WHO's European Region in Turkey (November 1998). Three polio-free countries reported imported polio cases in 1999 – China (from India), Iran (from Afghanistan) and Myanmar (from Bangladesh). These importations demonstrate the need to move forward as rapidly as possible towards global eradication and for countries free of polio to maintain high-level surveillance until eradication has been achieved.

Challenges for the Eradication Initiative

Acceleration

The success of the initiative is conclusive proof of the effectiveness of the WHO recommended strategies for eradicating polio. Poliovirus transmission has been stopped in the most- and least-densely populated areas on earth, from urban slums, jungles, mountains and deserts. To be effective, though, the strategies must be fully implemented with ALL children being reached during NIDs. AFP surveillance data show that the remaining polio-endemic countries have significant populations of children that have not been reached by either NIDs or routine immunization. WHO is working closely with the 30 remaining endemic countries to accelerate implementation of eradication strategies to be as close as possible to no cases at the end of the year 2000. In many endemic countries, extra rounds are being added to NIDs so children receive three to four doses of OPV per year. In other countries, either mopping-up campaigns or sub-national immunization campaigns are being targeted to high-risk populations.

India, for example, has adopted both approaches. During the period November 1999 to February 2000, four doses of OPV were delivered to all children in the country less than five years of age. In March and April 2000, two additional doses were delivered to all children living in six populous Northern states where almost all polio cases were concentrated in 1999. These states concentrated on a house-to-house approach to achieve the highest possible coverage. This effort was accompanied by improvements in the vaccine delivery system and increased supervision to increase the percentage of children reached. While these activities are taking place during 2000, much of the effect in reducing cases will not be seen until the year 2001. A similar level of activity will be required in 2001 in most remaining endemic countries to ensure that eradication is achieved.

Funding

Acceleration of the initiative has significantly increased costs. While a single dose of OPV costs less than US$0.08, 2.6 billion doses will be procured (1.275 billion by UNICEF) during the year 2000 for both routine immunization and NIDs. Operational costs are also increased both by the need to achieve the highest possible quality for NIDs, including distribution to remote regions and nomadic populations, and the increased number of rounds. Although many endemic countries have borne a significant portion of the costs of eradicating polio – China paid at least 90% of the cost itself – many of the remaining endemic countries are among the poorest and have many other health priorities. Accordingly, a greater proportion of the cost of polio eradication must be paid from external resources. From February 2000, the estimated total cost of the polio eradication initiative to the year 2005 was $ one billion. Of this $300 million remains to be raised. These resources must be secured in a timely manner so that strategies can be properly implemented. Delayed implementation will postpone the date when eradication will be achieved, increasing the cost by at least $100 million for every year's delay.

Political commitment

As the number of cases of polio falls, it is tempting to assume that the problem is solved and that funds and political support for the programme can safely be transferred to other health priorities. However, the approach of the last cases is precisely the time when maximum commitment is needed to ensure that the final chains of transmission are broken. NIDs must continue for a year or more after the last case and surveillance must function optimally until eradication is certified. For example, the most intense activity and highest costs were incurred in the Western Pacific Region during the 12 months after the last known case. Accordingly, both national and international leaders must maintain high levels of political and financial commitment for the programme until the last cases have been verified and all countries documented to be free of polio.

Conflict

Armed conflict remains an important challenge to the eradication initiative. The difficulty in reaching children in conflict zones, the destruction of the health, communication and transportation infrastructure and movements of civilian populations away from conflict zones act synergistically to create significant numbers of non-immunized children. These susceptible populations provide fertile soil for both continuing transmission and epidemics. For example, in 1999 an outbreak of 1100 cases of polio occurred in Angola, primarily among internally displaced persons crowded into improvised housing in Luanda without access to clean water or sewage systems [7]. In many countries, the challenges posed by armed conflict have been overcome through truces negotiated specifically for polio eradication [8]. Known as Days of Tranquillity, these truces call on all sides in the conflict to lay down their arms so that their children can be vaccinated. Days of Tranquillity for Polio have been used during NIDs in Afghanistan, the Democratic Republic of the Congo, El Salvador, the Philippines, Sierra Leone, Somalia, Sudan, Sri Lanka and Tajikistan. Informal truces for immunization have been observed in a number of other countries. The continuing conflicts in Afghanistan, Angola, DR Congo and Sudan will require that additional Days of Tranquillity be negotiated to protect the health of these most vulnerable children. Ultimate success of the initiative will also require that access be secured for comprehensive surveillance and appropriate mopping-up campaigns.

Conclusion

Although the exact target date – December 31 2000 – will not be met, continuous progress is being made in the countries that remain polio-endemic. The numbers of cases in India, Pakistan and other major reservoirs of wild virus are substantially less than in 1999. Barring unforeseen disruptions in the initiative, it is likely that polio will be eradicated by the end of 2002. Wild polioviruses should be contained one year later and global eradication will be certified in 2005. WHO projects that immunization against polio will stop some time before 2010. We can then look forward to the day when every child will be protected from the ravages of polio without the need for immunization.

References

1 Hull HF, Ward NA, Hull BP, Milstien JB, de Quadros C: Paralytic poliomyelitis: seasoned strategies, disappearing disease. Lancet. 1994;343:1331-1337.

2 John TJ: Antibody response of infants in tropics to five doses of oral polio vaccine. Br Med J 1976;I:812.

3 Patriarca PA, Wright PF, John TJ: Factors affecting the immunogenicity of oral poliovirus vaccine in developing countries: review. Rev Inf Diseases 1991;12:926-939.

4 Birmingham ME, Aylward RB, Cochi SL, Hull HF: National Immunization Days: State of the art. J Inf Diseases 1997;175:183-188.

5 Progress towards polio eradication, Nigeria, 1996-1998. Weekly Epidemiol Rec 1999;74:121-124.

6 Ghendon Y, Robertson SE: Interrupting the transmission of wild polioviruses with vaccines: immunological considerations. Bull World Health Organ 1994;72:873-883.

7 Valente F, Otten M, Balbina F, et al: Massive outbreak of poliomyelitis caused by type-3 wild poliovirus in Angola in 1999. Bull World Health Organ 2000;78(3):339-346.

8 Hull HF: Pax Polio. Science 1997;275:40-41.

Dr. H.F. Hull, Minnesota Department of Health, 717 Delaware, S.E., Minneapolis, MN 55414, USA.

Brown F (ed): Progress in Polio Eradication: Vaccine Strategies for the End Game.
Dev Biol. Basel, Karger, 2001, vol 105, pp 9-19

Progress Towards Polio Eradication: An African Perspective

B.D. Schoub[1], H.N. Gumede[1], T.G. Besselaar[1], N.K. Blackburn[1], E.M. Webb[2], O. Tomori[3], M. Otten[4]

[1] National Institute for Virology, Sandringham, South Africa
[2] Department of Health, Pretoria, South Africa
[3] Regional Virologist, WHO Afro, Harare, Zimbabwe
[4] Regional Epidemiologist, WHO Afro, Harare, Zimbabwe

Abstract: Despite daunting competing health priorities, Africa has made significant progress in polio control. Northern and Southern Africa appear to be polio-free and may shortly be certified as such; however, polio still remains endemic in West and Central Africa and the Horn of Africa. Countries «in difficult circumstances», wracked by major civil wars, have particularly low routine vaccine coverage, although NIDS have been carried out during negotiated days of tranquillity. AFP surveillance has also improved, although the quality of stool specimens is still far from ideal. There is, nevertheless, an extraordinary political commitment to the eradication campaign. Lessons from the history of polio in the continent need to be heeded in designing end-game strategies. Obstacles on the path to successful eradication are undoubtedly more formidable on the African continent – perhaps the most serious of all are the continuing wars. International political commitment and focussed and empowering developmental aid are urgently needed.

INTRODUCTION

The cover of a recent issue of the Economist (May 13th-19th, 2000) depicted an outline of the African continent on which was superimposed a picture of a heavily armed soldier under the caption «The hopeless continent» [1]. A number of articles in this controversial issue reflect on the feeling of hopeless resignation for the future of this hapless continent which is felt in some quarters of the industrialized world. Indeed, in recent times there have been natural disasters on a vast scale such as unprecedented flooding in Mozambique and Madagascar, together with desperate famine and poverty in much of the continent. Civil wars in West, Central and East Africa have displaced millions of civilians and caused severe disruption to primary health services. To compound all this, the toll of human disease often appears to have been so unfairly distributed to this continent – over two thirds of the world's population living with HIV/AIDS reside in sub-Saharan Africa, the great majority of whom cannot be afforded the privilege of any antiretroviral therapy. Moreover, the major portion of the world's TB burden and over 90% of the malaria death toll occur in sub-Saharan Africa.

However, even set against this horrendous backdrop, there is in essence no special or specific perspective from Africa on polio eradication, just obstacles and difficulties which are more formidable than elsewhere in the world. Africa, which was the last of the WHO regions to join the eradication initiative formally, will in all probability, as was the case with smallpox some 25 years ago, be the last region in the world where wild-type polio will circulate. It is clear that what is really relevant to the African continent is that special efforts will need to be made urgently which focus on the continent's particular difficulties. Notwithstanding, what this paper aims to demonstrate is that significant progress has taken place which does give cause for optimism that the global eradication target is both feasible and worthwhile.

Progress in Africa Towards Polio Eradication

The WHO African region consists of 48 countries/areas. These are divided into five epidemiological blocks – eastern, western, southern and central, in addition to a block called «countries in difficult circumstances». The last-named consist of three countries in conflict – Angola, the Democratic Republic of the Congo (DRC), and Ethiopia and Nigeria. Additional countries in difficult circumstances due to major outbreaks of hostilities include Sierra Leone, Liberia, Ethiopia/Eritrea, Sudan and Somalia (a country where no formal central governmental authority exists). Moreover, polio is endemic in Western and Central Africa and in the Horn of Africa.

Immunization coverage in Africa

Routine coverage with three doses of OPV varies from 65 to 75% for the eastern and southern blocks, drops to 50 to 55% for the western block, approximately 40% for the central block and in countries in difficult circumstances coverage is only around 30% [2]. However, supplementary immunization efforts were significantly enhanced during 1999 with some 133 million children receiving at least two supplementary doses of OPV – a 50% increase over the figures from 1998. National immunization days (NIDS) or subnational immunization days (SNIDS) were conducted in 35 countries between January 1999 and March 2000, with a coverage of over 80% in most countries.

AFP surveillance

Acute flaccid paralysis (AFP) surveillance improved considerably in 1999 with 4,999 AFP cases (0.8 non-polio AFP cases per 100,000 children less than 15 years of age) reported for 1999 compared to 1,754 (0.3 non-polio AFP cases per 100,000 children less than 15 years of age) for 1998. However, the adequacy of stool samples still remains a significant problem in Africa. The proportion of AFP cases with two stool samples collected within 14 days of the onset of paralysis declined somewhat from 39% in 1998 to 31% in 1999, considerably lower than the 68 to 86% reported from other WHO regions [3]. In addition, only 12 African countries reported that adequate specimens were taken from over 50% of their AFP cases in 1999 compared to 14 countries in 1998.

Given the heterogeneity of the African continent, an examination of two examples from either end of the spectrum of infrastructural development, the DRC and South Africa, may be useful to provide a further perspective on progress and the status of control programmes on the continent.

DRC

The DRC is a major global reservoir of polio due in large measure to the size of the country and the predominantly (70%) rural population, coupled to abject poverty, poor infrastructure and, in particular, a chronic and often intense civil war which has raged almost unabatedly since late 1996. Immunization coverage has been severely disrupted by hostilities; polio immunization coverage is estimated at 20% and 36% for OPV3 (three doses of OPV in children less than one year) for the western and eastern sectors of the country respectively [4]. The DRC was the last country in the African region to implement NIDS. These were planned for 1998 (following a few years of local immunization days) but were reduced to subnational immunization days (SNIDS) because of hostilities. Successful NID rounds were, however, conducted in 1999 during days of tranquillity following a United Nations brokered peace agreement. The formal ceasefire agreement is to be bolstered by an international corps of peacekeeping troops which will hopefully extend days of tranquillity to allow for NIDS during 2000.

AFP surveillance in the DRC, which is even more difficult to sustain than NIDS, is one of the lowest in the African continent – 0.18 cases per 100,000 population less than 15 years old. This is, however, expected to improve markedly after 11 national surveillance officers commenced active surveillance in April 2000, and a further 42 subprovincial officers commenced their activities in May 2000. In support of the anticipated enhanced AFP surveillance capacity the laboratory in Kinshasa has recently been accredited by WHO and is now a component of the global laboratory network.

South Africa

In contrast to the DRC, South Africa was one of the first countries in the world to manufacture both inactivated and oral polio vaccines and implement vaccination programmes in 1955 and 1960/61 respectively [5]. The country has a sophisticated First World medical service in the urban areas and a good primary healthcare infrastructure for much of the country. The National Institute for Virology in Johannesburg is one of three regional reference laboratories on the continent and also carries out sequencing and genotyping of isolates from the entire continent. The last known case of wild-type polio in the country occurred in 1989 [6]. Nevertheless, some recently acquired data regarding vaccine coverage and quality of surveillance gives some cause for concern even for this country. Routine immunization coverage figures have shown some worrying drop-out rates from OPV1 to OPV3; for example in 1998 there was a national drop-out rate of 19%, from 91% to 72% for OPV1 to OPV3. NIDS have been carried out in 1995, 1996, 1997 and 2000 (Table 1); however, in all years coverage for the second round was less than 80%, and in some provinces less than 66%.

AFP surveillance improved from 0.40 per 100,000 children under 15 years in 1998 to 0.90 for 1999, but the proportion of AFP cases with two stool samples collected within 14 days of onset of paralysis was only 31% in 1999.

Table 1: Mass immunization coverage: South Africa (expressed as percentages).

Province	1995		1996		1997*	
	1st Round	2nd Round	1st Round	2nd Round	1st Round	2nd Round
EC	70.0	57.7	86.7	49.1	78.6	70.2
FS	87.5	66.5	85.6	80.2	70.6	65.4
GA	104.6	110.2	84.7	95.3	74.0	67.6
KZ	84.5	71.5	81.4	70.6	71.8	85.6
MP	86.9	58.2	117.1	104.6	94.8	92.1
NC	65.9	69.1	114.3	54.7	65.7	49.5
NP	111.7	97.5	97.2	93.1	99.8	79.2
NW	81.3	78.4	87.1	54.4	70.8	68.6
WC	–	–	95.2	94.7	–	–
SA	89.6	78.0	90.0	77.2	79.1	75.6

* 1991 census

Reasons for Optimism

Progress towards eradication has undoubtedly been beset by major obstacles in delivery of vaccine and even more so by the inability to institute sustained surveillance systems. There are, nevertheless, solid reasons on which to base a rational optimism:-

Successful regional elimination

Southern and south-eastern Africa, together with North Africa, has not had wild-type polio for well over three years – the period specified by the Global Commission for the Certification of Polio Eradication. In some countries, wild-type polio has not occurred for over a decade. Provided that AFP surveillance is improved now and sustained at satisfactory levels, these regions may soon be certified polio-free.

A rough indication of the progressive decline in the number of countries circulating wild-type polio can be gauged from the countries of origin of wild-type polio isolates which were identified and sequenced at the National Institute for Virology in Johannesburg over the past five years (Table 2). In 1995 wild-type polio 1 came from some southern African countries such as Zambia and Namibia; from 1997 wild-type polio 1 came essentially only from Western, Central and East African countries. Wild-type 3 poliovirus from Africa was first identified at the National Institute for Virology in 1997 and has also been derived from the same regions of the continent as for wild-type 1 poliovirus. At the same time there has been a progressive increase in the number of Sabin-like viruses isolated, reflecting the increasing efficiency of AFP surveillance.

Molecular confirmation of increasing regional control

Phylogenetic analysis using the classical technique of partial genomic sequencing (150 nucleotides of the VP1/2A region of the virus) has demonstrated the stepwise reduction in the number of type 1 poliovirus genotypes (i.e. isolates which share greater than 85% sequence homology) until their ultimate disappearance. This was clearly shown in South Africa where three separate polio type 1 geno-

Table 2: Poliovirus isolations at the National Institute for Virology.

	Wild-type 1 poliovirus	Wild-type 3 poliovirus	Sabin-like poliovirus
1995	Namibia Tanzania Zambia	–	Zimbabwe SOA Tanzania
1996	Zambia Tanzania Angola	–	SOA Swaziland Zimbabwe
1997	Ghana CAR CIV DRC Nigeria NIE Senegal Togo CAE	CAR	CIV Uganda SOA Malawi Senegal Ghana
1998	Senegal Ghana Togo CIV NIE	NIE	SOA Uganda NIE
1999	CAR Angola CIV Ghana	CAR Angola Kenya DRC Ghana	CAR SOA Kenya Angola Uganda RDC CIV Ethiopia Zimbabwe Madagascar Ghana
2000 (early June)	CAR CIV DRC Angola Kenya Ethiopia	CAR DRC Kenya Angola	CAR SOA Kenya Angola Uganda Ethiopia Ghana CIV DRC

types circulated between 1980 and 1985, one of which was responsible for a large outbreak in 1982 [7]. A new genotype appeared in 1985 and displaced the other three. This genotype was also responsible for a very large outbreak in 1988 which eventually became the last known wild-type poliovirus to be isolated from an AFP case in South Africa in 1989.

Seven genotypes of type 1 poliovirus were shown to be circulating on the African continent over the past two decades [8]. In 1997, five African genotypes were demonstrated. At present it appears that what has remained of poliovirus type 1 is one Nigerian genotype and, because of continuing endemic circulation of the West

African genotype, this has now diversified into three separate clusters with less than 85% homology between them (Fig. 1). Full length sequencing of the VP1 gene (906 nucleotides) is currently being carried out and has demonstrated clustering into several lineages of isolates from West and Central Africa. It is anticipated that a clearer picture of the diversity of the remnant West/Central African wild-type 1 isolates will emerge when this analysis is completed.

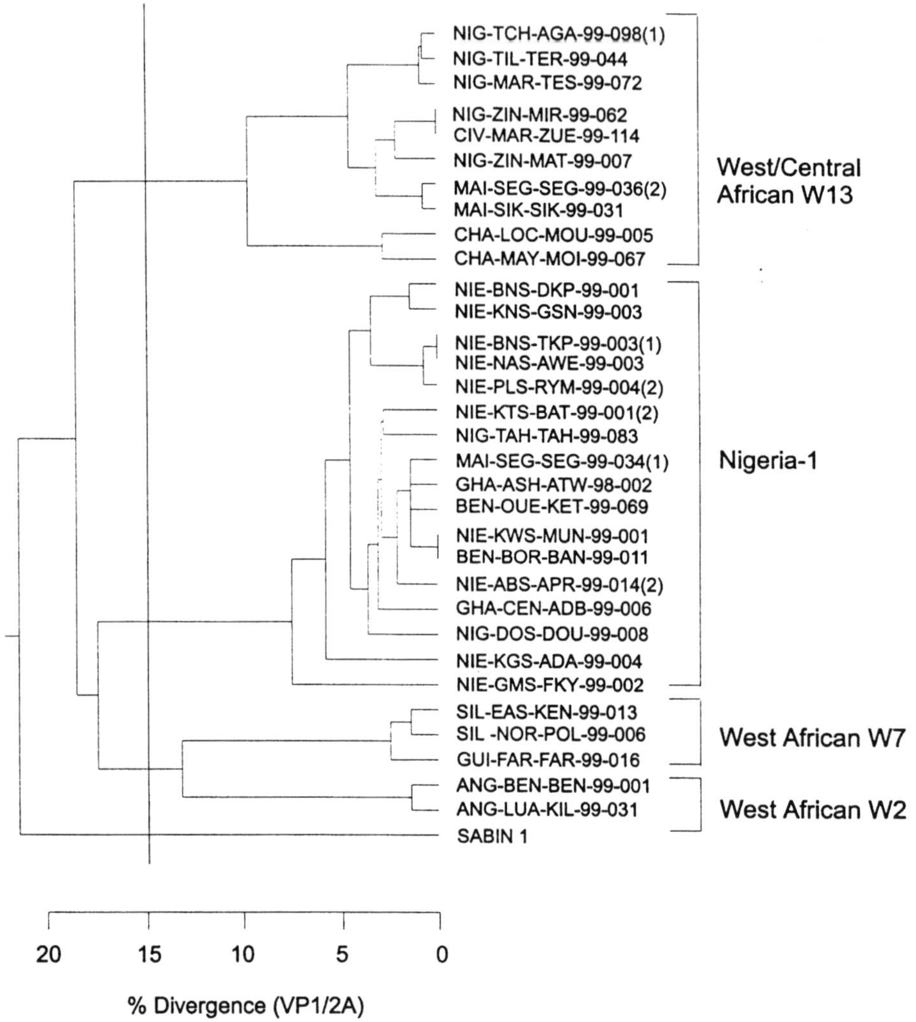

Fig. 1: Genetic relationships between type 1 polioviruses in sub-Saharan Africa 1999.

With regard to wild-type 3 polio, phylogenetic analysis of a relatively small number of isolates obtained since 1997, has shown three independent genotypes circulating in West and Central Africa (Fig. 2).

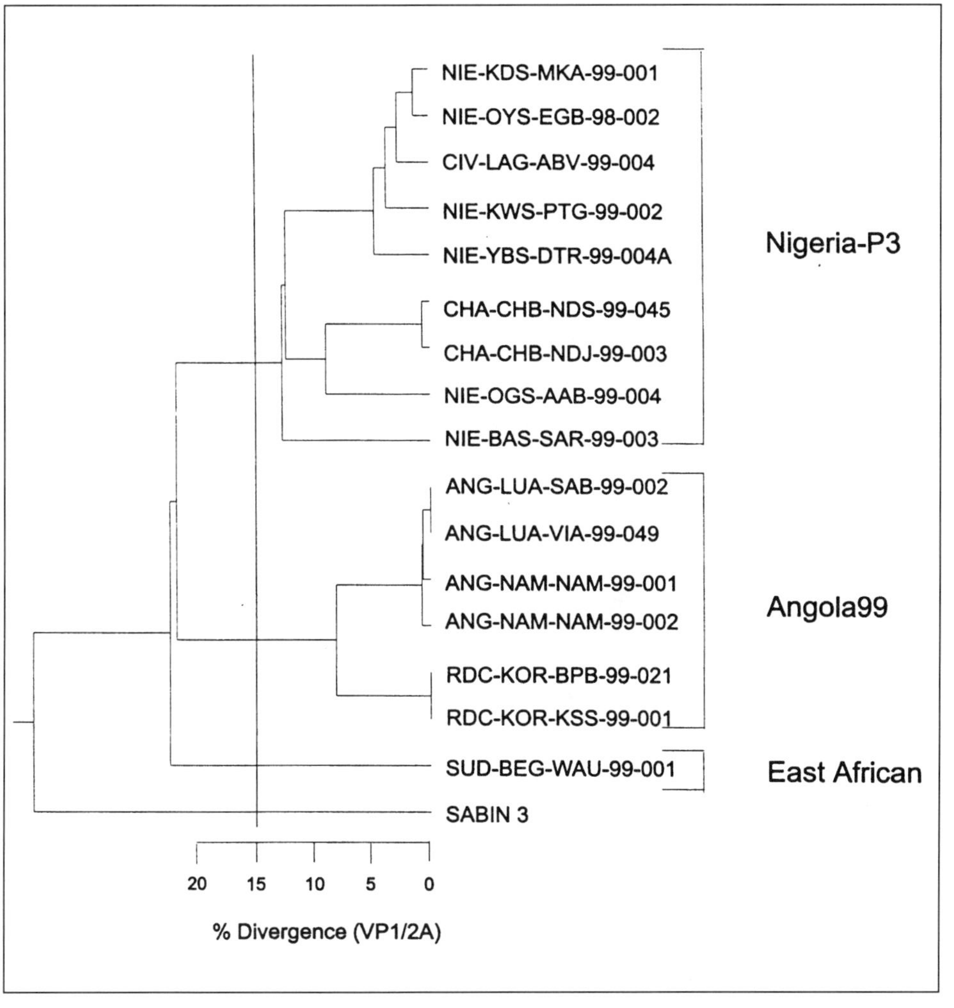

Fig. 2: Genetic relationships between type 3 polioviruses in sub-Saharan Africa 1999.

No evidence of spread from reservoir countries

Countries with good polio control programmes which border on reservoir countries such as Namibia, Botswana, Zambia and Tanzania, have not seen detectable cross-border importation of the virus.

Avoidance of anticipated outbreaks

In February and March 2000, Mozambique was devastated by the worst floods in its history – displacing some 300,000 to 500,000 people and causing widespread damage to water supplies and sanitation [9]. A substantial increase in diarrhoeal disease, including cholera, was reported, but no outbreak of polio materialized. In contrast, in 1988 the largest epidemic of polio recorded in South Africa followed extensive flooding [10].

Political commitment

Set against a background of competing public health emergencies on the vast scale of HIV/AIDS, tuberculosis and malaria, the extent of commitment by leaders of African countries to the polio eradication programme has indeed been remarkable. For example, South Africa, which is bedevilled by one of the most rapidly expanding HIV epidemics in the world as well as having one of the highest incidences of tuberculosis in the world (in the Western Cape Province of the country), saw its former President, Nelson Mandela, lend his enormous international stature to championing the control of a disease which ostensibly has not occurred in this country for over a decade, by accepting the patronage of the «Kick polio out of Africa» campaign.

Days of tranquillity

The days of tranquillity which played such an important role during the smallpox eradication campaign have been successfully negotiated for polio eradication activities in a number of African regions [11]. Universally there has not been anything other than encouragement for routine and supplementary immunization and surveillance activities by opposing sides in conflicts. There has also been a remarkable commitment by field workers, often operating in extremely dangerous conditions – some 19 NID staff and volunteers have already lost their lives in Africa as a result of hostilities.

African laboratory network

Gratifying progress has been made in expanding and accrediting the African laboratory network in spite of major logistical and financial difficulties as well as difficulties in retaining trained staff. Currently 37 of the 48 countries in Africa are serviced by the network of 12 national and three regional reference laboratories. During 1999, 13 of the 15 laboratories were accredited by the WHO.

Some African Perspectives on End-Game Strategies

Sensitivity of eradication criteria

The criteria for polio-free status – three year absence of wild-type polio in the presence of adequate AFP surveillance – may, as it stands, be inadequate to cover remote and inaccessible regions of Africa. Molecular analysis of type 3 polio isolates from the 1999 Angolan outbreak demonstrated this virus to be of a novel genotype, presumably circulating endemically for some time in a concealed focus

[12]. Such concealed foci are partly by infrastructural deficiencies which in some regions are abysmal, but largely by continuing wars and conflicts. The danger from concealed foci of infection which are undetected by routine AFP surveillance would be considerably greater for polio than was the case for smallpox.

Pressure to certify polio-free status

Examples from the African continent (Namibia, 1993/4 [13]) as well as elsewhere in the world, where outbreaks have occurred several years after apparent polio-free status, need to serve as a cautionary lesson against over-hasty certification of polio-free status.

War and displacement of civilians

The profound effect of war and displacement of civilians on polio outbreaks has been graphically illustrated in many countries in Africa and should not be underestimated. War not only severely interrupts vaccine delivery and surveillance, but causes mass migration of civilian refugees into underserved urban areas with poor sanitation facilities and water supplies. The largest outbreak of polio ever recorded in Africa, which took place in Angola in 1999, was in large measure due to civilian displacement [12]. Interestingly, this outbreak was due to poliovirus 3, generally not thought to have the same epidemic potential as type 1 poliovirus which was also co-circulating in that country at the same time. Civilian displacement and unregulated informal settlement in urban areas was similarly thought to be the prime contributing cause of the 1993/4 epidemic in Namibia, a country with good polio control and apparently free of polio for five years preceding the outbreak [13].

HIV/AIDS

Some preliminary investigations have indicated that children with HIV/AIDS do not persistently excrete poliovirus, which would be consistent with the predominant immunodeficiency being cellular rather than humoral [14]. However, even though humoral immuno-deficiency occurs in the later stages of the disease when survival is limited, the possibility may still exist that because of the vast population of children with HIV/AIDS in Africa a sufficient number of chronic excretors could perhaps sustain transmission and create a potential reservoir of poliovirus. Reassurance against this possibility still needs to be established.

Primate reservoir

There is an assumption that non-human primates, if they were naturally infected with human poliovirus, would only serve as an incidental host and, at worst, would not pose more of a risk than does monkeypox to smallpox eradication. However, given the extensive and often close contact between man and monkey in tropical Africa, this possibility, albeit remote, should not be summarily dismissed without further investigation.

Bioterrorism

Certainly the use of poliovirus as a biological weapon is a concern worldwide, and evil and perverted minds can be found in all four corners of the globe. There is also no cause for speculation that the spectre of polio as a biological weapon has any special African spin to it. In the context of bioterrorism perhaps mention should be made of the monstrous revelations now coming to light in South African law courts of the bizarre exploitations of chemical and biological weapons in the latter days of the apartheid era [15].

Conclusion

Given the extent of the obstacles which have been overcome, progress in polio control in the African continent has been truly remarkable. The final stages of the eradication initiative will, however, require substantial additional effort. This will need to come from international commitments and, most importantly, will need to be mediated through meaningful indigenous empowerment and ownership of the initiative.

An in-depth needs analysis for Africa must be carried out to pin-point exactly where developmental aid should be focussed, whether it be roads, communications (especially satellite technology) or appropriate transport systems. Lastly, it is clear that the most formidable obstacle to global polio eradication is war. Imaginative ways of safely maintaining routine and supplementary immunization and surveillance programmes in zones of conflict must be devised urgently at the highest international political level.

References

1 The Economist, London, 13th-19th May 2000.

2 World Health Organization. Progress towards poliomyelitis eradication. WHO African Region, January 1999 – March 2000. Wkly Epidemiol Rec May 2000;21:175-179.

3 World Health Organization. Progress towards global poliomyelitis eradication, 1999. Wkly Epidemiol Rec April 2000;17:134-143.

4 World Health Organization. Progress towards poliomyelitis eradication. Democratic Republic of the Congo, 1999. Wkly Epidemiol Rec March 2000;13:101-106.

5 Gear JHS: The history of the Poliomyelitis Research Foundation. Johannesburg, South Africa 1996;79-95.

6 Schoub BD, Chezzi C, Blackburn NK: Last virologically confirmed cases of wild-type poliomyelitis in South Africa. S Afr Med J 1995;85:55.

7 Chezzi C, Blackburn NK, Schoub BD: Molecular characterization of type 1 polioviruses associated with epidemics in South Africa. J Med Virol 1997;52:42-49.

8 Chezzi C, Blackburn NK, Schoub BD: Molecular epidemiology of type 1 polioviruses from Africa. J Gen Virol 1997;78:1017-1024.

9 Anon: Flooding in Mozambique. Bull World Health Organ 2000;78:562.

10 Schoub BD, Johnson S, McAnerney JM, van Middelkoop A, Kustner HGV, Windsor I, Vinsen C, McDonald K: Poliomyelitis outbreak in Natal/KwaZulu, South Africa, 1987-1988. 2. Immunity aspects. Trans Roy Soc Trop Med Hyg 1992;86:83-85.

11 Tangermann RH, Hull HF, Jafari H, Nkowane B, Everts H, Aylward RB: Eradication of poliomyelitis in countries affected by conflict. Bull World Health Organ 2000;78:330-338.

12 Valente F, Otten M, Balbina F, van de Weerdt R, Chezzi C, Eriki P, van-Dunnen J, Okwo Bele J-M: Massive outbreak of poliomyelitis caused by type-3 wild poliovirus in Angola in 1999. Bull World Health Organ 2000;78:339-346.

13 Van Niekerk ABW, Vries JB, Schoub BD, Chezzi C, Blackburn NK: Outbreak of paralytic poliomyelitis in Namibia. Lancet 1994;344:661-664.

14 Wood DJ, Sutter RW, Dowdle WR: Stopping poliovirus vaccination after eradication: issues and challenged. Bull World Health Organ 2000;78:347-357.

15 Bjornsdottir US, Smith D: South African religious leader with hyperventilation, hypophosphataemia, and respiratory arrest. Lancet 1999;354:2130.

Dr. B.D. Schoub, National Institute for Virology, Private Bag X4, Sandringham 2131, South Africa.

Brown F (ed): Progress in Polio Eradication: Vaccine Strategies for the End Game.
Dev Biol. Basel, Karger, 2001, vol 105, pp 21-31

The Efficiency and Reliability of Polio Surveillance

T. Hovi

National Public Health Institute (KTL), Enterovirus Laboratory, Helsinki, Finland

Key words: Poliovirus, surveillance, transmission, acute flaccid paralysis, environmental specimens, enterovirus diagnostics.

Abstract: Surveillance for acute flaccid paralysis (AFP) in children younger than 15 years, and careful investigation of the cases, are the cornerstones for monitoring the progress of the poliomyelitis eradication programme. However, its sensitivity to detect wild type poliovirus (wtPV) circulation decreases when the incidence of true polio cases approaches zero. Under these conditions, only about one in 100,000 children is being investigated for poliovirus excretion. No real alternative approach which is generally exploitable has been developed. Environmental surveillance may in optimal conditions be at least as sensitive in detecting poliovirus circulation as AFP surveillance. However, optimal conditions, i.e. converging sewage systems, are not used by most people in the remaining endemic countries. Enterovirus surveillance, based on isolation of poliovirus in the routine diagnostic services, is only applicable in a few countries, where the diagnostic activity covers the entire population. Whichever approach is used, we will never reach 100% certainty of complete elimination of wtPV circulation. However, by applying all these approaches optimally, we may eventually reach a probability level allowing the safe cessation of immunisation.

Introduction

The goal of the polio eradication initiative is to stop circulation, and to prevent re-emergence of wild type poliovirus (wtPV) in human populations all over the world. All the biological criteria that are needed for global eradication to be possible are unquestionable in the case of poliomyelitis, and the success of the initiative has been dramatic [1]. Although a substantial amount of work remains to be done, the global eradication of poliomyelitis and that of wtPV is indeed possible within a few years.

Poliovirus infections occur 100-1000-fold more frequently than clinically recorded paralytic poliomyelitis. Therefore, to monitor the progress of the programme and to document eventually the completion of the eradication, we can only rely on virological surveillance, i.e. on a systematic search for wtPV excreted by infected individuals. The problem of the efficiency and reliability of poliovirus surveillance in this context could also be designated as the population sensitivity of the surveillance, and can be transformed into the following simple question: if the surveillance does not find wtPV anywhere, can we believe that the virus really has been eliminated from the human population?

Poliovirus surveillance can be based on two separate approaches. In the clinical case-driven surveillance, such as the WHO gold standard, acute flaccid paralysis (AFP) surveillance [2], the assumption is that if circulating in a population, wtPV is likely to be found in patients with a disease typically caused by poliovirus. The direct virus-targeted surveillance is based on the view that all poliovirus-infected individuals, whether symptomatic or not, excrete relatively large amounts of the virus in the stools for several weeks. Hence, putative circulation of wtPV in a population could be detected by screening the excreta.

This article deals with different approaches to virological surveillance, factors influencing the efficiency of the approaches at the population level, the reliability of information obtained by them, and discusses the level of certainty of eradication that we can reach best by exploiting the different approaches.

Background and Definitions

Poliovirus infection and poliomyelitis

Depending on the causative serotype and the strain, some 1-0.1% of wtPV-infected unimmunised individuals develop the typical paralytic disease, perhaps almost as many show aseptic meningitis, and up to 10% may have non-specific common cold like symptoms. Hence, the «typical» paralytic disease could also be considered a complication of the usually benign wild type poliovirus infection. In partially immune populations, the case:infection rate may be much lower than the 0.1% [3], and the length of excretion and amounts of virus are likely to be even more variable than in the non-immune individuals. The case:infection rate is important in the case-derived surveillance but has no significance in the direct virus-targeted surveillance.

All poliovirus-infected individuals, irrespective of the possible clinical consequences of the infection, excrete the virus in the stools for a relatively long time, usually six to eight weeks, and during the early phase of the infection, in the oropharyngeal excreta as well. The concentration of poliovirus in the excreta varies; that in the stools may be 10^5 cell culture infecting units ($CCID_{50}$) per gram of stool during the first two weeks, lower and highly variable thereafter [4]. The amount of virus excreted in the oropharynx is much smaller. The amount of excreted virus is relevant to the direct virus-targeted surveillance systems.

As long as wtPV circulation exists, there is a risk of its transportation to other parts of the world, including populations that have been polio-free for long periods. One can expect that, in vaccinated populations, most of the imports lead to abortive chains of transmission [5], because of the small number of susceptible host individuals within reach. However, it is not known how long an imported wtPV could continue silent circulation in a vaccinated population before causing notified paralytic cases and becoming recognised. Likewise, it is not known how long after the last notified polio case due to wtPV infection, there could still be silent wtPV circulation in a population.

Efficiency of virological surveillance

Examining every individual in a population for poliovirus excretion is a practical impossibility. Our knowledge on the frequency of poliovirus-excreting individuals in a given population is always indirect and often based on examination of a small sample of people. Hence, we cannot entirely exclude the possibility that the virus could exist in the unexamined part of a sampled population. Efficiency of surveillance could be defined as the probabilty to uncover existing virus circulation, i.e. to detect the virus in the examined specimens if there are virus excretors in the population. This requires good geographical and demographic coverage of the sampling procedures, timely collection and immediate analysis of the specimens, as well as prompt reporting and correct interpretation of the data generated.

Reliability of surveillance

The reliability of surveillance data is affected by several factors, starting from the feasibility of the rationale of the surveillance approach and extending to the reporting and analysis of the surveillance data. The surveillance could be considered optimally reliable if we could believe that a positive finding indeed means presence of the virus in the population, and that a negative finding means the opposite. Detection of poliovirus in a clinical specimen usually means that infections still occur in the population. However, a negative surveillance finding should not be immediately interpreted to document absolute absence of poliovirus. Rather, even if technically reliable, it simply means that the virus has not been found by the methods used. In theory, it could still be present.

In principle, the reliability of the surveillance data is largely dependent on the quality of the primary laboratory data, and that of data collection and analysis. Quality criteria have been defined, and are being strictly monitored, in the established surveillance system of the WHO Polio Eradication Programme. Any alternative approach should allow designation of similar criteria, in order to assess the reliability of the results obtained.

Clinical Case-Driven Surveillance (also called event-driven surveillance)

Brief description

Acute flaccid paralysis surveillance (AFP surveillance) is the gold standard in the WHO coordinated polio eradication campaign. It comprises an active search for acutely paralytic children in the community, virological examination of their faecal specimens, and centralized data collection and analysis. Factors influencing efficiency and reliability of the data are shown in Figure 1. Good quality AFP surveillance means that the annual rate of non-polio AFP cases in children younger than 15 years is at least 1:100,000, and at least 80% of the cases have been investigated in detail [2]. If this situation continues for three years, WHO considers that poliovirus circulation in the population has ceased.

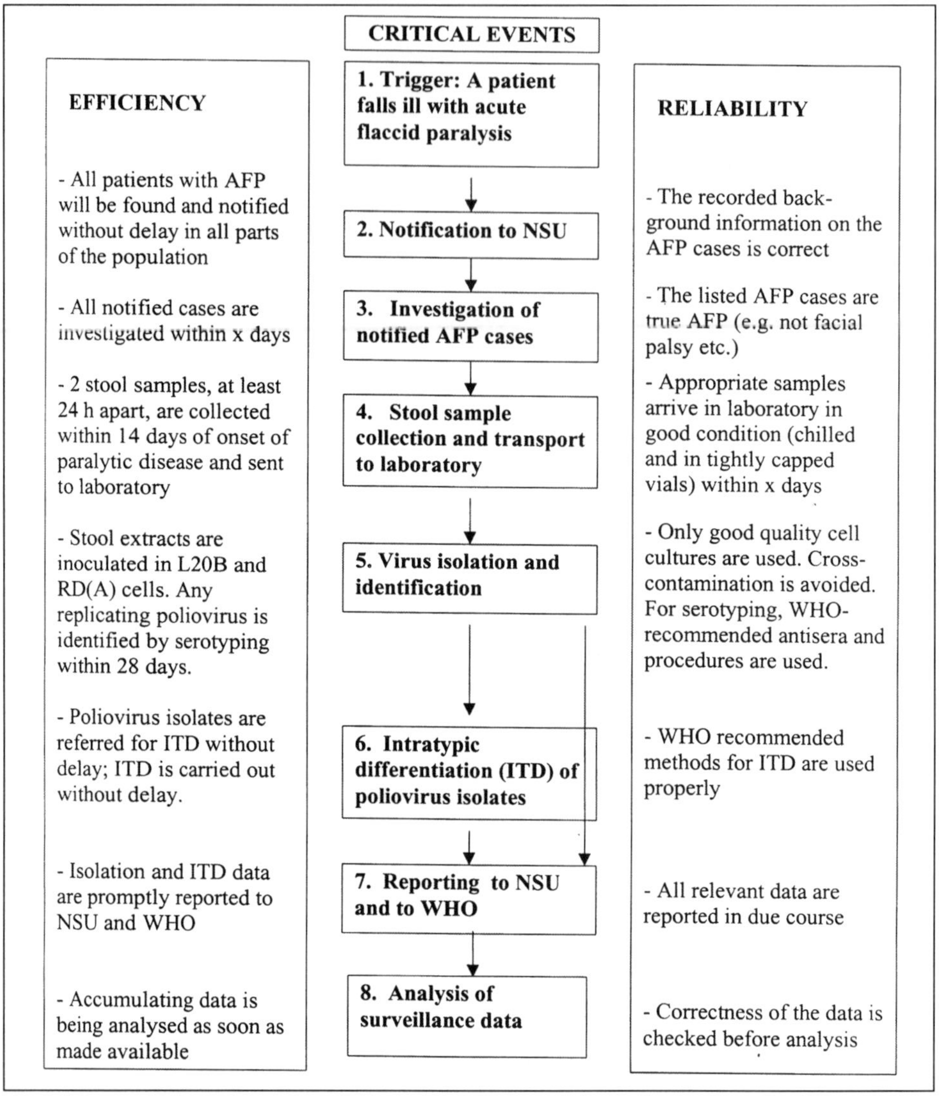

Fig. 1: Factors influencing efficiency and reliability of acute flaccid paralysis (AFP) surveillance. L20B, a murine recombinant cell line expressing human poliovirus receptor, relatively selective for polioviruses; RD(A), a human rhabdomyosarcoma cell line susceptible to non-polio enteroviruses; ITD, intratypic differentiation; NSU, national surveillance unit.

Limitations

Theoretically, in spite of failure to detect poliovirus infection in properly examined specimens collected from all children with AFP, relatively extensive poliovirus circulation could still occur in the community. Good quality AFP surveillance means that as few as 1: 100,000 children are annually examined for wtPV excretion. This is not a very tight screen [6], especially if we assume that the morbidity:infection ratio is clearly below the generally held 1:100 - 1:1,000, as it could be in vaccinated populations. Furthermore, because 80% peformance is accepted in each of the several individual quality parameters [2], the proportion of specimens that fulfil all the criteria might be significantly less than 80%. This view has been one of the arguments in the western countries that have decided not to try to establish a proper AFP surveillance system. In several countries that have established an AFP surveillance a long time after the elimination of poliomyelitis, the proportion of virologically examined cases has remained very low [7]. The clinicians tend to think that there is no reason to take specimens from those with obvious non-polio diseases, e.g. cases of Guillain-Barré syndrome (GBS), which is the most frequently occurring true diagnosis in the designated AFP. Difficulties in applying the criteria for good quality AFP surveillance in small populations were discussed recently [8]. It should be noted that this limitation is relevant not only in the case of small countries, but also if a larger country is divided into areas with small sub-populations.

Alternative events as starting points

Because of the difficulties in encouraging the clinicians to collect faecal specimens from all cases of AFP, a definition often considered irrelevant in everyday work, alternative clinical entities have been suggested as potential starting points in case-driven poliovirus surveillance. To be more easily accepted than AFP surveillance, the entities selected should be clearly defined and generally suspected to be caused by polio- or other enteroviruses. Aseptic meningitis (AM) is the most likely candidate, and has an incidence that is much higher than that of non-polio AFP. In countries with an established mumps immunisation programme, the most common cause of AM is an enterovirus infection. Cell cultures generally applied for isolation of non-polio enteroviruses are usually highly susceptible to poliovirus infection also. However, the routine practices to attempt aetiological diagnosis in individual cases of AM vary from country to country, and in many countries from hospital to hospital. Moreover, many milder cases are not even referred to hospitals. Therefore, to guarantee the use of standard methods comparable to those of AFP surveillance, one would need a specific organisation actively looking for, and investigating, all cases of AM. It is unlikely that this kind of organisation would be readily established only for the sake of polio surveillance. One severe confounding factor would also be the strongly epidemic nature of enterovirus AM. It would be practically impossible to determine a constant background level as a quality indicator of surveillance, similar to that of the critical non-polio AFP incidence of at least 1:100,000 in children younger than 15 years of age.

In conclusion, it seems very unlikely to me that any alternative clinical entities could be found to replace AFP in case-driven poliovirus surveillance. AFP surveillance is the only form of case-driven poliovirus surveillance that in practice can be applied to all populations in a standardised fashion and with good coverage.

Direct Virus-Targeted Surveillance

Environmental surveillance

Rationale

Poliovirus excreted into the stools enters the environment, usually in sewage, and may survive there under suitable conditions for several months. The survival time is sufficiently long to enable monitoring of poliovirus excretion by analysing sewage samples. Analysis of sewage samples has been used to monitor the extent of polio epidemics and OPV campaigns in both geographical and temporal terms [3,9,10]. Excretion of poliovirus into the faeces does not depend on the case: infection rate and, therefore, search for poliovirus in environmental specimens is an independent and potentially very powerful approach to poliovirus surveillance. Stool surveys could also be used for the same purpose, but because of the considerable working load, they can be targeted to relative small populations only.

Possibilities and limitations

Factors influencing the efficiency and reliability of the data are given in Figure 2. "Transportation" of poliovirus in the sewage may be complicated but experiments carried out with intentionally introduced OPV virus suggest that the recovery of poliovirus at a remote downstream sampling site can be more than 10% in a city sewage system [Hovi T, Stenvik M, Salonen H, Kangas A, submitted]. By mathematical modelling it was demonstrated that the population sensitivity of this approach is increased greatly by repeated sampling. Furthermore, analysis of one litre samples collected at a single site representing one million people twice a month might reveal poliovirus circulation faster than optimally working AFP surveillance [Ranta J, Hovi T, Arjas E, submitted].

One of the problems of environmental surveillance is the difficulty in obtaining high population coverage for sampling. It might be technically possible in industrialised countries but would mean a very high working load. Furthermore, in most parts of the world, conventional converging sewage systems are serving only small parts of the population. Therefore, sampling must be targetted to sites that can be considered to represent faeces contaminated sewage derived from major risk populations.

Technical aspects

Two different approaches have been used for sampling: (i) grab sampling, which means collecting a moderate volume, e.g. one litre, of raw sewage, and testing the sample for presence of virus after concentration, and (ii) trap sampling, which can be achieved by immersing an absorbant in the sewage, e.g. a cotton gauze pad or ground glass in a virus-permeable bag, and then eluting bound materials and assaying the eluent for poliovirus. The former approach may sound more feasible because it allows direct quantification of the virus in the sewage sample, while one would expect that various solid materials suspended in the sewage might block the absorbant trap and interfere with the binding of poliovirus. However, both types of traps have been used successfully to demonstrate wild type poliovirus in the sewage [3, 9,11,12]. Proper comparative studies assessing relative sensitivities of the two approaches have not been published.

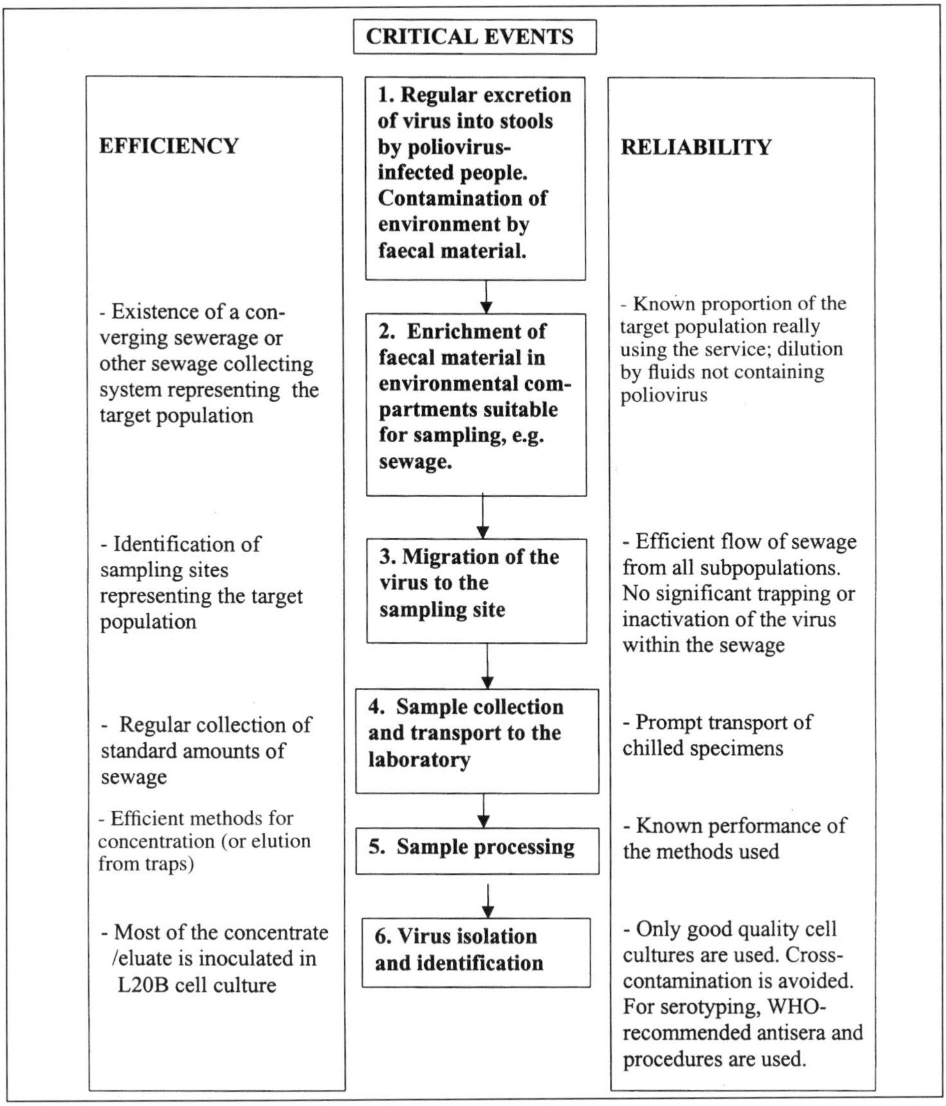

Fig. 2: Factors influencing efficiency and reliability of environmental surveillance. Later steps are similar to those of AFP surveillance.

Several different methods have been described for the concentration of the grab samples [9]. Relatively little comparative work has been carried out, and therefore, whatever method is being used, it is important that the laboratory determines its own sample sensitivity with spiked sewage specimens. Cell culture is still the only generally applicable method for demonstrating wild type poliovirus in environmental specimens. The two cell lines already established in the WHO Polio Laboratory Network for use on clinical specimens, (i) the human poliovirus receptor-expressing recombinant murine cell line L20B, and (ii) the human rhabdomyosarcoma-derived RD cell line, are suitable for this purpose.

Coping with an excess of OPV-derived viruses

Regular cell culture systems do not distinguish wild type poliovirus from OPV-derived strains, which may be abundant in the environment, reflecting use of OPV in the respective populations. However, the use of OPV in general immunisation does not necessarily prevent detection of wild type poliovirus in the environment [12]. This can be further facilitated by incubation of the cultures at elevated temperatures that are selective for the wild type virus [13]. This approach would require an incubator with a tightly controlled thermostat unit. Alternatively, if a specific genotype is suspected, genotype-specific RT- PCR can be designed and used successfully to detect wtPV in the presence of Sabin-like virus, in an excess of several orders of magnitude [14]. Yet another possibility is to block the excess of the OPV-derived strains by Sabin strain-specific monoclonals in cell culture [15]. None of these selective means is widely used at the moment.

Possible quality criteria

Since non-polio enteroviruses frequently occur in sewage waters [10], an environmental surveillance project should detect non-polio enteroviruses regularly and, in populations recently immunised, OPV-derived viruses in a significant proportion of the specimens examined. Other quality criteria could be the demonstration of logical reasons that were used for selecting the sampling sites and sampling frequencies, follow-up of standard operation procedures with known sample sensitivity, and timeliness aspects similar to those applied for clinical specimens.

Enterovirus surveillance

Enterovirus surveillance is here designated to mean thorough analysis of data generated in a population through routine enterovirus diagnostics by examining stool specimens in cell culture. The reason for collecting a faecal specimen for enterovirus isolation is usually aseptic meningitis but all the the data accumulated from results of faecal culture for enteroviruses, for any reason, can be used. Factors influencing the efficiency and reliability of results obtained through this system are shown in Figure 3. A factor limiting the coverage of this approach is the lack of uniformity in triggering sample collection, similar to that discussed above in regard to AM surveillance. An important aspect is the quality of the often numerous laboratories carrying out the primary diagnosis in a country. A quality assurance system should be organised to guarantee the reliability of the results. It is important to confirm that the laboratories do not use insensitive isolation techniques and consequently miss wtPV. Likewise, they should not miss poliovirus by mis-identifying it for non-polio enteroviruses in serotyping. They should also promptly refer all poliovirus isolates, and all non-typable enteroviruses, to the NPL for further characterisation.

It is obvious that enterovirus surveillance may be a useful supplementary approach for poliovirus surveillance in a limited number of industrialised coun-

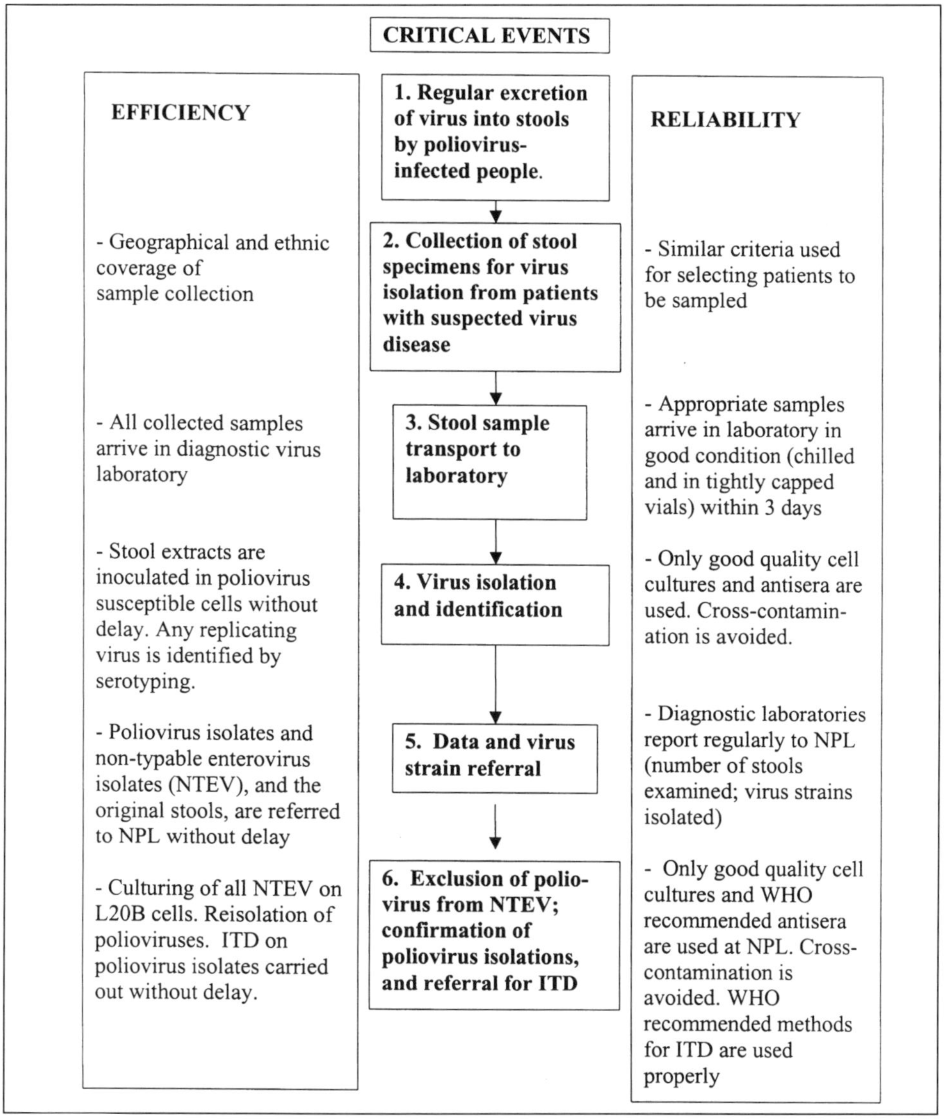

Fig. 3: Factors influencing efficiency and reliability of enterovirus surveillance.

tries where the population coverage of sampling can be considered sufficient. It has not yet been determined what kind of sampling frequency (e.g. per 1000 children under 15 years) could be acceptable for a national certification document.

General Conclusions

It is unequivocally clear that AFP surveillance should be globally preferred as the main approach for surveillance of wtPV circulation, in spite of the fact that its sensitivity is not optimal at low level wtPV circulation in vaccinated populations [6]. In practice, no other system can be applied at the same level in every population. It appears equally unquestionable that if the AFP surveillance is not working optimally in a population, supplementary approaches should be used in the search for the potentially circulating wtPV. Environmental and enterovirus surveillance may be useful alternatives under suitable conditions. In both cases, general criteria should be established to assess the sensitivity of the approaches and to monitor the quality of the procedures. It is important to remember, however, that whatever the surveillance system used, we can never scientifically prove that wtPV has been completely eradicated from mankind and nature. Even at best, we have to be satisfied with a statement such as «We have looked for the virus with reliable methods in x individuals and y environmental specimens, and did not find it. Therefore, it cannot exist at this level of prevalence» (modified from Mark Pallansch). For poliovirus circulating in human populations, time and continuing surveillance may help us to uncover even low level silent circulation. For wtPV possibly hidden in the environment under conditions which maintain the infectivity, e.g. in the permafrost, we have no means of coping. We can simply hope that if existing, these viruses remain in the frozen state. Global risk assessment based on known facts, mathematical modelling and common sense will be necessary when considering the eventual stopping of polio vaccination.

References

1 Anonymous: Progress towards global poliomyelitis eradication, 1999. Weekly Epid Rec 2000;75:134-143.

2 Birmingham ME, Linkins RW, Hull BP, Hull HF: Poliomyelitis surveillance: The compass of eradication. J Infect Dis 1997;175(Suppl. 1):S146-S150.

3 Hovi T, Cantell K, Huovilainen A, Kinnunen E, Kuronen T, Lapinleimu K, Pöyry T, Roivainen M, Salama N, Stenvik M, Silander A, Thodén C-J, Salminen S, Weckström P: Outbreak of poliomyelitis in Finland: Widespread circulation of antigenically altered poliovirus type 3 in a vaccinated population. Lancet 1986;1:1427-1432.

4 Piirainen L, Stenvik M, Roivainen M, Eskola J, Beuvery EC, Hovi T: Randomised, controlled trial with the trypsin-modified inactivated poliovirus vaccine: assessment of intestinal immunity with live challenge virus. Vaccine 1999;17:1084-1090.

5 Conyn-van Spaendonck MA, Oosvogel PM, van Loon AM, Wijngaarden JK, Kromhout D: Circulation of poliovirus during the poliomyelitis outbreak in The Netherlands in 1992-1993. Am J Epidemiol 1996;143:929-935.

6 Gary HE, Sanders R, Pallansch MA: A theoretical framework fort evaluating the sensitivity of surveillance for detecting wild poliovirus: Factors affecting detection sensitivity in a population with circulating wild poliovirus. J Infect Dis 1997;175(Suppl 1):S141-S145.

7 Oostvogel PM, Spaendonck MA, Hirasing RA, van Loon AM: Surveillance of acute flaccid paralysis in The Netherlands. Bull WHO 1998;76:55-62.

8 Hovi T, Stenvik M: Patients with acute flaccid paralysis and polio surveillance in Finland Bull WHO 2000;78:298-304.

9 Metcalf TG, Melnick JL, Estes MK: Environmental virology: from detection of virus in sewage and water by isolation to identification by molecular biology - a trip over 50 years. Annu Rev Microbiol 1995;49:461-487.

10 Pöyry T, Stenvik M, Hovi T: Viruses in sewage waters during and after a poliomyelitis outbreak and subsequent nationwide oral poliovirus vaccination campaign in Finland. Appl Environm Microbiol 1988;54:371-374.

11 Böttiger M, Herrstrom E: Isolation of polioviruses from sewage and their characteristics: experience over two decades in Sweden. Scand J Infect Dis 1992;24:151-155.

12 World Health Organization. Environmental surveillance of wild poliovirus circulation in Europe. WHO/EURO, Copenhagen, 1992. EUR/ICP/EPI 019/8000B:3.

13 Manor Y, Handsher R, Halmut T, et al: Detection of poliovirus circulation by environmental surveillance in the absence of clinical cases in Israel and the Palestinian authority. J Clin Microbiol 1999;37:1670.

14 Tambini G, Andrus JK, Marques E, Boshell J, Pallansch M, de Quadros CA, Kew OM: Direct detection of wild poliovirus circulation by stool surveys of healthy children and analysis of community wastewater. J Infect Dis 1993;168:1510-1514.

15 van der Avoort HGAM, Hull BP, Hovi T, Pallansch MA, Kew OM, Crainic R, Wood DJ, Mulders MN, van Loon AM: Comparative study on five methods for intratypic differentiation of polioviruses. J Clin Microbiol 1995;33:2562-2566.

Dr. T. Hovi, National Public Health Institute (KTL), Enterovirus Laboratory, Mannerheimintie 166, FIN-00300 Helsinki.

Brown F (ed): Progress in Polio Eradication: Vaccine Strategies for the End Game.
Dev Biol. Basel, Karger, 2001, vol 105, pp 33-40

A Scenario for Polio Eradication

I. Arita

Agency for Cooperation in International Health (ACIH), Kumamoto, Japan

Key words: Polio eradication, population density, surveillance, immunisation, smallpox eradication, AFP (acute flaccid paralysis)

Abstract: Polio eradication has entered the phase operating in the Asian sub-continent and in sub-Saharan Africa, where polio is still endemic in 30 countries. These countries are apparently most resistant to the eradication effort. The WHO polio panel held in May, in Geneva, discussed a scenario to stop transmission by 2002 and thereafter three years for certification. This paper discusses the scenario based on experience with smallpox eradication from the viewpoint of impact of population density on immunisation. The programme in the Indian sub-continent, which has the world's highest population density, may require a more rigorous surveillance-containment type strategy than that in sub-Saharan Africa which, with its lower density of population in many countries, may be relatively susceptible to the eradication effort. However, countries with higher population density and/or with political trouble may pose substantial difficulties. Also briefly discussed are measures to be taken after interruption of polio transmission world-wide. These still require intensive studies. The goal is foreseeable and with intensified mobilisation of global resources.

Introduction

When it met in Geneva in May 2000, the WHO polio eradication panel discussed a scenario in which the programme interrupts polio transmission worldwide in 2002 and thereafter a three years' certification programme would follow. We supported such a scenario in our publication in March [1]. As of May 2000, there are 30-polio endemic countries in the Indian sub-continent and sub-Saharan Africa, a reduction from 125 polio endemic countries in five continents in 1988. They are, though, hard-core countries which have been resistant to the eradication effort. In this paper, we discuss a few factors relevant to future progress, in the hope that it would shed light on how to make the above scenario real.

Method of Analysis

Eradication of diseases was comprehensively reviewed in the Dahlem Conference, Berlin, held in 1997 [2]. Among many diseases, smallpox and polio, being acute viral infections, have many common features when eradication is specifically considered. Firstly, effective vaccination coverage is expected to reduce the number of individuals susceptible so that transmission dies out. Secondly, surveillance is the basis on which strategy is built, requiring a special standard method, namely, search for rash and fever cases in smallpox and for acute flaccid paralysis (AFP) in polio. Thirdly, and most important, disease eradication requires strong leadership, mobilisation of global resources and high productivity. These are essential to complete eradication within a short period of time because it is impossible to sustain global co-ordination and resource mobilisation over a long period [3].

Unlike smallpox, polio has subclinical infections, which may cause difficulty in surveillance, but the Sabin vaccine can infect contacts, increasing coverage. Thus, the two diseases share common basic features with some technical differences. This paper discusses the scenario in comparison with the smallpox experience. In fact, current polio eradication strategies, such as mass immunisation campaigns, active search, certification, containment of laboratory virus stocks, etc., have all followed the experiences in smallpox eradication.

Results

Impact of population density on immunisation

The principal strategy for eradication is to reduce those susceptible by intensive immunisation programmes in a given area so that transmission among groups of susceptibles dies out. Population density plays a distinct role in terms of the number of susceptibles in a unit area [4]. Table 1 illustrates this concept, namely a high immunisation coverage of even 90% will leave 100 susceptibles in a densely populated area of 1000 persons per km. This implies that an immunisation programme would have substantial difficulty in reducing the susceptibles in such an area. In contrast, there is no such difficulty in an area of low population density. Mindful of this, if we compare the eradication status of smallpox and polio, there is a striking resemblance of persistent transmission in the Indian sub-continent between the two diseases.

Table 1: Number of susceptibles per km^2 by immunisation coverage.

Density population per km^2	Immunisation coverage		
	50%	**80%**	**90%**
1000	500	200	100
500	250	100	50
200	100	40	20
100	50	20	10
50	25	10	5

Figure 1 shows the smallpox eradication status in 1973, six years after the start of the intensified global smallpox eradication programme. Endemic countries remained in the Indian sub-continent, where the population density is one of the highest in the world. Figure 1 also shows the polio eradication status in January 2000, 12 years after the start of the global polio eradication programme. Similarly,

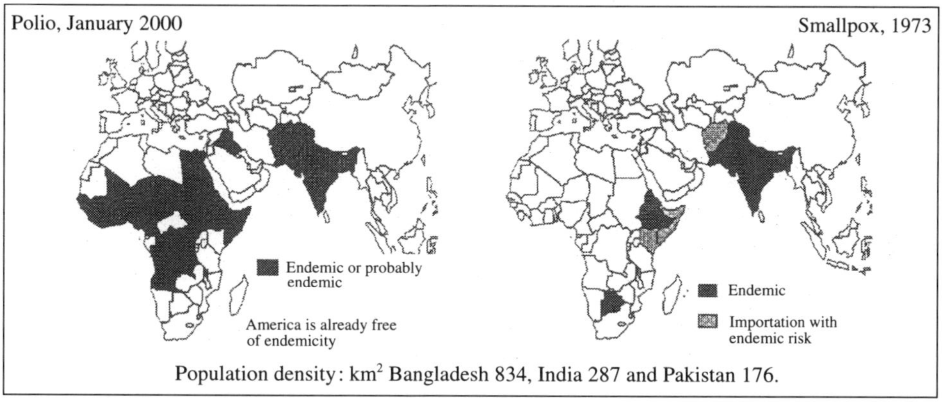

Fig 1: Status of eradication.

endemic polio remains in the Indian sub-continent. While we shall discuss sub-Saharan Africa in the next section, we believe the high population density in the Indian sub-continent plays a significant role in the persistent transmission of

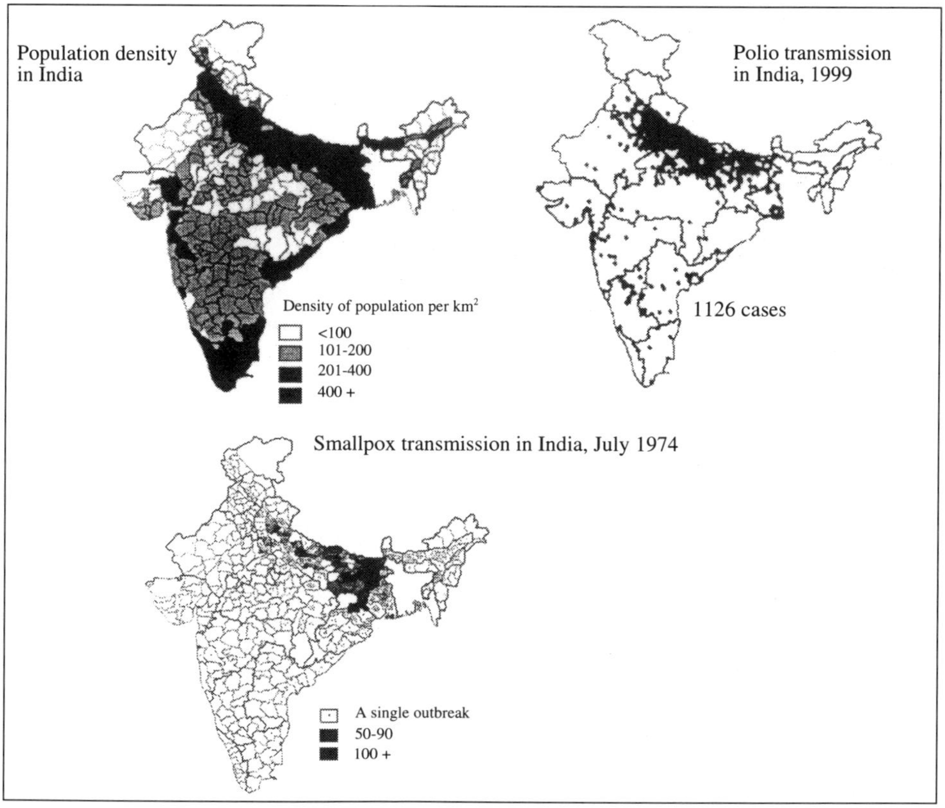

Fig. 2: Population density and transmission.

smallpox or polio. Close observations in India also substantiate this observation. (Fig. 2). In all India, the three northern states with the highest density population, Uttar Pradesh, Bihar and West Bengal were or have been resistant to the eradication effort both in both smallpox and polio.

To overcome this problem would require «100% immunisation coverage», which is impossible. The following episode is indicative. From 1962 to 1972, the Indian national smallpox eradication programme was conducted nation-wide with 100% target coverage. Despite their most intensive efforts, the incidence just continued without any reflection of the effort. In 1973, in recognition of the failure of this nation-wide campaign, the mass-campaign was discontinued and instead an active search for cases and containment of discovered cases was conducted, with mobilisation of all Indian health centres staff. After 18 months, the incidence reached zero (Fig. 3). The conclusion from this is that because of the high population density, high vaccination coverage, such as 95%, left a substantial number of susceptibles and only an active search detected hidden cases, which were rapidly contained by a limited area immunisation action. In addition, use of the smallpox vaccine was greatly reduced with this new strategy.

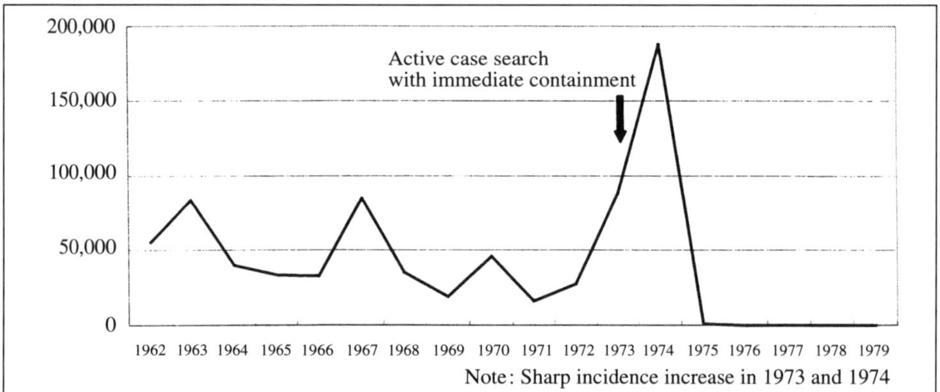

Fig. 3: Number of smallpox cases reported by year in India.

Currently, polio eradication in the Indian sub-continent depends mainly upon repeated NID (mass immunisation vaccination of the 0-5 age group) and ultimately a "final" immunisation campaign in high-risk areas to stop transmission – "mop-up". It is hoped that this strategy works, as it did in Cambodia (population density 52 per km), where the last polio case occurred in 1997. However, if the current strategy is unable to circumscribe effectively the transmissions in 2000, the strategy, NID combined with active search for cases and subsequent outbreak containment may be needed – a modified strategy of surveillance-containment measures used in smallpox eradication. It would be best to start this before the epidemic season of summer 2001. Practical modus operandi should be prepared, including concise definition of (i) AFP requiring containment, (ii) timing, (iii) population group for the containment vaccination, (iv) formation of teams, (v) logistics and (vi) mobilisation of necessary resources. As already mentioned, smallpox and polio differ in terms of manifestation of infection, and effectiveness of immu-

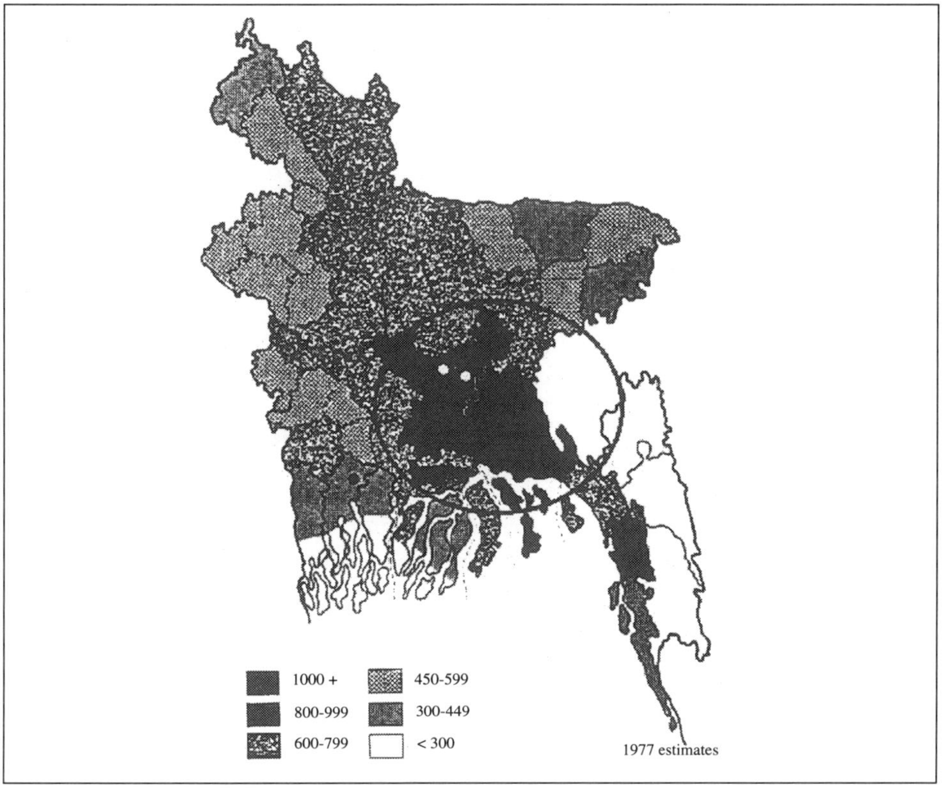

Fig. 4: Population density in Bangladesh.

nisation. Nevertheless, we should consider that the density of population plays a vital role and 100% vaccination, as experience has shown, is impossible.

The current situation in Bangladesh appears to be relevant and is intriguing. In 1999, 28 isolates of wild polio virus were discovered. Of these, 26 were found in the area roughly circled (Fig. 4). As of May 2000, one wild virus has been reported in 2000. Incomplete surveillance? Or diminishing transmission? In either case, why not focus on this area with surveillance-containment measures in addition to NID. Pakistan should receive the same treatment as India.

Guarded optimism, yet epidemic risk in sub-Saharan Africa

Low density of population, at the same time, may explain why some national programmes have rapidly stopped polio transmission by rather mediocre immunisation programme and surveillance. The best examples have been in Bolivia, Papua New Guinea and Southern African countries. The density of population in most of these countries is extremely low, being less than 10-30 per km. Likewise, many countries in sub-Saharan Africa have a low population density. (Table 2) Thus, sub-Saharan Africa may enjoy a guarded optimism for stopping polio transmission by 2002. Sometimes, transmission may die out naturally. The current

Table 2: Population density and wild polio virus isolates[1] in Sub-Saharan Africa, 1999.

	Density of population km^2	Polio virus
West		
Benin	52	8
Burkina Faso	40	0
Chad	5	34
Côte d'Ivoire	44	9
Gabon	4	0
Gambia	103	0
Ghana	77	3
Guinea	31	4
Guinea Bissau	31	0
Liberia	26	11
Mali	9	4
Mauritania	2	1
Niger	7	7
Nigeria	125	94
Senegal	45	0
Sierra Leone	62	1
Togo	76	1
East/Central		
Burundi	224	0
Cameroon	29	1
CAR	5	0
Congo	8	0
DRC	20	2
Eritrea	29	0
Ethiopia	54	0
Kenya	57	0
Rwanda	223	0
Somalia	16	0
Sudan	11	9
Uganda	85	0
South		
Angola	9	53
Botswana	3	0
Malawi	88	0
Mozambique	23	0
Namibia	2	0
South Africa	35	0
Tanzania	36	0
Zambia	11	0
Zimbabwe	29	0

[1] Data only for preliminary review requiring more information in 2000.

eradication strategy in this region would be workable. However, there are some circumstances, which might cause delay. For example, the density of population in Nigeria is 125 per km, the highest in sub-Saharan Africa. As of May 2000, the disease was highly endemic there. The country may require treatment similar to that used in India. In smallpox eradication, Nigeria was also the last endemic country in the entire West Africa despite its relatively better health system [4].

Risk of importation establishing transmission

In any poor country with inefficient surveillance and mediocre immunisation, the above risk exists as long as transmission is continuing in the region. If political disturbance occurs, the risk becomes greater as happened in Angola and DRC. Poor surveillance in the Horn of Africa also poses the risk. Further, slow laboratory confirmation may delay the action for detection and containment. Thus, continuing vigilance, namely surveillance, and response in all the nations in sub-Saharan Africa will be needed. Intensified mobilisation of resources (personnel and transport) is the key. It is clear, the sooner the transmission is interrupted, the smaller the risk.

Mobilisation of world resources

The greatest benefits of eradication will be to save human burden and the health budget by finally discontinuing immunisation programmes. This second benefit is greatest in industrialised countries. It is important for such highly developed countries to assist the endemic countries in terms of expertise, transport, vaccine and laboratory services. In smallpox eradication for the last three years of the campaign (so to speak – "the end game" here) in the Indian sub-continent as well as the horn of Africa, WHO and bilateral collaboration invested around 150 to 200 international personnel with an adequate supply of transport into the last endemic countries – India, Bangladesh, Pakistan, Ethiopia and Somalia. These actions accelerated and safeguarded the success. In polio eradication, much greater personnel investment than at present in key countries such as Nigeria would be most desirable.

Measures after zero incidence world-wide

How can we assure no transmission? Studies on the South American experience (last case in 1991) may help to set up the strategy. In smallpox eradication, pockmark survey in school children was extremely useful for certification in Africa. Also, vigorous nationwide search for hidden smallpox cases, house-to-house, was conducted three times in India and eight times in Bangladesh during the two year certification period, to ensure no hidden transmission [5]. In polio eradication, sub-clinical infection may pose problems in sub-Saharan Africa where sometimes surveillance would have been poor and necessary visits restricted due to political unrest. International commitment would be the key word to do the job. The results of surveillance on vaccine-associated poliomyelitis are important.

As with smallpox virus stocks, international registration of laboratories with wild poliovirus is planned for final destruction of the virus. This may pose difficulties since there are many laboratories worldwide which have the virus, unlike the situation with smallpox virus stocks at that time. Even today, smallpox virus stocks have not been destroyed despite repeated recommendations by WHO.

For those countries where no polio has been reported for a long time, use of IPV has already been initiated or suggested, while continued use of OPV for the rest of the world could also be envisaged. OPV is affordable. However, vaccine-associated polio paralysis occurs in one in a million vaccinees. How long these dual immunisations will continue depends upon how post-eradication measures are successfully implemented. WHO started a study on the fate of vaccine virus in vaccinated population, in the context of polio eradication. The study should be promoted. Reserve stocks of vaccines should also be prepared. Perhaps, global development of "surveillance, alert and response" would be the key, to be undertaken simultaneously, while these measures are being processed.

Stopping polio immunisation is the final target

To realise this, satisfactory results of the measures mentioned above are required so that all nations are assured that stopping polio immunisation is safe. Parenthetically, the measures taken for post-eradication of smallpox were in fact by "hindsight", by evaluating how global stoppage of transmission had been convincingly achieved. Perhaps it would be worthwhile for WHO to have a policy meeting at the end 2002 when the world incidence will be reaching zero.

Conclusion

The global programme has now entered a most critical phase. It requires continuous analysis of programme strategy and its adjustment. The smallpox eradication programme altered its strategy several times, in the course of 10 years, shifting from mass immunisation to surveillance-containment, for example. The goal is foreseeable following the scenario, but we need redoubled efforts supported by global mobilisation of resources.

Acknowledgement

I am grateful to Dr. Geoffrey Schild, who invited me to prepare this report. My thanks are to Prof. Teigi Yamamoto, Dr. Kohei Toda and Dr. Takashi Nakano, medical advisors to JICA, for their valuable comments.

References

1 Arita I, Nakane M: Does polio eradication succeed meeting the target year of 2000? Japanese Journal of Infectious Diseases, National Institute of Infectious Disease, Tokyo, Japan, 2000;53:6-10.

2 Report of the Dahlem Workshop on the Eradication of Infectious Diseases, Berlin, March 16-22, John Wiley & Sons, 1997.

3 Arita I: Are there better global mechanisms for formulating, implementing, and evaluating eradication programs? Report of the Dahlem Workshop on The Eradication of Infectious Diseases, Berlin, March 16-22, John Wiley & Sons, 1997, pp 177-186.

4 Arita I, Wickett J Fenner F: Impact of population density on immunisation programmes. Journal of Hygiene 1986;96:459-456.

5 Arita I: Virological evidence for the success of the smallpox eradication programme. Nature 1979;279:293-298.

Dr. I. Arita, Agency for Cooperation in International Health (ACIH), 4-11-1 Higashi-machi, Kumamoto-City, Kumamoto, 862-0901 Japan.

Brown F (ed): Progress in Polio Eradication: Vaccine Strategies for the End Game.
Dev Biol. Basel, Karger, 2001, vol 105, p 41

SESSION II

The Biology and Molecular Biology of Polioviruses

Chairperson: *Jeff Almond*

Brown F (ed): Progress in Polio Eradication: Vaccine Strategies for the End Game.
Dev Biol. Basel, Karger, 2001, vol 105, pp 43-50

Some Problems of Molecular Biology of Poliovirus Infection Relevant to Pathogenesis, Viral Spread and Evolution

V.I. Agol, G.A. Belov, E.A. Cherkasova, G.V. Gavrilin, M.S. Kolesnikova, L.I. Romanova, E.A. Tolskaya

M.P. Chumakov Institute of Poliomyelitis & Viral Encephalitides, Russian Academy of Medical Sciences, Moscow, Russia

Key words: Poliomyelitis, pathogenesis, epidemiology, genetic drift, recombination

Abstract: Molecular mechanisms of poliovirus reproduction in the human gut remain largely unexplored. Nevertheless, there are grounds to believe that the virus spreads from cell to cell, like that from person to person during natural circulation, and involves a relatively small proportion of the highly heterogeneous viral population generated by the previous host. This mechanism of random sampling is responsible for the majority of fixed mutations, and contributes to the maintenance of a certain level of viral fitness (virulence). In the long term, random sampling may lead to the decrease in fitness and even to extinction of some viral evolutionary branches, explaining cases of self-limiting poliovirus infection in immunodeficient patients. A low propensity of the Sabin viruses for natural circulation may also be a related phenomenon. The trend to decrease in fitness may be interrupted by the appearance of rare, fitter (more virulent) variants, which may be responsible for poliomyelitis outbreaks caused by wild type virus, and for the development of paralytic disease in chronic carriers of the Sabin vaccine. All these evolutionary events are largely stochastic and hence are unpredictable in principle.

At a meeting devoted to polio eradication, it seems appropriate to discuss primarily those molecular mechanisms of poliovirus reproduction that are relevant to the eradication programme. In this context, there are two important issues, (i) the factors controlling the level and duration of poliovirus excretion and (ii) the properties of the excreted virus. With regard to item (i), the key questions concern the nature and abundance of the target cells, the character of cellular responses to the infection (in particular, infection with virulent and attenuated strains), the level and rate of viral reproduction in these cells, and the mechanisms of viral clearance. For obvious reasons, there are few, if any, direct approaches for investigating the cellular and molecular aspects of poliovirus reproduction in the human gut. Our current understanding of these aspects is based primarily on more or less justified extrapolations from animal and in vitro experiments.

Variability of Cell Responses to Poliovirus Infection

It is well known that only the cells expressing appropriate receptors which mediate entry of the viral genome into the cytoplasm can be susceptible to poliovirus. Unfortunately, the presence and abundance of poliovirus receptors in tissues of a human organism, and in particular, in the cells of alimentary tract (the place of primary infection) are not adequately characterized. Nevertheless, there is reason to believe that expression of the functional poliovirus receptor is restricted to relatively few cell types.

The presence of the receptor is a condition necessary but not sufficient for poliovirus reproduction. The host cell-specific intracellular variability of poliovirus reproduction is a well-known phenomenon. Thus, the duration of a single reproduction cycle and the yield of infectious viral progeny may vary significantly among cell lines. Sometimes this variation is especially prominent for attenuated poliovirus strains. For example, the yield of Sabin 1 virus is dramatically suppressed and the length of the reproductive cycle markedly prolonged in human neuroblastoma cells compared to HeLa cells [1].

Theoretically, different molecular mechanisms may be responsible for variations in the intracellular capacity to support poliovirus reproduction. Several host proteins appear to be involved in the IRES-dependent initiation of translation of picornavirus RNAs, and it is likely that expression of at least some of these proteins is controlled in a tissue-specific fashion. It was suggested long ago that different cells may possess somewhat different, but perhaps overlapping, sets of accessory translation initiation factors (for example, neural cells may be unique in this respect) [2, 3], and accumulating data tend to support this notion. Intracellular restrictions on poliovirus growth may operate also on steps other than translation initiation. These restrictions may impose additional significant limitations on poliovirus reproduction in certain cells of the human organism. However, no adequate information is available about the nature and tissue distribution of such factors in the human alimentary tract.

Another important, though not yet adequately appreciated, factor of poliovirus pathogenesis concerns the type of cellular response to the infection. Poliovirus is generally cytocidal but it may kill its host cell in two different ways: (i) by inducing the canonical cytopathic effect (CPE) or (ii) by triggering the apoptotic response [4, 5]. Several poliovirus proteins result in severe damage of cellular functions, which is recognized by the cell as an intervention requiring an apoptotic response. Examples of such stresses include suppression of host translation and transcription mediated by the viral proteinases 2A [6] and 3C [7].

Apoptosis is a kind of defensive suicidal reaction of the infected cell. It may result in its premature death and consequently in a decrease in the virus yield. In addition, a portion of the progeny may be sequestered in the "apoptotic bodies" and thus prevented from further spread. On the other hand, poliovirus is equipped with several functions able to counteract the apoptotic response [4, 8, N. Neznanov et al., in preparation]. HeLa cells become committed to apoptosis very early after infection but the implementation of the apoptotic programme is normally interrupted by the turn-on of the viral anti-apoptotic functions [8]. This, however, is not a universal scenario.

Depending on the balance of host pro-apoptotic and anti-apoptotic factors, the time-course and vigour of the intracellular reproduction, and on some external conditions, poliovirus infection may result in either CPE or apoptosis. The outcome is highly host cell-specific, as judged by experiments with different cell lines [L. I. Romanova et al., in preparation], but we know very little, if anything, about the character of the cellular response to poliovirus infection in the human organism. On the basis of some indirect and admittedly weak considerations we may expect that apoptosis may play a significant role in the pathogenesis.

Thus, we have at most only a very vague idea about what is going in the poliovirus-infected human gut. Nevertheless, the general impression is that under natural conditions poliovirus is not as aggressive as one may infer from experiments using the standard laboratory models. The very rare incidence of overt paralytic disease among non-immune infected persons may be largely due to the relatively innocuous nature of the virus itself. This innocuousness may hypothetically be caused, at least in part, by a limited capacity of the virus to grow in the human gut due to a low abundance of susceptible cells and/or their low capacity to support viral reproduction. This point is important for the consideration of the nature of poliovirus evolution.

The Nature of Poliovirus Evolution

For the eradication programme, the evaluation of the evolutionary potential of poliovirus is of uppermost importance. Genome sequencing during poliomyelitis outbreaks demonstrates that the virus usually evolves at a rate of a few percent of nucleotides per year [9]. The molecular events underlying the viral evolution are relatively well understood. Copying of the poliovirus genome is accomplished by the error-prone viral RNA-dependent RNA polymerase, which is devoid of the proof-reading capacity (ability to remove erroneously incorporated nucleotides). The rate of error is so high that, on the average, each progeny RNA molecule differs from its template by at least one mutation. As a result, any, even a plaque-purified, population of poliovirus is represented by a highly heterogeneous "swarm" of genomes, or a quasispecies [10].

The abundance of mutants in a viral population is a necessary but not sufficient condition for the evolution to occur. Those who for some reason have sequenced fragments of poliovirus RNA already sequenced in other labs have been undoubtedly impressed by the absence of substantial differences in spite of numerous passages separating the objects of sequencing. Thus, under constant conditions the poliovirus genome is generally quite stable. A mutation is fixed only if there is a good reason for this. There are two major "good reasons": (i) if the mutation confers a selective advantage through fitness increase; and (ii) if the infecting viral sample represents a relatively small portion of the quasispecies population and therefore just does not contain more competitive variants. In the latter case, the mutation is fixed regardless of its phenotypic value.

For a practical perspective, it is very important to assess the contributions of adaptation (Darwinian evolution) and random sampling (neutral evolution) to the changes occurring in poliovirus properties upon natural circulation of the virus. Indeed, the former is expected to result in the selection of fitter and perhaps more virulent variants, whereas the viral fitness may be maintained at a more or less constant level or it may even decrease as a result of the latter. There are strong enough arguments that the majority of random mutations in any genome are phenotypically neutral, some are detrimental and only a tiny minority may increase the fitness. Therefore, a decrease in fitness or even self-extinction are likely results of long-term random sampling. This phenomenon is known as the Muller's ratchet [10].

Again, there are serious obstacles for studying this problem directly in the case of poliovirus: no adequate approach for the evaluation of fitness of viral isolates for their natural ecological niche, the human gut, is available. Nevertheless, investigation of viral properties, and in particular sequencing of portions of the viral genome, permit reasonably accurate assessments to be made.

The adaptive evolution of poliovirus certainly does occur, for example, in the gut of vaccinees fed with the oral poliomyelitis vaccine. Some of the attenuating mutations present in the Sabin strains appear to decrease virus fitness for the gut. Viruses isolated from faecal samples soon after vaccination very often demonstrated loss of such mutations, e.g. those located in the 5'-untranslated region [11]. Another example of adaptive evolution is represented by changes in the antigenic determinants, helping the virus to escape the host immunity [12]. Nevertheless, the results of sequencing of the genomes of evolving poliovirus lineages strongly suggest that the most important quantitative factor in poliovirus evolution appears to be random sampling [13].

How can conclusions of this sort be derived from the sequencing results? There are two indicators, the presence of which is strongly suggestive of a significant contribution of neutral evolution: (i) the predominance of synonymous mutations (nucleotide substitutions that do not change the sense of codons), and (ii) the constant rate of mutation fixation. Indeed, synonymous mutations may be less likely to affect the level of fitness

We have studied two evolving poliovirus lineages [13]. The first corresponded to 11 wild type strains isolated from poliomyelitis patients over the territory of the FSU in 1991 to 1995 and comprising a distinct cluster of the T geotype [14]. These strains indeed belonged to a common lineage, as inferred not only from the close similarities of their genomic sequences but also from the fact that the first isolate, which came from Tajikistan, was very close to a strain isolated the same year in Pakistan, a close neighbour of Tajikistan. The other set of viruses was represented by five vaccine-related strains isolated successively from an immunodeficient patient with paralytic poliomyelitis [15]. About 2500 nucleotides corresponding to the VP1, 2A, 2B genes and portions of the 2C and 3D regions in each of the consecutive isolates were sequenced. In both lineages, the overwhelming majority (around 75%) of accumulated mutations turned out to be synonymous substitutions, and the fixation of both total and synonymous mutations occurred at constant rates (with linear regression coefficients being ≥ 0.95). Thus, the character and the rate of genetic changes occurring during evolution of the two poliovirus populations are consistent with a major role of random sampling.

For the circulating wild type poliovirus, a plausible scenario of such a mode of evolution is easy to conceive. Person-to-person transfer appears to involve relatively small viral samples, representing only a small proportion of the variants generated in the previous host. This situation is to some extent reminiscent of plaque-to-plaque passages. Mechanistically, the random sampling of poliovirus in the gut of immunodeficient patients is more difficult to imagine. However, the character of mutation accumulation forces us to propose that in this case the mechanism is essentially the same. It seems likely that the ratio between the virus titre in the intestinal content and the number of susceptible cells is such that the spread of infection is again similar to plaque-to-plaque transfer.

If genetic drift is accepted as a major factor of poliovirus evolution, we may discuss some possible biological consequences. Since the evolution is not directed toward a specific destination(s), it should result in a significant diversification of the viral genome. This fact may be illustrated by remarkable differences between the sets of mutations accumulated in the viral RNA during the long-term reproduction of the Sabin 1 vaccine in the gut of different immunodeficient patients [13, 16]. Although the choice of specific mutations to be fixed is unpredictable in principle, the random sampling mode of evolution is expected to maintain viral fitness at a relatively constant level or it may even result in its decline. This corollary follows from the relative proportion of phenotypically neutral, debilitating and adaptive mutations among the multitude of random substitutions. The possibility of a decrease in virus fitness, the Muller's ratchet, is of particular interest. It may result in self-extinction of some evolutionary branches, explaining known cases of self-limiting poliovirus infection in immunodeficient patients. This phenomenon may also contribute to a low propensity of the Sabin viruses for natural circulation.

Being responsible for the overwhelming part of fixed mutations, neutral evolution is certainly not the only mechanism of poliovirus variability in nature. We have already mentioned some examples of adaptive changes known to occur during poliovirus evolution. The adaptive mutations are expected to accumulate even more frequently in populations with a significantly decreased fitness. This could occur just because a greater proportion of random mutations of a debilitated genome are expected to increase fitness. The selective value of such adaptive mutations is also expected to increase. Thus, the trend to self-extinction may be counteracted by stochastic appearance of mutations increasing the fitness [17].

Disturbances in the purely neutral mode of poliovirus evolution could also be readily revealed by analysis of mutation fixation. Typical disturbances consist of varying rates of evolution of different parts of the viral genome and in an uneven rate of viral evolution in time (deviations from the molecular clock). Both these phenomena were observed during the evolution of real poliovirus populations [13].

Occurrence of Poliovirus Recombinants and its Biological Meaning

In addition to the fixation of nucleotide substitutions, another powerful mechanism of poliovirus evolution is recombination. The mechanism(s) of recombination is beyond the scope of the present discussion. The biological significance of this phenomenon however, merits a few remarks.

Intertypic poliovirus recombinants are abundant among isolates from healthy vaccinees [18] and cases of vaccine-associated poliomyelitis [19, 20]. These observations raised the possibility that recombinants might have some selective advantage over the non-recombinant parents, perhaps by possessing increased levels of neurovirulence. Although such a hypothesis cannot be ruled out, we favour another explanation. As argued in the preceding section, poliovirus reproduction in the human gut involves random sampling and as a consequence accumulation of debilitating mutations. Recombination may be considered as a kind of proofreading mechanism serving to negate the effects of such errors through rescuing "healthy" portions of the progeny RNA molecules. In other words, replication is accompanied by such a load of adverse mutation, and the number of particles used for viral propagation is so small, that recombination is the easiest way to save viable virus. According to this proposal, the intertypic recombinants, for example between Sabin strains, should not necessarily be more virulent compared to their monotypic parents. Experiments are underway to check the validity of this prediction.

Interestingly, there is a strong bias, among the natural intertypic poliovirus recombinants, with regard to the donors of the portion of the viral genome encoding capsid proteins. For example, we have observed preferential abundance of recombinants belonging to serotype 2 [19]. There is no obvious reason why recombination between two viral parents should occur non-reciprocally. Therefore, we propose that preponderance of a certain serotype among intertypic poliovirus recombinants is a secondary phenomenon, reflecting the negative selection related to the immune status of the particular virus excretor. According to this explanation, the abundance of, say, type 2 recombinants was merely due to a relatively low immunity to type 2 poliovirus in the guts in which these recombinants have been generated.

Concluding Remarks

Although the molecular biology of poliovirus reproduction in the human gut remains largely unexplored, the virus spread from cell to cell and from person to person during natural circulation appears to involve a relatively small portion of the highly heterogeneous viral population generated by the previous host (cell or organism, respectively). This mechanism of random sampling is responsible for the majority of fixed mutations, and results in maintenance of a certain level of viral fitness (virulence). In long terms, random sampling may lead to fitness decrease (the Muller's ratchet). Theoretically, it may even result in extinction of some evolutionary branches of the virus, explaining known cases of self-limiting poliovirus infection in immunodeficient patients. A low propensity of the Sabin viruses for natural circulation may also be a related phenomenon. The trend to fitness decrease may be interrupted by the appearance of rare, fitter (more virulent) variants, which may be responsible for poliomyelitis outbreaks caused by wild type viruses, and the development of paralytic disease in chronic carriers of the Sabin vaccine derivatives.

An unpleasant feature of this scenario is that it is largely based on stochastic events and is unpredictable in principle. Therefore, one should be cautious with calculations assuming that such epidemiological parameters as secondary attack rate, basic reproduction number and critical populations' size [21] are represented by constant values. Any evolutionary branch may disappear or may give rise to a new flowering outgrowth. The only way to get rid of the virus is to cut the roots – to eradicate the whole tree. However, the questions remain (i) how many roots does the tree possess and (ii) how deep are these roots in the soil?

Acknowledgement

Collaboration with Galina Lipskaya (WHO, Copenhagen), Kurt Bienz and Denis Egger (Basel University) and Olen Kew (CDC, Atlanta) is gratefully acknowledged. Experimental work in the authors' laboratory on which the paper is based was supported by grants from the Russian Foundation for Basic Research and the European Union grants Copernicus and INTAS.

References

1 Tolskaya EA, Kolesnikova MS, Ivannikova TA, Drozdov SG, Korolev MB, Agol VI: Restricted growth of attenuated poliovirus strains in cultured cells of a human neuroblastoma. J Virol 1989;63:4034-4039.

2 Svitkin YV, Maslova SV, Agol VI: The genomes of attenuated and virulent poliovirus strains differ in their in vitro translation efficiencies. Virology 1985;147:243-252.

3 Svitkin YV, Pestova TV, Maslova SV, Agol VI: Point mutations modify the response of poliovirus RNA to a translation initiation factor: a comparison of neurovirulent and attenuated strains. Virology 1988;166:394-404.

4 Tolskaya EA, Romanova LI, Kolesnikova MS, Ivannikova TA, Smirnova EA, Raikhlin NT, Agol VI: Apoptosis-inducing and apoptosis-preventing functions of poliovirus. J Virol 1995;69:1181-1189.

5 Agol VI., Belov GA, Bienz K, Egger D, Kolesnikova MS, Raikhlin N, Romanova LI, Smirnova EA, Tolskaya EA: Two types of death of poliovirus-infected cells: caspase involvement in the apoptosis but not cytopathic effect. Virology 1998;252:343-353.

6 Goldstaub D, Gradi A, Bercovitch Z, Grosmann Z, Nophar Y, Luria S, Sonenberg N, Kahana C: Poliovirus 2A protease induces apoptotic cell death. Mol Cell Biol 2000;20:1271-1277.

7 Feduchi E, Carrasco L: Poliovirus protease 3C(pro) kills cells by apoptosis. Virology 2000;266:352-360.

8 Agol VI, Belov GA, Bienz K, Egger D, Kolesnikova MS, Romanova LI, Sladkova LV, Tolskaya EA: Competing death programs in poliovirus-infected cells: Commitment switch in the middle of infectious cycle. J Virol 2000;74:5534-5541.

9 Kew OM, Mulders MN, Lipskaya GY, Da Silva EE, Pallansch MA: Molecular epidemiology of polioviruses. Semin Virol 1995;6:401-414.

10 Domingo E, Escarmis C, Menendez-Arias L, Holland JJ: Viral quasispecies and fitness variations, in Domingo E, Webster R, Holland JJ (eds): Origin and Evolution of Viruses. San Diego, Acad Press, 1999, pp 141-161.

11 Minor PD, Dunn G: The effect of sequences in the 5' non-coding region on the replication of polioviruses in the human gut. J Gen Virol 1988;69:1091-1096.

12 Minor PD: Antigenic structure of picornaviruses. Curr Top Microbiol Immunol 1990;161:121-154.

13 Gavrilin GV, Cherkasova EA, Lipskaya GY, Kew OM, Agol VI: Evolution of circulating wild poliovirus and of vaccine-derived poliovirus in an immunodeficient patient: a unifying model. J Virol 2000; 74:7381-7390.

14 Lipskaya GY, Chervonskaya EA, Belova GI, Maslova SV, Kutateladze TN, Drozdov SG, Mulders M, Pallansch MA, Kew OM, Agol VI: Geographical genotypes (geotypes) of poliovirus case isolates from the Former Soviet Union: relatedness to other known poliovirus genotypes. J Gen Virol 1995;76:1687-1699.

15 Kew OM, Sutter RW, Nottay BK, McDonough MJ, Prevots DR, Quick L, Pallansch MA: Prolonged replication of a type 1 vaccine-derived poliovirus in an immunodeficient patient. J Clin Microbiol 1998;36:2893-2899.

16 Bellmunt AG, May G, Zell R, Pring-Akerblom P, Verhagen W, Heim A: Evolution of poliovirus type 1 during 5.5 years of prolonged enteral replication in an immunodeficient patient. Virology 1999;265:178-184.

17 Escarmis C, Davila M, Domingo E: Multiple molecular pathways for fitness recovery of an RNA virus debilitated by operation of Muller's ratchet. J Mol Biol 1999;285:495-505.

18 Cammack N, Phillips A, Dunn G, Patel V, Minor PD: Intertypic genomic rearrangements of poliovirus strains in vaccinees. Virology 1988;167:507-514.

19 Lipskaya GY, Muzychenko AR, Kutitova OK, Maslova SV, Equestre M, Drozdov SG, Perez Bercoff R, Agol VI: Frequent isolation of intertypic poliovirus recombinants with serotype 2 specificity from vaccine-associated polio cases. J Med Virol 1991;35:290-296.

20 Furione M, Guillot S, Otelea D, Balanant J, Candrea A, Crainic R: Polioviruses with natural recombinant genomes isolated from vaccine-associated paralytic poliomyelitis. Virology 1993;196:199-208.

21 Fine PE, Carneiro IA: Transmissibility and persistence of oral polio vaccine viruses: implications for the global poliomyelitis eradication initiative. Am J Epidemiol 1999;150:1001-1021.

Dr. V.I. Agol, Institute of Poliomyelitis, Kievskoye shosse 27 km., Moscow Region 142782, Russia.

Brown F (ed): Progress in Polio Eradication: Vaccine Strategies for the End Game.
Dev Biol. Basel, Karger, 2001, vol 105, pp 51-58

The Molecular Basis of Poliovirus Neurovirulence

S. Ohka, A. Nomoto

Department of Microbiology, Graduate School of Medicine,
The University of Tokyo, Tokyo, Japan

Key words: Poliovirus receptor, transgenic mice, viral dissemination, blood brain barrier, axonal transport, neurovirulence

Abstract: Species specificity of poliovirus (PV) is mostly governed by host cellular molecules that serve as the PV receptor (PVR). Molecular cloning of the gene and cDNAs of human PVR and the subsequent development of PV-sensitive transgenic (Tg) mice carrying the human PVR gene made it possible to investigate molecular mechanisms for PV-specific dissemination in the whole body. After intravenous inoculation which makes artificial viremia, poliovirus appears to enter the central nervous system (CNS) at a fairly high rate via the blood brain barrier, suggesting existence of a specific permeation system for PV. This main dissemination process does not require PVR. After intramuscular inoculation, PV appears to be incorporated by endocytosis at synapses, and the endosomes containing PV transported through axons to neuron cell body, where viral replication occurs. Efficiency of viral multiplication in the CNS probably determines the neurovirulence level, which differs between PV strains. An important determinant for neurovirulence phenotype resides in the internal ribosomal entry site (IRES). This has led us to a concept of «IRES-dependent virus tropism».

INTRODUCTION

Poliomyelitis is an acute disease of the central nervous system (CNS) that is caused by poliovirus (PV), a human enterovirus that belongs to the *Picornaviridae*. The poliovirion is an icosahedral, non-enveloped particle that is composed of 60 copies of each of four capsid proteins, VP1, VP2, VP3, and VP4, and a single-stranded RNA genome of positive polarity. The three-dimensional structure of the virion particle (Hogle et al, 1985) has revealed depressions ('canyon') on the surface of the virion, which have been suggested to be attachment sites for the PV receptor (PVR) [1,2].

PVR, a member of the immunoglobulin superfamily, functions to bind virus and to convert its conformation, and is thought to be the only molecule that is involved in the uncoating process of PV. In fact, the interaction between PV (160S) and purified soluble PVR leads to a conformational change of the virion that manifests itself as 135S and 80S particles [3].

Phenomenalism of PV pathogenesis was first described in the 1950s [4,5]. In humans, after oral ingestion of PV, the virus multiplies in the alimentary mucosa, moves into the blood through the tonsils and Peyer's patches, and then invades the CNS probably through the blood brain barrier (BBB) (Fig. 1). Although it may not be the main dissemination pathway, a neural pathway has been reported for humans and monkey (Fig. 1) [6,7]. However, understanding the molecular basis of PV neurovirulence was hampered by the restricted host range of a virus that infects only primates.

Species specificity of PV is mostly governed by PVR. Indeed, transgenic mice that carry the human PVR gene have been shown to be susceptible to all three serotypes of PV. The development of PV-sensitive transgenic (Tg) mice [8,9] made it possible to study in detail the mechanisms of viral dissemination in the whole body. Actually, many comparative neurovirulence tests with various inoculation routes have revealed that the Tg mice are an excellent animal model for the study of PV neurovirulence.

Here we describe the establishment of experimental systems to study PV dissemination and replication in a body of the Tg mouse.

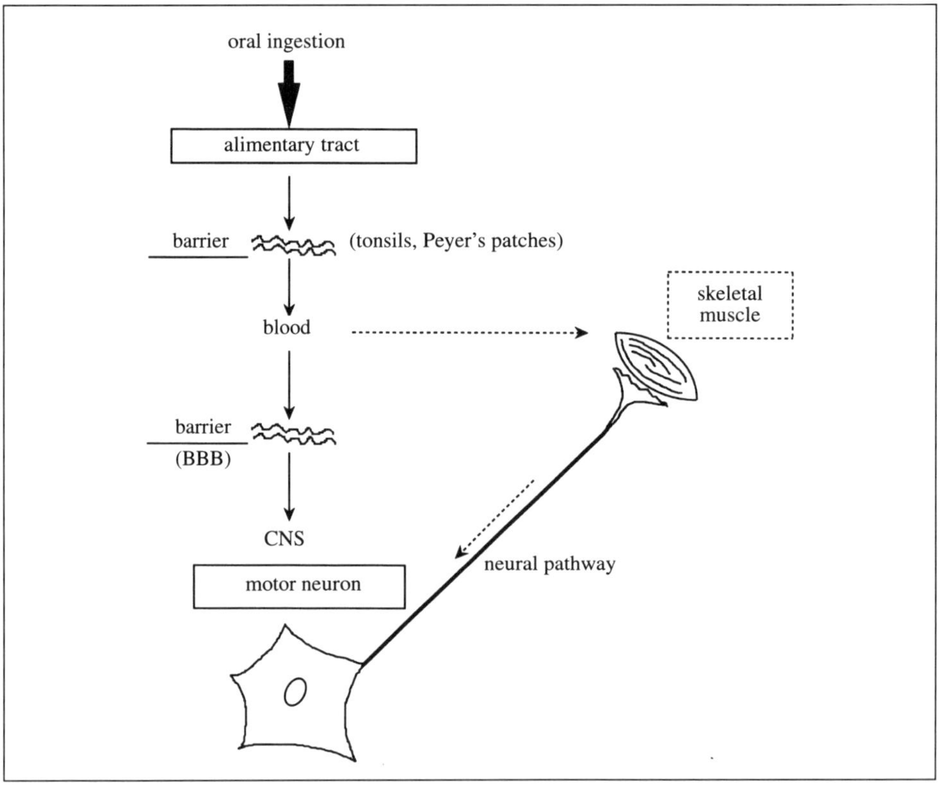

Fig. 1: Dissemination pathways of PV in humans. Dissemination pathways are shown by arrows. Of these, possible minor pathways are indicated by dotted arrows.

Materials and Methods

Transgenic mice

The Tg mouse line ICR-PVRTg21 [8], in the hemizygous stage of six to ten weeks of age, was used as an animal model. ICR or IQI mice were used as non-Tg mice. All mice used were free from specific pathogens.

Viruses and cells

The virulent Mahoney strain and the attenuated Sabin 1 strain of type 1 poliovirus were derived from infectious cDNA clones pOM1 [10] and pVS(1)IC-O(T) [11], respectively.

Suspension-cultured HeLa S3 cells were maintained in RPM1 1640 medium supplemented with 5% newborn calf serum (NCS) and used for preparation of viruses. African green monkey kidney (AGMK) cells were grown in Dulbecco modified Eagle medium supplemented with 5% NCS and used for plaque assays.

Purification of viruses

Viruses in cytoplasmic extracts of infected HeLa cells were purified by chromatography on DEAE-Sepharose CL-6B, followed by two cycles of CsCl equilibrium centrifugation in a buffer containing 10 mM Tris-HCl (pH 7.4), 10 mM NaCl, 20 mM EDTA and 1% Brij 58. For the preparation of (^{35}S)methionine-labelled viruses, virus was grown in methionine-free medium in the presence of (^{35}S)methionine.

Virus inoculation and tissue sampling

For intravenous (IV) administration, each mouse was inoculated with approximately 6.5×10^6 PFU containing 0.4 mCi of labelled virus via tail vein under mild ether anaesthesia. Mice were dissected five hours later. The tissues were weighed, minced, and dissolved with a tissue solubilizer, and 10 ml of liquid scintillation cocktail were then added. Accumulation rates of viruses to the brain were calculated by using the methods of pharmacokinetics [12].

For intramuscular (IM) administration, five ml of a virus solution (10^6 PFU) were inoculated into the left calf of each mouse under anaesthesia. For analysis of the materials in the sciatic nerve, the nerve was ligated tightly with silk thread near the junction of the thighbone and pelvis as described previously [13], and ^{35}S-labelled or non-labelled PV was inoculated into the calf.

Antibodies

To determine whether PVR is involved in PV dissemination, mouse anti-human PVR monoclonal antibody (mAb), p286, was used [12]. For IV inoculation, two nmol of the mAb were intravenously administered to Tg mice five hours before the virus inoculation. For IM inoculation, up to 42.2 mg of the mAb were co-injected with 10^6 PFU.

To detect PV antigens, the sections of the sciatic nerve, fixed with acetone-methanol (3:2) at room temperature, were reacted with rabbit hyperimmune serum against poliovirus type 1, and then treated with goat anti-rabbit IgG conjugated with fluorescein isothiocyanate [14]. The sections were observed with a confocal laser scanning microscope (Bio Rad).

Sucrose density gradient centrifugation

Seven and a half hours after IV inoculation, ^{35}S-labelled materials in the parenchyma fraction of the brain were analysed by centrifugation on 15-30% sucrose density gradient in a buffer containing 0.1% bovine serum albumin (BSA) and phosphate-buffered saline (8g of NaCl, 0.2g of KCl, 1.15g of Na_2HPO_4, and 0.2g of KH_2PO_4 per liter). Centrifugation was at 200,000g for two and a half hours at 4°C in a Beckman rotor SW41.

One and a half hours after the IM inoculation of [^{35}S]methionine-labelled Mahoney virus, the sciatic nerve that had been ligated was homogenized at 4°C in phosphate-buffered saline containing 1% Nonidet P40 and 0.1% BSA. After centrifuging the homogenate to remove the debris, the supernatant was analysed by sucrose density gradient centrifugation.

Results

Neurovirulence of IV-inoculated virus

The 50% lethal dose (LD_{50}) and minimum LD_{100} have been calculated to be 8.5×10^4 and 4.0×10^6 PFU/mouse, respectively, when the Tg mice are IV-inoculated with the virulent Mahoney strain. These doses are approximately 400 times higher than those using intracerebral inoculation [12]. The data suggest that about 0.25% of IV-inoculated virus has to invade the brain. Considering the fact that approximately 0.3% of the total amount of IV-inoculated virus is distributed to the cerebrum, most of the virus distributed should move into the brain [12]. This suggests that BBB permeation of PV is very efficient.

Accumulation of IV-inoculated virus in the CNS

To determine the rate of PV movement from the circulating blood to the CNS, Tg mice were IV-inoculated with ^{35}S-labelled Mahoney or Sabin 1 virus, and the time course of PV accumulation in the CNS tissues was measured up to seven and a half hours after the inoculation (data not shown) [12]. The data shown by integration plot indicate that the virus accumulates linearly in the CNS tissues up to seven and a half hours after the inoculation. The rate in the cerebrum was estimated to be 0.164 ml/min/g tissue. In tissues other than the CNS, linear accumulation was not seen, and the rates reach a plateau during the duration of the experiment (data not shown). These results strongly suggest the existence of a BBB permeation mechanism specific for PV.

Comparative study of PV accumulation in the brain

Similar accumulation experiments were carried out on the brain by using non-Tg mice to determine the contribution of human PVR to accumulation rates of viruses. As shown in Table 1, the rates observed in Tg mice resemble those in non-Tg mice. Thus, human PVR seems not to play an important role in delivering circulating PV to the brain. The accumulation rate was also examined for the Sabin 1 strain to determine the contribution of virion surface characteristics to the rate. The accumulation rates of the Sabin 1 virus in both Tg and non-Tg mice were slightly higher than that of the Mahoney virus, although the difference was in a range of negligible values. It should be noted that the accumulation rates observed for PVs are more than 100 times higher compared with that of albumin (Table 1), which is known to exhibit significantly restricted permeability across the BBB. Accumulation rate of cationized rat serum albumin, which is known to have an efficient BBB permeability, is similar to those of PVs (Table 1). These data strongly suggest that

Table 1: Accumulation rate of IV-inoculated PV into the mouse brain.

Virus or control material	Tg mouse	Non-Tg mouse	Rat
Mahoney	~ 150[a]	~ 150	
Sabin 1	~ 250	~ 250	
Albumin		1	
Cationized rat serum albumin			~ 150

[a] Approximate comparative value of accumulation rate of the Mahoney virus when that of albumin (0.001 µl/min/g tissue) is regarded as 1.

PVs permeate the BBB at a fairly high rate, independently of PVR and virus strains.

Since the possible permeation of PV through the BBB is not mediated by human PVR, it is possible that intact infectious PV particles exist in the parenchyma fraction of the brain. Accordingly, ^{35}S-labelled materials recovered in the parenchyma fraction at seven and a half hours after the inoculation were analysed by centrifugation on sucrose density gradients [12]. The majority of the radioactivity was associated with materials at 160S (data not shown). Indeed, this fraction had plaque forming activity.

Neurovirulence of IM-inoculated virus

To study mechanisms for viral transportation from the skeletal muscle to the CNS, 10^6 PFU of the virulent Mahoney strain were inoculated into the left calf of the Tg mice. This condition causes initial paralysis in all the infected mice within 48 hrs of inoculation [14]. No paralysis was observed when non-Tg mice were used in a similar experiment. The initial paralysis was inhibited by transection of the sciatic nerve before IM inoculation. This indicates involvement of the sciatic nerve in development of the initial paralysis.

As a way of measuring the velocity of PV transport through the sciatic nerve, we cut the sciatic nerve at a distance of 2 cm from the inoculation point at increasing times after the inoculation. Cutting at two, four and six hours after the inoculation protected all six mice, four of six mice, and two of six mice, respectively. The results indicated that at least a part of IM-inoculated PV reaches the transection point within four hours of inoculation. This means that some of the IM-inoculated virus moves faster than 12 cm/day. Thus, the velocity of the PV transport fell into the classification of fast retrograde axonal transport because the rate of slow retrograde axonal transport is <0.6 cm/day. Since materials that are transported by the fast retrograde axonal transport system are usually enclosed by endosomes, PV may be incorporated at synapses by endocytosis.

To confirm the contribution of PVR to the development of initial paralysis, the calves of Tg mice were inoculated with mixtures of PV and various amount of mAb p286, and observed for paralysis 48 hr after the inoculation. Co-injection of mAb p286 with PV protected the mice from paralysis in a dose-dependent manner (data not shown). The data indicate that PVR plays an important role(s) in the development of paralysis that include virus incorporation into synapses and virus transport through the sciatic nerve.

Virus-related materials in the sciatic nerve

Immunohistochemical analysis was used for detection of PV antigens in the sciatic nerve. Transverse sections of the sciatic nerve were prepared from the transection points at three to six hours after IM inoculation of the Mahoney virus, and examined for PV antigens. These were detected in many myelin-sheathed axons of the infected Tg mice (data not shown). The data proved that PV antigens exist in axons of the sciatic nerve. A similar result was obtained when the attenuated Sabin 1 strain was used.

Involvement of PVR in the retrograde axonal pathway of PV suggested the possibility that PV-related materials in the sciatic nerve are not intact 160S particles because of the virion conformational conversion activity of PVR. Accordingly, the form of PV-related materials recovered from the sciatic nerve were analysed by sucrose density gradient centrifugation. The data indicated that a majority of PV-related materials in the sciatic nerve had a sedimentation coefficient of 160S. Thus, the intact virion particle appears to be transported through the axon.

Discussion

Using PV-sensitive Tg mice, we have established experimental systems for the study of two dissemination pathways of PV toward the CNS (Fig. 1). One is the BBB permeation of circulating PV, and the other the retrograde axonal transport of IM-inoculated PV. The latter system with Tg mice was also reported by Ren and Racaniello [15] and Gromeier and Wimmer [16].

Ren and Racaniello [15] proposed the possibility that circulating PV replicates in the muscle and is transported to the CNS through the axons. However, the Mahoney virus, after IV inoculation of 6.5×10^6 PFU/mouse, multiplied in the muscle to a maximum of 10^4 PFU/muscle of Tg mice. On the other hand, lethal doses of IM-inoculated Mahoney virus were more than 10^6 PFU (data not shown). These observations strongly suggest that BBB permeation of circulating PV is the main pathway for the virus, and that the axonal pathway from the skeletal muscle is not mainly involved in the dissemination to the CNS [12]. Both the pathways, however, are used by many neurotropic viruses. Therefore it is very important to elucidate the molecular basis of these dissemination pathways of PV as a model of neurotropic virus.

Our data involving IV inoculation of PV support the notion that the virus permeates the BBB at a fairly high rate without virus replication and involvement of human PVR. Some host cellular molecules other than PVR must be involved in BBB permeation of PV. Identification of such a molecule will be important for understanding PV neurovirulence.

During retrograde axonal transport, PV may be enclosed by endosomes because it is known that these are involved in the fast retrograde transport system. This, in turn, led us to an idea that PV is incorporated at synapses by endocytosis which should probably be inhibited by anti-human PVR mAb. Thus, it is possible that PVR-dependent endocytosis is the main way for IM-inoculated PV to enter motor neurons in vivo. Recent preliminary result showed that the cytoplasmic domain of PVR has an affinity to TCTEL-1 which is a human homologue of mouse cytoplasmic dynein light chain-1. The same molecule was identified also in Eckard Wimmer's laboratory (personal communication). PV-containing endosomes may interact with the dynein motor molecule via the cytoplasmic domain of PVR, resulting in retrograde transport to the neuron cell body.

It should be noted that the bulk of PV-related materials in the sciatic nerve showed a sedimentation coefficient of 160S. This suggests that lytic replication of PV including the uncoating step begins in the neuron cell body after retrograde axonal transport. It is totally unknown, at present, why PV can take the form of intact 160S particles during PVR-dependent neural pathway.

It is of interest that the virulent and attenuated PV strains do not show any significant difference in efficiency in both the dissemination pathways. Therefore, the neurovirulence level with different PV strains seems to be determined mainly by the multiplication capacity of PVs in neurons of the CNS. Molecular genetic analysis has been carried out to identify determinants for strain specific neurovirulence. As a result, an important determinant(s) was mapped within the internal ribosomal entry site (IRES) of the RNAs of all three serotypes of PV [17]. The result suggests that the replicating capacity of PV in the CNS reflects, in part, efficiency of the translation initiation derived from PV IRES. This finding is the beginning of a general concept of "IRES-dependent virus tropism".

Acknowledgements

We thank Y. Sasaki, and K. Iwasaki for expert technical assistance, and E. Suzuki, and Y. Matsushita for help in preparation of the manuscript. This work was supported in part by a grant from the Ministry of Education, Science, Sports, and Culture of Japan, the Ministry of Health and Welfare of Japan, and the Science and Technology Agency of Japan.

References

1 Mendelsohn CL, Wimmer E, Racaniello VR: Cellular receptor for poliovirus: Molecular cloning, nucleotide sequence, and expression of a new member of the immunoglobulin superfamily. Cell 1989;56:855-865.

2 Koike S, Horie H, Ise I, Okitsu A, Yoshida M, Iizuka N, Takeuchi K, Takegami T, Nomoto A: The poliovirus receptor protein is produced both as membrane-bound and secreted forms. EMBO J 1990;9:3217-3224.

3 Arita M, Koike S, Aoki J, Horie H, Nomoto A: Interaction of poliovirus with its purified receptor and conformational alteration in the virion. J Virol 1998;72:3578-3586.

4 Bodian D: Emerging concept of poliomyelitis infection. Science 1955;122:105-108.

5 Sabin AB: Pathogenesis of poliomyelitis: Reappraisal in the light of new data. Science 1956;123:1151-1157.

6 Howe H, Bodian D: Neuronal Mechanisms in Poliomyelitis, Milford H (ed): Commonwealth Fund, New York, NY, Oxford University Press, London, England.

7 Nathanson N, Bodian D: Experimental poliomyelitis following intramuscular virus injection. I. The effect of neural block on a neurotropic and a pantropic strain. Bull Johns Hopkins Hosp. 1961;108:308-319.

8 Koike S, Taya C, Kurata T, Abe S, Ise I, Yonekawa H, Nomoto A: Transgenic mice susceptible to poliovirus. Proc Natl Acad Sci USA 1991;88:951-955.

9 Ren R, Costantini F, Gorgacz EJ, Lee JJ, Racaniello VR: Transgenic mice expressing a human poliovirus receptor: A new model for poliomyelitis. Cell 1990;63:353-362.

10 Shiroki K, Ishii T, Aoki T, Kobashi M, Ohka S, Nomoto A: A new cis-acting element for RNA replication within the 5' noncoding region of poliovirus type 1 RNA. J Virol 1995;69:6825-6832.

11 Kohara M, Abe S, Komatsu T, Toga K, Arita M, Nomoto A: A recombinant virus between the Sabin 1 and Sabin 3 vaccine strains of poliovirus as a possible candidate for a new type 3 poliovirus live vaccine strain. J Virol 1988;62:2828-2835.

12 Yang W-X, Terasaki T, Shiroki K, Ohka S, Aoki J, Tanabe S, Nomura T, Terada E, Sugiyama Y, Nomoto A: Efficient delivery of circulating poliovirus to the central nervous system independently of poliovirus receptor. Virology 1997;229:421-428.

13 Hirokawa N, Sato-Yoshitake R, Yoshida T, Kawashima T: Brian dynein (MAP1C) localizes on both anterogradely and retrogradely transported membranous organelles in vivo. J Cell Biol 1990;111:1027-1037.

14 Ohka S, Yang W-X, Terada E, Iwasaki K, Nomoto A: Retrograde transport of intact poliovirus through the axon via the fast transport system. Virology 1998;250:67-75.
15 Ren R, Racaniello VR: Poliovirus spreads from muscle to the central nervous system by neural pathways. J Infect Dis 1992;166:747-752.
16 Gromeier M, Wimmer E: Mechanism of injury-provoked poliomyelitis. J Virol 1998; 72: 5056-5060.
17 Nomoto A: Recombinant polioviruses as candidates for oral live poliovaccines. Microbiol Immunol 1993;37:169-174.

Dr. A. Nomoto, Department of Microbiology, Graduate School of Medicine, The University of Tokyo, 7-3-1 Hongo, Bunkyo-ku, Tokyo 113-0033, Japan.

Brown F (ed): Progress in Polio Eradication: Vaccine Strategies for the End Game.
Dev Biol. Basel, Karger, 2001, vol 105, p 59

SESSION III

Current Poliovirus Vaccines

Chairperson: *David Wood*

Brown F (ed): Progress in Polio Eradication: Vaccine Strategies for the End Game.
Dev Biol. Basel, Karger, 2001, vol 105, pp 61-66

Strengths and Weaknesses of Current Polio Vaccines – A View from Industry

F.E. André

SmithKline Beecham Biologicals, Rixensart, Belgium

Key words: Polio, eradication, vaccine, manufacturer

INTRODUCTION

The strengths and weaknesses of the currently available polio vaccines – the Sabin live oral (OPV) and the Salk inactivated injectable (IPV) trivalent vaccines – have been abundantly debated, from the scientific and technical points of view, since their introduction four decades ago. These are well known to all vaccinologists [1] and need not be detailed here. However, with the imminent eradication of all three types of wild polioviruses and the hoped-for discontinuation of vaccination, it is appropriate to re-examine these from the point of view of a vaccine manufacturer who has been producing both vaccines from their beginning. For planning purposes, vaccine manufacturers need to know, well in advance, what the mid-term and long-term requirements for vaccines will be. In particular, the issues that need to be agreed upon by international vaccinologists are what vaccines will be required in the three eras spanning a short 10-year period that are in front of us, namely, pre-eradication, post-eradication and post-vaccination. There should also be a clear consensus on how, when and where these vaccines will be used. This will allow advanced planning on the quantities to be produced, distributed and stockpiled for each vaccine. The overall plan should aim at achieving and proving complete interruption of wild poliovirus transmission as soon as possible while at the same time reducing to acceptable levels the risk of re-emergence of these viruses from revertant vaccine strains, the environment or laboratory stocks. Contingency plans should also be made to detect and stop quickly this re-introduction should it occur either naturally or maliciously. International agreement and commitment, at the highest level, of all stakeholders, with strict monitoring of the implementation of plans, is essential to achieve and maintain cessation of poliovirus transmission in Nature. It is only when this can be guaranteed that stopping vaccination, which is the ultimate goal, should be considered. The pros and cons of OPV and IPV in each of the three coming eras will be discussed against the background of relevant scientific knowledge and politico-economic considerations.

Current Situation

Although the systematic use of IPV has led to the elimination of poliomyelitis in a few industrialised countries, the spectacular progress made in the control of poliomyelitis in the world during the last few years has been achieved through the rational use of OPV alone. The vaccination strategies and programmes that have now been put in place in all countries rely on two main immunisation approaches – routine high vaccine coverage of infants and National Immunisation Days (NIDs) targeting all under-fives – either in combination or separately, complemented by "mop-up" operations in high risk groups identified by close surveillance for wild poliovirus circulation. Transmission of wild poliovirus in human populations is best studied by laboratory-based surveillance and investigation of cases of acute flaccid paralysis (AFP) among children less than 15 years of age which occur at a rate of one per 100,000 per year on average. Generalisation of these strategies, pioneered in Latin America in the 1980s, has led to interruption of wild poliovirus transmission in all but 30 countries situated in South Asia and West and Central Africa. Endemic polio has been absent since early 1999 or earlier (since 1991 in the Americas) in three of the six WHO Regions [2]. It is doubtful that this could have been obtained with IPV which has never been routinely used in developing countries.

Characteristics of OPV

The positive attributes of OPV that have made possible that feat are listed in Figure 1. The most important one is the fact that annual world production capacity currently stands at two billion doses which is sufficient to achieve eradication. This huge capacity makes possible an average selling price of 10 dollar cents per dose due to the resulting economies of scale. Another tremendous advantage of OPV is its oral administration which allows implementation of NIDs. The effectiveness of OPV is enhanced by its spread from vaccinated to unimmunised close contacts

STRENGTHS	WEAKNESSES
• Huge production capacity (2 billion doses/year) • Oral administration • Low selling price (10 cents/dose) • Better herd immunity (intestinal immunity and transmission to non-vaccinees) • Bulk can be stored frozen	• Reversion to virulence (1VAPP / million doses) • Thermolabile • Requires 3 administrations (more in LDC's) for full efficacy • Possible persistent transmission leading to re-emergence of wild viruses

Fig. 1: Relevant scientific, logistic and operational attributes of live attenuated (SABIN) oral polio vaccine.

thus surreptitiously immunising them. As OPV replicates in intestinal mucosa, it provides stronger local immunity to infection with wild poliovirus. For the above two reasons, OPV gives better herd immunity than IPV. Thus not everyone has to be vaccinated to interrupt virus transmission in a population.

The main disadvantage of OPV is that the attenuated strains easily revert to neurovirulence causing vaccine associated paralytic poliomyelitis (VAPP) in vaccine recipients and their close contacts. However, this adverse side effect is very rare, occurring at a rate of about one case per million doses distributed. Whether OPV- derived revertant strains will evolve back into true wild polioviruses and thus lead to their re-emergence after eradication is a theoretical possibility that cannot be ignored. OPV is thermolabile and requires storage and transport in a refrigerated environment that can be maintained relatively easily in a functioning and well-maintained cold chain. The use of individual Vaccine Vial Monitors is a safeguard against the administration of sub-potent vaccine. To be fully efficacious OPV has to be administered on at least three separate occasions in industrialised countries and possibly more than five times in developing countries. This problem can be solved by annual NIDs with OPV which is possible due to its oral administration. OPV can be stored in a frozen state for extended periods of time which would be of practical advantage for stockpiling in bulk form but the shelf-life of OPV ready-for-use in final containers will be only a couple of years. Apart from the rare occurrence of VAPP and the worrying possibility of reversion to wild viruses, through back mutation or recombination with other vaccine-derived strains or enteroviruses, the positive characteristics of OPV described above – plentiful supply, low price, ease of administration and better herd immunity – would seem to make it almost the ideal vaccine, certainly in the pre-eradication era and possibly (if backward evolution of the Sabin strains proves to be only a theoretical fear) also in the post-eradication era. In the post-vaccination era, OPV would also be the preferred vaccine to stockpile because it can be stored longer in bulk, is accepted to be the vaccine of choice to stop an epidemic should this occur and will require less stringent containment during production than IPV (see below).

Characteristics of IPV

Figure 2 shows the strengths and weaknesses of IPV. The great advantage of IPV is that it does not cause VAPP. Because of ethical, safety and medico-legal considerations, accentuated by public opinion demanding safety at all costs, this attribute is forcing an increasing number of developed countries to switch from OPV to IPV. This change of policy has cost implications. In the U.S. it was estimated that implementation of a sequential IPV/OPV vaccination schedule would cost three million dollars for prevention of each case of VAPP [3] a price that is unaffordable for less developed countries. The development of combined vaccines incorporating IPV with diphtheria, tetanus, pertussis (DTP), hepatitis B and *Haemophilus influenzae* type b protective antigens may improve the cost-effectiveness of preventing VAPP but production capacity for these combined vaccines, often using acellular pertussis vaccines [4], is currently too low to effect significant economies of scale. The biggest disadvantage of IPV, in the context of polio eradication, is the fact that the existing world annual production capacity, though not precisely known, almost certainly does not exceed 100 million doses. The selling

STRENGTHS	WEAKNESSES
• No VAPP • Easier to combine with DTP, HEP.B, Hib ... • ? More thermostable • Fewer administrations required	• Limited production capacity (? 100 million doses/year) • Parenteral administration • High price (1-5 USD/dose) • Poorer herd immunity • Wild viruses used in production • Cannot be stored frozen

Fig. 2: Relevant scientific, logistic and operational attributes of killed (SALK) injectable polio vaccine.

price of IPV varies in different countries but is at least one order of magnitude higher than OPV with an estimated range of one to five dollars per dose. This price could be brought down if production capacity was greatly increased but this will require significant investments in new production facilities. As it will take at least five years for these facilities to come on stream and discontinuation of polio vaccination is scheduled to take place by 2010 the time to recoup any investments will be very short. Under these circumstances it is not surprising that vaccine manufacturers are unanimous in their reluctance to make such investments unless credible guarantees are given by the international community that there will be a viable market for the billions of doses of IPV that will be needed up to the post-vaccination era. Another big disadvantage of IPV is the fact that it has to be administered parenterally by specially trained personnel, which significantly complicates the logistic and operational aspects of vaccination programmes. NIDs would become "impossible". However, they may not be necessary as three spaced doses of enhanced IPV are sufficient to give optimal protection. However, the protection conferred by IPV is almost exclusively to the vaccinated individual since intestinal immunity after IPV is less solid and of shorter duration than after OPV. To obtain herd immunity with IPV a higher vaccine coverage than is currently obtained in most developing countries with DTP will be required. This will be another "impossible" task in the foreseeable future. Thus it can be concluded that IPV cannot be used alone in the pre-eradication era. In any case it is quite likely that this era will end before sufficient quantities of IPV to replace OPV completely can be produced in view of the limited existing capacity.

However, it must be admitted that in the pre-eradication and post-eradication eras it would be easier to establish that eradication has indeed been obtained. If only IPV is used, OPV will not circulate (unless persistent transmission occurs). OPV use could mask the continued transmission of wild viruses. All poliovirus isolates have to be typed as vaccine-derived or not if OPV is used to prove that eradication has been obtained. If OPV is not used, all poliovirus isolates will be wild viruses. Production of IPV in the post-eradication and post-vaccination eras will require increased containment safeguards because the seed viruses currently used are wild viruses. If these "escape" from production facilities they could start wide epidemics in unvaccinated and non-immune populations. It has been suggested by a WHO taskforce that BSL4 containment facilities would be required for this purpose, a recommendation that all manufacturers regard as "unrealistic".

One way around this problem is to use attenuated viruses – like the Sabin strains – to produce IPV when less stringent containment (e.g. BSL2+) would be sufficient. However, such an IPV has, as yet, not been developed in spite of long-standing efforts. Finally, stockpiling of IPV in the post-vaccination era will require maintaining a continuous large production because IPV bulk cannot be stored frozen for long periods (as is the case for OPV) in order to replace continually expired stocks. The attributes reviewed above do not make IPV an attractive vaccine in the context of polio eradication. Its widespread use would be justified (and necessary) only if reversion of Sabin strains to wild viruses that cause epidemics is proven beyond doubt. On the other hand, in industrialised countries with good surveillance, switching to IPV, although not cost-effective, is safe and can be justified on ethical and socio-political grounds, particularly if polyvalent paediatric vaccines are used (to reduce the number of injections) and high vaccine coverage rates can thus be maintained. However, worldwide switch to IPV would not be practical or effective, would be expensive and would almost certainly delay attainment of polio eradication by many years.

Politico-Economic Considerations

There is currently considerable socio-political support internationally for polio eradication and the mood is optimistic. However, if attainment of this praiseworthy goal is delayed for too long, pessimism will set in and this prize could slip away from our grasp. Vaccine manufacturers – and there are only a handful still engaged in polio vaccine production – also support eradication not only for ethical reasons but also because polio vaccines, in particular OPV, are not as profitable as more recent vaccines. Owners of vaccine manufacturers – their shareholders – will be glad when polio vaccines are produced in limited quantities only for stockpiling, provided of course, the cost of this production and stockpile is borne from public funds. The situation in the post-vaccination era will be analogous to that of maintaining a battle-ready army in peacetime except that the army will not be national but global. Unusual political collaboration will be required internationally but this will not, in the health field, be unprecedented. After all, smallpox has been and remains eradicated. Polio eradication is a war that mankind should wage together. We must win it and succeed in keeping the peace thereafter. The dividends, both in terms of international political goodwill and economic benefits, will be enormous.

Summary and Conclusions

Polio eradication is within our grasp and, unless something terribly wrong and unexpected happens, the three types of wild polioviruses will cease to circulate in human populations within the next few years. This achievement will be a result of the rational use of OPV. A momentous global decision – discontinuation of vaccination – will then have to be taken. The most important uncertainty that will weigh upon that decision is whether wild polioviruses can re-emerge after "eradication", defined as "complete interruption of wild polioviruses transmission", has been obtained. It is important to realise that "eradication" does not mean "extinction" in the sense that the dodo is extinct. After eradication, wild polioviruses will still lurk in laboratory specimens and in protected environmental sites (like glaciers) and may even “re-emerge” by back mutation or recombination of Sabin-derived strains that may continue to circulate even after OPV use is discontinued. Theoretically, the risk of re-emergence of wild polioviruses would be lessened if IPV was used for a number of years to immunise all those born after cessation of OPV usage. But the question is “by how much?”. Vaccination with IPV will reduce the risk that persistent OPV-derived strains (e.g. in immunodeficient patients) will have the chance to establish permanent transmission after vaccination is totally discontinued. However, the risk of re-emergence will not be changed since this will be determined by the risk of accidental re-introduction. Whether the expense of switching completely from OPV to IPV globally can be justified will depend upon the relative risks of wild poliovirus re-emergence from either OPV-derived sources or other environmental sources including “escape” of virulent seed viruses from IPV production facilities. This balance of probabilities and risks will be very difficult to determine. In any case, it is likely that the decision to upscale IPV production to required levels has already been delayed too long so that polio eradication will be achieved by the use of OPV in developed as well as in less developed countries that cannot afford to use IPV at a high enough vaccine coverage rate to make it safe. Wild poliovirus transmission has been interrupted with OPV in the Western Hemisphere. There is no reason why this cannot be done in the rest of the world. In industrialized countries that can afford it and where vaccine coverage is sufficient to prevent wild virus circulation, IPV, in combined vaccines, will be increasingly used. Let us hope that politicians in developing countries and zealous ethicists in the developed world will understand why, in the present and foreseeable future circumstances, OPV is better than IPV in the poorer countries and will not demand, in the name of equity in health, a total switch to IPV. For eradication, IPV cannot, and hopefully need not, replace OPV. At this stage it should not.

Acknowledgements

The author would like to thank colleagues in industry, in particular Pierre Thysman of SmithKline Beecham Biologicals, in national and international health organisations and academia for frank discussions that have led to the opinions expressed in this article. However, he accepts full responsibility for any defects, either factual or logical, in these opinions.

References

1 Melnick JL: Advantages and disadvantages of killed and live poliomyelitis vaccines. Bulletin of the World Health Organization 1978;56(1):21-38.

2 Hull HF: Progress towards global polio eradication, in Brown F (ed): Progress in Polio Eradication: Vaccine Strategies for the End Game. Dev Biol. Basel, Karger, 2001, vol 105, pp 3-7.

3 Miller MA, Suter RW, Strebel PM, Hadler SC: Cost-effectiveness of incorporating inactivated poliovirus vaccine into routine childhood immunization schedule. J Am Med Assoc 1996;276 (12):967-971.

4 André FE: Development and clinical application of new polyvalent combined paediatric vaccines. Vaccine 1999;17:1620-1627.

Dr. F.E. André, SmithKline Beecham Biologicals, 89, rue de l'Institut, B-1330 Rixensart.

Brown F (ed): Progress in Polio Eradication: Vaccine Strategies for the End Game.
Dev Biol. Basel, Karger, 2001, vol 105, p 67

SESSION IV

When and How Can we Stop Vaccination?

Chairperson: *John Furesz*

Brown F (ed): Progress in Polio Eradication: Vaccine Strategies for the End Game.
Dev Biol. Basel, Karger, 2001, vol 105, pp 69-72

The Scientific Basis for Stopping Polio Immunisation – Issues and Challenges

D.J. Wood

National Institute for Biological Standards and Control, Potters Bar, U.K

Key words: Polioviruses, vaccines, polio eradication, public health policy, review

Abstract: Eradication of polio is in sight. Once this is finally achieved there is general agreement that the world should move from the current policy of universal childhood immunisation, mostly with the oral poliovirus vaccine (OPV), to no immunisation. The challenge ahead is to build consensus on how and when this is achieved. The major area of scientific uncertainty is whether OPV-derived strains excreted by vaccinees will establish chains of transmission in communities, especially in settings of poor hygiene, when population immunity levels begin to fall after immunisation ceases. Evidence from several sources suggests that this may not occur. Most convincing are studies that show polioviruses are not detected beyond three months after mass OPV campaigns in at least two countries that only use OPV in this way. However it is clear that there are significant gaps in our knowledge. These include the transmissibility of OPV-derived strains under certain ecological settings, the potential for persistently infected individuals to re-seed viruses into a community, and the molecular basis of transmissibility. Research in these areas is underway and will help develop and refine strategies for stopping polio immunisation. The potential risks and benefits of ceasing polio immunisation are such that the best available science is required to reach an informed decision.

INTRODUCTION

The almost total eradication of wild type polioviruses has been achieved largely through widespread use of the OPV, developed by Dr Sabin. Although the most important short-term goal is to achieve eradication, the World Health Organisation (WHO) convened a meeting in March 1998 to review the scientific basis for stopping immunisation against polio and to determine whether stopping immunisation should be a longer-term goal. The consensus from that meeting was that vaccination with OPV should stop and that immunisation with IPV may stop when the following criteria are met:

(i) there is assurance of the global eradication of polioviruses;

(ii) there is suitable containment of wild polioviruses;

(iii) there is evidence that the only poliovirus strains in the population when conditions (i) and (ii) are fulfilled, namely OPV-derived strains, will circulate for only a limited period in the post vaccination era.

Assurances of global eradication and of proper containment of laboratory stocks are huge challenges. However, the major area of scientific uncertainty identified at the meeting was what would happen to the circulation of OPV-derived strains excreted by the last cohorts of immunised children into a rapidly expanding susceptible population. The issues and challenges for the future have recently been reviewed [1] and this paper summarises the current state of knowledge.

Transmissibility and Persistence of OPV-Derived Strains

Person-to-person transmission of OPV-derived polioviruses is well documented and has been reviewed recently [2]. The Sabin type 2 strain in OPV is the most transmissible of the three vaccine strains. Even though this transmissibility is well known, several lines of evidence suggest that OPV-derived strains tend to circulate for only a limited time in populations if not constantly re-introduced through new vaccinations. The most convincing data are from countries where mass OPV campaigns are the only means of providing OPV (with no supplemental doses between campaigns). Since 1962, Cuba has administered OPV only in mass campaigns in February and April of each year. Stool and serological studies in children born after April in one year and before February in the next show circulation of virus for no longer than three months [3]. Similar conclusions have been drawn from virological studies after mass campaigns using monovalent OPV in Hungary [4].

Indirect evidence for the limited circulation of OPV-derived strains in various populations is provided by the observation that outbreaks of poliomyelitis are invariably associated with wild-type rather than OPV-derived strains, even in partially immunised populations [5]. These data suggest that the vaccine-derived strains are less transmissible than wild type strains. However, it should be noted that currently available data are limited and there are important gaps in our knowledge of the transmissibility and persistence of OPV-derived strains [6]. In this context recent studies that have suggested the possibility that the Sabin type 2 strain, at least, may revert to wild-type transmissibility characteristics are important and need to be extended.

Persistent Infections in Immunocompromised Persons

Patients with primary B cell immunodeficiencies appear to be at most risk for prolonged poliovirus infection. These deficiencies may be profound and rare, such as X-linked agammaglobulinaemia and in industrialised countries usually diagnosed in infancy. More subtle and more prevalent are common variable immunodeficiency or selective IgA deficiency, not diagnosed until later childhood, if at all. In industrial countries these persons have a high chance of survival and a high chance of being immunised against polio before their immunodeficiency diagnosis is made. A total of nine immunodeficient patients with prolonged poliovirus excretion have been described [reviewed in 1]. All three serotypes of OPV have been involved and five of the nine patients have not had paralysis. The longest period of continued excretion of an OPV-derived strain recorded so far is in excess of 10 years. The viruses undergo extensive molecular changes during the prolonged period of replication in the human gut and those that have been tested have been neurovirulent in animal models [7]. At least one antiviral agent, pleconaril [8], is available for treatment but its efficacy for eradicating a persistent poliovirus gut infection remains to be determined. The transmissibility of these drifted OPV-derived viruses is not known nor is the frequency of such persistent infections. Systematic studies are underway to address this question and it may be expected that the pool of persistently infected individuals will reduce, at least in industrialised countries, as more of those countries switch to use of the inactivated poliovirus vaccine. However the fact that long-term infections may occur will have to be taken into account when strategies are devised for stopping immunisations.

There are very limited data on secondary immunodeficiencies, such as HIV infection or malnutrition, as risk factors for prolonged poliovirus infections. Given the importance of these conditions in some parts of the developing world, such information is urgently needed.

Will the Polio Niche Remain Vacant if OPV Immunisation is Stopped?

A theoretical concern about stopping OPV vaccination is that another enterovirus would evolve to fill the ecological niche left by the disappearance of polioviruses. An important question that needs to be answered is what exactly is the "polio niche". A reasonable definition would be a virus that uses the human cellular poliovirus receptor, a member of the immunoglobulin super family of unknown function [9]. Only viruses with the antigenicity of polioviruses are known to use this particular cellular receptor. Therefore, if a virus were to evolve to fill the niche it would probably have poliovirus antigenicity. As there are only three serotypes of poliovirus, there seems to be a restriction on the number of distinct antigenic configurations that can use the receptor and yield viable polioviruses. There has been no emergence of a new poliovirus serotype since the definition of the poliovirus serotypes almost 50 years ago. Thus the risk of the evolution of a new poliovirus to occupy the polio niche once polio immunisation has stopped can be considered as highly unlikely.

Contingency Plans

A pre-requisite for stopping polio immunisation is that contingency plans are made for the unlikely re-emergence of polio by, for example, a bioterrorist release of the virus in the polio-free area. If wild polioviruses or vaccine-derived polioviruses that had reverted to wild-type transmissibility were detected then the consensus view, developed by a group of WHO consultants meeting in January 2000, is that monovalent OPV should be used to control such an outbreak. This would produce a faster type-specific immune response than trivalent OPV and would also avoid the unnecessary seeding of additional viruses into what may be a population with low levels of immunity to polio. This plan means it will be necessary to develop a stockpile of monovalent OPV and that some of the stockpile be filled into vials for immediate distribution. Further study is needed to define the size of the stockpile.

In addition to a stockpile for emergency use the WHO Consultation also recommended that research be continued into new vaccines for polio. This is required so that we have in our arsenal all the weapons that we may possibly need in the post-vaccination era. In particular, emphasis was placed on the need to develop an inactivated vaccine from the Sabin strains rather than the current wild type seed viruses. This is to minimize biosafety concerns for future production of IPV. Secondly, alternative live attenuated vaccines, preferably based on the Sabin strains, but engineered to be less transmissible than the current strains, should also be evaluated in at least phase 1 and 2 clinical trials.

Conclusions

The pace of progress towards the goal of polio eradication is such that there is an urgent need to identify and conduct the research that will inform the decision-making process of how and when to stop immunisation against polio. This includes not only the virological and epidemiological issues identified here and in this scientific meeting but also the means by which the political will and co-operation can be achieved to conduct a co-ordinated world-wide cessation of polio immunisation.

References

1 Wood DJ, Sutter RW, Dowdle WR: Stopping poliovirus vaccination after eradication: issues and challenges. Bull WHO 2000;78:347-357.

2 Fine P, Carneiro IAM: Transmissibility and persistence of oral poliovirus vaccine viruses; implications for the global poliomyelitis eradication strategy. Am J Epidem 1999;150:1001-1021.

3 Mas Lago P: Eradication of poliomyelitis in Cuba. Bull WHO 1999;77:681-687.

4 Domok I et al: Enterovirus survey in children after mass vaccination with live attenuated polioviruses. Brit Med J 1962;1:743-746.

5 Patriarca PA, Sutter RW, Oostvogel PM: Outbreaks of paralytic poliomyelitis, 1976-1995. J Inf Dis 1997;175(Suppl.1):S165-S172.

6 Fine PEM: Gaps in our knowledge about transmission of vaccine derived polioviruses. Bull WHO 2000;78:358-359.

7 Minor PD: Characteristics of poliovirus strains from long-term excretors with primary immunodeficiency in Brown F (ed): Progress in Polio Eradication: Vaccine Strategies for the End Game. Dev Biol. Basel, Karger, 2001, vol 105, pp 75-80.

8 Win-63843. Drugs of the future 1997;22:40-44.

9 Mendelsohn CL, Wimmer E, Rocaniello VR: Cellular receptor for poliovirus: molecular cloning, nucleotide sequence and expression of a new member of the immunoglobulins superfamily. Cell 1989;56:855-865.

Dr. D.J. Wood, N.I.B.S.C., Blanche Lane, South Mimms, Potters Bar, Herts EN6 3QG, U.K.

Brown F (ed): Progress in Polio Eradication: Vaccine Strategies for the End Game.
Dev Biol. Basel, Karger, 2001, vol 105, p 73

SESSION V

Risks of Reintroduction of Polio Post Eradication

Chairperson: *Tapani Hovi*

Brown F (ed): Progress in Polio Eradication: Vaccine Strategies for the End Game.
Dev Biol. Basel, Karger, 2001, vol 105, pp 75-80

Characteristics of Poliovirus Strains from Long-Term Excretors with Primary Immunodeficiencies

P. Minor

National Institute for Biological Standards and Control, Potters Bar, U.K.

Abstract: Individuals who are deficient in humoral immunity are particularly at risk from infection with enteroviruses, and poliovirus in particular, where antibodies are the main source of protection from disease. Long-term excretion of vaccine strains of poliovirus has been documented for many years and instances of paralytic poliomyelitis in hypogammaglobulinaemic patients who were subsequently found to have been excreting virus for prolonged periods have been reported in the U.S.A., Germany and Japan. The identification of a healthy immunodeficient patient in the U.K. who has probably been excreting type 2 poliovirus for 15 years will be described, with the characteristics of the virus and the results of attempts at treatment so far. Such individuals pose a significant risk to the eradication programme unless they can be identified and treated.

Introduction

It was shown in the 1950s that passively administered immunoglobulin was able to prevent the development of poliomyelitis if given before or soon after infection [1]. Neutralising antibody is therefore a sufficient condition for protection from disease, and it has been recognised that deficiencies in humoral immunity render patients particularly liable to contract poliomyelitis, notably vaccine-associated poliomyelitis where the incidence is considered to be at least 3000-fold greater in hypogammaglobulinaemic than in immunocompetent individuals. It is not clear whether HIV infection and the resulting immunodeficiency can have the same effect. It is known, however, that in some instances hypogammaglobulinaemic patients can excrete poliovirus for very long periods with or without detectable symptoms. This paper reviews the properties of poliovirus strains from several such cases.

Excretion of Virus by Immunocompetent Individuals

Immune competent individuals rarely excrete the vaccine strains of poliovirus for longer than 10 or 12 weeks and none for longer than six months. About 50%

excrete virus for six weeks and 1% for 10 [2]. In this period the virus is able to change very rapidly and effectively by mutation and recombination, adapting to conditions in the gut by losing or suppressing the mutations known to attenuate the virus in animal models. The Sabin vaccine strains are generally considered poorly transmissible. The reason for this is not known but may be related to the titre of excreted virus and the duration of excretion which is determined by factors which are not clear. Long-term excretion would increase the chances of transmission in any event, but also increase the opportunity for the virus to acquire better transmission characteristics for which there would be a strong selection pressure in a post-eradication, post-immunisation world.

Viruses from Paralytic Cases

There are several reports of isolates from hypogammaglobulinaemic patients who suffered paralytic poliomyelitis. Hara et al [3] reported the case of a three year old boy with agammaglobulinaemia with undetectable level of serum IgG and IgA who developed poliomyelitis 553 days after being fed oral poliovaccine. Type 2 poliovirus was isolated from 23 stool specimens, including one taken 348 days before the illness and 213 days after the last vaccination. Excretion of virus continued for 684 days after the development of paralysis, and the child was therefore known to have been producing virus for 1032 days based on isolations, and presumably for a total of 1237 days since the last vaccination. The titres of virus in 20% stool suspensions were between 10^4 and $10^{5.5}$ $TCID_{50}$ per ml, and excretion of virus stopped without the development of detectable antibody in the faeces between 1237 and 1259 days post immunisation.

All 23 strains isolated differed significantly in their antigenicity from the Sabin 2 strain by the polyclonal antibody-based Wecker and MacBride tests available at the time, but were also distinct from available wild type strains. Using absorbed sera the isolate taken 348 days before illness was intermediate in character while all subsequent isolates were non-vaccine like. The strain isolated one week after onset of paralysis was highly virulent in primates. The conclusion reached was that the strains, at least one of which was virulent, were derived from the Sabin type 2 vaccine. The patient had frequent diarrhoea, and the sample taken 348 days before illness was taken to investigate possible rotavirus infection. The gastrointestinal symptoms did not seem to affect poliovirus excretion.

Kew et al [4] described a patient who developed poliomyelitis in 1981, at the age of 16, having been diagnosed as hypogammaglobulinaemic at the age of 12 with low but detectable levels of serum IgG and IgA. He had received several doses of oral poliovaccine, the last at age 10, and remained ventilator-dependent from 1981 until his death in 1990. Isolates and stool specimens were available at days 11, 23, 48, 126, 158 and 200 after the onset of paralysis but none before or after that period, so that it is not known if the patient stopped excreting virus before death. The titre of virus in the stool specimens is also not known, and might have been of interest.

Sequencing studies of the isolates were undertaken covering the complete region of the genome encoding VP1 (nucleotides 2480 to 3385) and a part of the region encoding VP1/2A (nucleotides 3296 to 3445). The first isolate obtained 11 days after onset of paralysis was a mixture of two separate strains which differed at 50 positions in a sequence of 906 bases and were present in a ratio of approximately two to one. Both populations resembled the Sabin vaccine in sequence rather than wild-type strains. The minority population was not detectable in subsequent isolates. Over the period for which isolates were available the rate of mutation in the whole of VP1 at third base positions where there is assumed to be no selective pressure, was estimated at 3.3% substitutions per year. This is close to the estimated evolution rate in epidemics of 3.06% per year. On this basis the patient was estimated to have been excreting virus for 9.3 years before paralysis developed, two years earlier than the time of administration of the last dose of OPV, thought to be the initiation of the infection. The two populations in the first isolate were estimated to have diverged 2.5 years before the sample was taken. Over the period studied several coding changes appeared in the VP1 sequence of the major variant. At day 11 there were 16, five in the region spanning neutralisation site 1, one in site 2. Three other coding changes accumulated over the next 189 days, two in antigenic sites and one at VP1 residue 56.

Bellmunt et al [5] described a third case of prolonged excretion of poliovirus by a hypogammaglobulinaemic (common variable immune deficient patient) also of type 1. Forty-four isolates were made over a 5½ year period, starting four days after the onset of paralysis, and including one isolate from a throat wash. Excretion of virus stopped spontaneously. Isolates from throat wash and faecal specimens four days after onset of paralysis were antigenically distinct. The throat-wash isolate and the last faecal isolate were sequenced in their entirety, and shown to be closest to the Sabin 1 strain from which they were presumed to have been derived, but from which they differed by 5.4 and 8.3% respectively. Based on the overall sequence, including coding changes, the rate of mutation was estimated at 0.97% per year, and the time between infection and the first isolate estimated at 5.4 years. Using third base substitutions in VP1/2A, or changes in the sequence of the highly variable section of the 5' non-coding region from bases 640 to 743, the estimates were 7.7 and 4.2 years respectively. The patient had received three doses of OPV in 1984 and in 1986, six and four years respectively before the onset of paralysis. The data from VP1/2A third base changes gave a rather earlier time of infection than expected. There were 48 and 57 nucleotide changes in the 744 bases of the 5' non-coding region for the first and last isolates compared to Sabin 1, and 33 compared to each other. The predicted structure for the region was maintained, with most substitutions in loops rather than base paired stems. Amino acid changes were particularly prevalent in VP4 and in VP1 in the region of Nag1 and P2A. There were 47 amino acid differences between the first and last isolates. Both had reverted at bases 481 and 6203, which have been implicated in attenuation [6] although this was not confirmed by site-directed mutation [7].

Viruses from Healthy Patients

While excretion of poliovirus by hypogammaglobulinaemics is most obviously indicated by the development of poliomyelitis there are several well documented examples of long term excretion without apparent adverse effects. MacCallum [8] described a study initiated in 1961 in which 30 patients were deliberately immunised with monovalent oral poliovaccine. Of the thirty patients most shed virus for only a short period. However, one, a three year old boy, shed type 1 poliovirus for about 3.5 years, terminated by a Shigella infection, while another, a teenage girl, shed type 3 virus for a period of 637 days, after which virus excretion stopped. This is the only instance so far where isolates are available throughout the period of shedding from the known time of infection, although the first isolate was made at 36 days post infection. The amount of virus shed is reported as less than 100 $TCID_{50}$ per gram of stool, which is a very low level compared to the normal figure of about 10^5 per gram. Martin et al [9] has reported studies on all seven strains still available from intervals throughout the period of virus shedding, including their complete genomic sequence. Isolates arose which were shown to be antigenic variants in sites 2, 3 and 4 by their reactivity with monoclonal antibodies, but over a more prolonged time course than for immune competent vaccine recipients. While the viruses rapidly directly reverted the two mutations identified as attenuating the Sabin type 3 vaccine strain relative to its virulent precursor strain Leon, the virulent phenotype for animals was only partially regained. Changes in the 5' non-coding region were consistent with the predicted secondary structure, in that base pairs were maintained and the overall thermodynamic stability was kept fairly constant, while other changes occurred in non-base paired loop regions. In the capsid region mutations occurred in known antigenic sites consistent with the findings with monoclonal antibodies, but mutations in other loci involved in capsid uncoating or assembly or close to the proposed receptor site also occurred, sometimes independent of antigenic changes and presumably reflecting adaptation to changes in the condition of the gut. Other major areas for coding changes included P2C and P3CD, where a protease cleavage site absent in the Sabin type 3 strain but present in all other unrelated viruses examined so far was regenerated. The simultaneous selection in 2C and 3CD might explain the frequency with which type 3 recombinant viruses are generated in vaccinees [2], although the reason for the selection is not known. The rate of evolution of the virus away from the Sabin type 3 sequence, when expressed in terms of numbers of differences at a particular time point was extraordinary constant. Considering all changes over the whole genome the figure was 1.28% per year, similar to that reported in the type 1 case by Bellmunt et al [5], and the rate for third base changes in the capsid region was 3.4% per year, identical to the figure reported for the third base changes in VP1 of the type 1 case described by Kew et al [4].

Misbah et al [10] described isolates of type 2 poliovirus from a male nurse with common variable immunodeficiency, who was found to excrete virus over a one year period when subject to virological investigation following a bout of gastroenteritis. Shedding of virus stopped spontaneously, and sequence studies (J. Martin, pers. comm.) have shown that the virus is a recombinant. The variation relative to the Sabin strains is consistent with the view that the patient was infected by a child on the paediatric ward where he was a nurse. The virus is virulent (J. Martin, pers. comm.).

A second serendipitous series of isolates from a healthy hypogammaglobulinaemic patient was found as a result of studies of isolates made by clinical virology laboratories in the U.K. as part of the process to certify the U.K. as polio free. A series of isolates was obtained in 1995, with a difference of about 10% from the Sabin type 2 sequence (G. Dunn, in preparation). On identifying the individual from whom the isolates came, it was found that he was still excreting virus through 1999 and to the present (June 2000). Sequence data showed that the attenuating mutations in the 5' non-coding region, in VP1 at amino acid 143, and in the region of VP4 had all been lost along with many other changes by 1999 and the virus was virulent for animals. The virus clusters with the Sabin type 2 strains by sequence, and the patient who is in excellent health and on regular intravenous immunoglobulin, continues to excrete virus at a titre of about 10^4 to 10^5 pfu per gram of stool. Continued isolation and sequencing studies are underway as treatments including oral immunoglobulin and antivirals have been or may be attempted, so that if the treatment is only partially effective it may be detected by a switch in the sequence of the predominant excreted strain. Based on the current data the individual is definitely known to have been excreting virus for 5.5 years, and based on the sequence data, it is likely to be nearer to 16 years, consistent with his last immunisation at age 11 before immunodeficiency was diagnosed.

The Nature of Immunodeficiency and the Termination of Virus Shedding

There are a range of immunodeficiencies with respect to humoral immunity. The best understood is x-linked agammaglobulinaemia which has a known lesion in a signal transducing molecule preventing the differentiation of the pre B cell, and so preventing synthesis of immunoglobulin of any class. It occurs at a frequency of about 1 in 700,000 Caucasians. Hyper 1gM syndrome is a defect in class switching, preventing the maturation of the IgM response to IgG, IgA and IgE. The most common form of humoral immune deficiency is common variable, which may affect one in 50,000 Caucasians and whose aetiology is not well defined. The incidence in non-Caucasians of any of these deficiencies is unknown.

The cause of termination of shedding of poliovirus is not clear. Savilahti et al [12] reported that IgA deficient individuals shed poliovirus for longer periods than normal controls after vaccination, although none of the eight examined excreted virus at six months post infection. It is highly plausible that an IgA response plays a part in the normal clearance of infection, but it is not clear why long term excretion in hypo and gammaglobulinaemic patients is relatively rare. MacCallum reported two of 30 patients and studies in a treatment clinic in London have identified no individuals excreting poliovirus although over 100 have now been examined (G. Dunn, pers. comm.). The reason for the cessation of shedding in this type of patient is not clear, and conversely the number who may be susceptible to long term shedding is unknown. It is clear however, that the virus may sometimes, but not always, evolve to a virulent form, shed at high titres, which can infect both the throat and the intestine, leading to the possibility of transmission by the respiratory as well as the faecal-oral route. The individuals concerned are presumably well protected currently by intravenous immunoglobulin rather than the less easily administered intramuscular presentation of the past. Provided treatment is given regularly, one hopes they are at little risk. However, they represent a reservoir of infection and opportunity for virus evolution which has serious implications for the cessation of vaccination. It seems clear that the numbers of such individuals should be determined and treatments to clear the virus be developed.

References

1 Hammon WMcD, Coriell LL, Wehrle PF, Stokes J: Evaluation of Red Cross gamma globulin as a prophylactic agent for poliomyelitis. F. Final report of results based on clinical diagnoses. JAMA 1953;151:1272-1285.

2 Minor PD, John A, Ferguson M, Icenogle JP: Antigenic and molecular evolution of the vaccine strain of type 3 poliovirus during the period of excretion by a primary vaccinee. J Gen Virol 1986;67:693-706.

3 Hara M, Saito Y, Komatso T, Kodama H, Abo W, Chiba S, Nakao T: Antigenic analysis of poliovirus isolated from a child with agammaglobulinaemia and paralytic poliomyelitis after Sabin vaccine administration. Microbiol Immunol 1981;25:905-910.

4 Kew OM, Sutter RW, Nottay BK, McDonough MJ, Prevols DR, Quick L, Pallansch MA: Prolonged replication of a type 1 vaccine derived poliovirus in an immunodeficient patient. J Clin Microbiol 1998;36:2893-2899.

5 Bellmunt A, May G, Zell R, Pring A, Kerblom P, Vergagen W, Heim A: Evolution of poliovirus type 1 during 5.5 years of prolonged enteral replication in an immunodeficient patient. Virology 1999;265:178-184.

6 Christodoulou C, Colbere-Garapin F, Macadam A, Taffs LF, Marsden S, Minor PD, Horaud F: Mapping of mutations associated with neurovirulence in monkeys infected with Sabin 1 poliovirus revertants selected at high temperature. J Virol 1990;64:4922-4929.

7 McGoldrich A, Macadam AJ, Dunn G, Rowe A, Burlison J, Minor PD, Meredith J, Evans DJ, Almond JW: Role of mutations G-480 and C-6203 in the attenuation phenotype of Sabin type 1 poliovirus. J Virol 1995;69:7601-7605.

8 MacCallum FO: Hypogammaglobulinaemia in the United Kingdom, VII. The role of humoral antibodies in protection against and recovery from bacterial and virus infections in hypogammaglobulinaemia. Spec Rep Ser Med Res Counc 1971;310:72-85.

9 Martin J, Dunn G, Hull R, Patel V, Minor PD: Evolution of the Sabin strain of type 3 poliovirus in an immunodeficient patient during the entire 637-day period of virus excretion. J Virol 2000;74:3001-3010.

10 Misbah SA, Lawrence PA, Kuriz JB, Chapel HM: Prolonged faecal excretion of poliovirus in a nure with common variable hypogammaglobulinaemia. Post grad Med J 1991;67:301-303.

11 Rosen FS, Cooper MD, Wedgewood RJP: The primary immunodeficiencies. New England Journal of Medicine 1998;333:431-440.

12 Savilahti E, Klemola T, Carlsson B, Mellander L, Stenvik M, Hovi T: Inadequacy of mucosal IgM antibodies in selective IgA deficiency: excretion of attenuated polioviruses is prolonged. J Clin Immunol 1988;8:89-94.

Dr. P.D. Minor, N.I.B.S.C., Blanche Lane, South Mimms, Potters Bar, Herts EN6 3QG, U.K.

Brown F (ed): Progress in Polio Eradication: Vaccine Strategies for the End Game.
Dev Biol. Basel, Karger, 2001, vol 105, p 81

Poster Session I

Brown F (ed): Progress in Polio Eradication: Vaccine Strategies for the End Game.
Dev Biol. Basel, Karger, 2001, vol 105, pp 83-92

Risks of Reintroduction of Polio after Eradication: the Vaccine Origin of an Outbreak of Type 3 Poliomyelitis

J. Martín, G.L. Ferguson, D.J. Wood, P.D. Minor

Division of Virology, National Institute for Biological Standards and Control, Potters Bar, Hertfordshire, U.K.

Key words: Live-attenuated poliovaccines, polio eradication, poliovirus transmissibility

Abstract: Sabin live-attenuated strains, which have proved to be the most effective tools for poliovirus eradication, could also be the source of reintroduction of polio epidemics after global eradication of wild poliomyelitis is achieved. There are still considerable gaps in our knowledge about the persistence of vaccine-derived viruses in the population and the mechanisms involved in poliovirus transmissibility, both of which are essential factors in assessing the risks posed by such strains and in designing effective strategies for the cessation of polio immunisation. In this report, we have examined virological and epidemiological aspects of an epidemic of poliomyelitis in 1968 in Poland that was shown to be associated with the use of the USOL-D-bac live-attenuated vaccine strain. Possible causes of the origin and progress of the outbreak included the pattern of virus excretion from vaccinees, mutations identified in epidemic viruses and the unique vaccination policies in Poland during the years preceding the epidemic.

Introduction

As we approach the complete eradication of wild poliomyelitis new public health and scientific issues arise, particularly those concerning the risks of reintroduction of polio epidemics after the hypothetical cessation of polio immunisation that will follow eradication [1].

Sabin live-attenuated strains replicate in the gut of vaccinees and often give rise to strains of increased neurovirulence that very rarely cause poliomyelitis in the vaccinees or their contacts [2]. Sabin-derived strains have never been reported to be responsible for poliomyelitis outbreaks, not even in unvaccinated groups of individuals within well-vaccinated communities, where wild strains have been shown to spread rapidly and cause epidemics [3]. However, it is very difficult to predict whether vaccine-derived viruses, which will be the only poliovirus strains in the community after wild poliovirus eradication, will pose a threat to unvaccinated children in the post-eradication era. Various studies suggest that persistence of vaccine-derived strains in the population is of limited duration [1], but some experts consider that the available information is still insufficient to justify that conclusion [4]. Of greater concern is the identification of several cases of long-term virus excretion by immunocompromised vaccinees who have been shown to excrete poliovirus strains for periods of up to 10 years after vaccination [1]. Despite some ongoing studies in different countries, the prevalence of long-term excretion among immunodeficient individuals is currently unknown [1]. In addition, very little is known also about the molecular basis of poliovirus transmissibility, but since few mutations differentiate the vaccine strains from their wild parents [2], it is not inconceivable to assume that vaccine-derived strains of increased transmissibility will be selected during person-to-person virus passage, particularly in conditions of low population immunity and in the absence of wild poliovirus competitors.

The USOL-D-bac Live-Attenuated Vaccine Strain

The USOL-D-bac strain was among a number of type 3 live-attenuated poliovirus strains that were developed in the late 1960s as alternative vaccine candidates to Sabin 3, which had shown genetic instability and raised doubts about the duration of the immunity they provided [5]. Although all three serotype Sabin vaccine strains have proved to be very efficient during the last 30-40 years, the low risk of vaccine-associated paralytic poliomyelitis (VAPP) linked to the use of Sabin 3 is still of significant concern. Sabin 3 is the strain most commonly found in cases of VAPP [2], which is the major cause of poliomyelitis in countries where wild poliovirus has long been eradicated. The possible need for safer attenuated strains to be used during the latest stages of world polio eradication and to be maintained as emergency vaccine stocks for the post-vaccination era has revived research in this field [6].

The USOL-D-bac strain was developed in 1962 from a type 3 poliovirus strain, USOL-D, isolated in 1960 in Czechoslovakia from a paralytic patient [7]. USOL-D was initially amplified by three serial passages in rhesus monkey kidney cells. The virus was then subjected to 17 rapid passages in the same cell substrate using large amounts of virus inocula (100 PFU/cell) at alternative temperatures (four passages at 35°C followed by one passage at 33°C, seven at 35°C and five at 33°C). Four virus lines were then derived by plaque purification followed by preparation of virus stocks at low multiplicity of infection (0.001) in rhesus monkey kidney cells. The USOL-D-b virus progeny was selected on the basis of in vitro genetic markers that were known to correlate with loss of neurovirulence and was then subjected to two identical plaque purification processes. The USOL-D-bac variant was chosen following the same selection criteria as above. No neurotropic activity was detected in monkeys that were inoculated intracerebrally with this strain (in doses exceeding 10^7 $TCID_{50}$). Intraspinal inoculation of doses approximating 10^6 $TCID_{50}$ did not produce any clinical signs of poliomyelitis. Mild histological lesions were detected in the lumbar cord of some animals but there was no evidence of spread of virus to the upper parts of the central nervous system. The USOL-D-bac seed preparation was freed from SV40 virus at the Institute of Poliomyelitis and Viral Encephalitis, Moscow, where a batch of vaccine (lot 283) was prepared in green monkey kidney cells to be used in field trials [8]. Between 1963 and 1967, the neurotropic activity of the virus was tested in six different laboratories in Czechoslovakia, USSR, Germany, Italy, UK and Romania. All these studies indicated that the USOL-D-bac strain possessed a higher degree of attenuation than that seen with the Sabin 3 vaccine strain [9].

The USOL-D-bac vaccine virus (lot 283) was given to children in small-scale trials in Czechoslovakia, USSR and Switzerland [5, 8-11]. The conclusions of these trials (detailed in Table 1) were as follows. No untoward reactions associated

Table 1: Results from small-scale vaccine trials for the characterisation of the USOL-D-bac strain. a) Virus excretion and immunogenicity after vaccination. b) Genetic stability after multiplication in vaccinees.

A

Trial	Ref.	Vaccination schedule			Virus excretion[b] (% of vaccinees)		Antibody response[c]			
			No. of vaccinees[a]				Pre-immune		Non-immune	
		Strain	Pre-immune	Non-immune	Pre-immune	Non-immune	Positive sera (%)	Antibody titre (log_2 GMT)	Positive sera (%)	Antibody titre log_2 GMT)
Czechoslovakia	[10]	USOL	8	2	75.0	100	87.5	11.4	100	8.1
Czechoslovakia	[11]	USOL	16	34	87.5	100	93.7	10.9	88.2	8.0
		Sabin 3	22	39	59.0	92.3	54.5	7.2	84.6	7.6
USSR	[8]	USOL		19		100			100	8.5
		Sabin 3		17		100			100	7.6

a The numbers of previously immunised vaccinees who had type 3 antibodies and non-immune vaccinees are indicated.
b Percentage of vaccinated children who excreted the virus in at least one stool.
c Antibody response against type 3 poliovirus measured 4-6 weeks after vaccination.
GMT: Geometric Mean Titre.

B

Trial	Ref	Vaccine/No. of vaccinees	Properties of progenies from vaccinees[a]					
			Temperature sensitivity		Neurovirulence[c]			
			No. of progenies tested	Change in rct/40 character (% of progenies)[b]	No. of progenies tested	No. of monkeys inoculated	Clinical signs[d]	Histological signs[e]
Czechoslovakia	[10]	USOL/10	26	19.2	9	18	0 (2)	4 (2)
Czechoslovakia	[9]	USOL/50	108	21.3	29	57	0 (5)	11 (25)
		Sabin 3/61	72	69.4	20	38	10 (5)	14 (15)
USSR	[8]	USOL/19	54	85.2	10	17	9[f]	6 (3)
		Sabin 3/17	47	87.2	9	13	6[f]	4 (2)
Switzerland	[5]	USOL/NK	10	10	NK			

a Viruses isolated during 10 weeks of sampling after vaccination.
b Percentage of isolates with [log_{10} titre at 36°C-log_{10} titre at 40°C] <5.0.
c Analysed by intracerebral inoculation of monkeys with 6.5-7.5 log_{10} PFU virus doses.
d No. of monkeys with paralysis, in brackets no. of monkeys with muscular weakness.
e No. of monkeys with wide-spread histological signs, in brackets no. of monkeys with mild histological signs.
f Severity of clinical signs not specified.
NK: Not Known.

with vaccine administration were reported. The virus replicated well in the intestine of both non-immune children and those previously fed with Sabin 3 virus who were known to have type 3 antibodies. The patterns of virus excretion from USOL-D-bac and Sabin 3 vaccinees were similar, but in some circumstances, USOL-D-bac vaccinees were reported to excrete virus more frequently, for longer periods of time, and in higher titres than their Sabin 3 counterparts [8, 9]. Virus replication of the USOL-D-bac strain in vaccinees was associated with the development of a serum antibody response that was as good or better than that induced after Sabin 3 feeding [Table 1a, 5, 8, 10, 11]. Furthermore, the level of serological immunity in children receiving the USOL-D-bac strain as the second dose was significantly higher than that in children fed twice with Sabin 3. Results from studies on the stability of this virus were discrepant (Table 1b). In two studies in Czechoslovakia, USOL-D-bac virus progenies were found to be more attenuated than Sabin 3 progenies [9-11]. In a study in the USSR, a high rate of reversion was observed for both type 3 strains and no significant differences were identified between USOL-D-bac and Sabin 3 progenies [8]. The results of another study in Switzerland indicated a high degree of stability of the rct/40 character of the USOL-D-bac virus; however, only a small number of isolates was examined and no comparison was made with Sabin 3 progenies [5].

A massive vaccine trial with the USOL-D-bac strain followed these studies [11]. Approximately 22,000 persons living in one region of Czechoslovakia were fed with the vaccine. Of the vaccinated persons, more than 9,500 were children aged two-14 months receiving their primary vaccination, nearly 11,000 were children aged 15-72 months who had been vaccinated previously with all three types of Sabin vaccine, and more than 1,700 were adults. No untoward reactions in any of the vaccinees or their contacts were reported. Extensive serological surveillance carried out five weeks and nine months after vaccination confirmed the potent immunogenicity of the USOL-D-bac vaccine strain.

The above data came to the attention of WHO experts who recommended that a number of small-scale trials should be carried out in different countries under WHO's auspices [5]. The objectives of the trials were to obtain more information on the USOL-D-bac strain regarding its immunogenicity in seronegative children and the genetic stability following multiplication in the gut of vaccinated children and susceptible contacts, and to compare the results with those obtained from feeding similar groups of children with the Sabin 3 strain. A batch of the USOL-D-bac vaccine was prepared at the Istituto Sieroterapico Milanese, Milan, from the original vaccine batch (lot 283) prepared in the USSR. The new vaccine batch (lot 2/66.01.12) was subjected to exhaustive quality tests in the production laboratory, the Institute of Poliomyelitis and Viral Encephalitis, Moscow, and the National Institute for Medical Research, London [5]. All tests in all three laboratories were satisfactory and consistent with the low neurovirulence characteristic of the USOL-D-bac parent strain. Institutes in seven countries (France, Hungary, Japan, Poland, Romania, the United Kingdom and the USSR) agreed to co-operate in the studies. Altogether, 163 children between three and 26 months of age were vaccinated with USOL-D-bac vaccine and 112 of similar ages with Sabin 3 between September 1967 and March 1968. Children in closed or semi-closed communities were fed the vaccines in Hungary, Japan, Poland, Romania and the USSR and children in families were given the vaccines in France and the United Kingdom. No pathological symptoms were observed in the vaccinated children or their contacts during 12 weeks of careful surveillance after vaccination in five of the seven countries, but in two, Romania (four cases) and the USSR (one case), paralytic cases occurred in contacts of children immunised with the USOL-D-bac strain. Although the evidence from studies in the USSR and Romania was not entirely conclusive, it was considered sufficient to abandon further investigation of the strain. The results from the trials, however, indicated that the USOL-D-bac vaccine was superior to the Sabin 3 vaccine in terms of implantation in the gut, immunogenicity and genetic stability [5].

In Poland, one of the countries in the studies, a large outbreak due to type 3 poliovirus occurred four months after trials with the Sabin 3 and the USOL-D-bac had been completed [12]. The description of the 1968 poliomyelitis epidemic in Poland and evidence of its association with the use of USOL-D-bac vaccine strain are presented in the next section.

The 1968 Epidemic of Type 3 Poliomyelitis in Poland

In accordance with the programme of the vaccine trials in Poland, on 3 November 1967, eight children in a weekly nursery in Poznán were vaccinated with USOL-D-bac virus, whereas on 15 November 1967, 10 children in a children's home in Bialystok were fed with the Sabin 3 strain. In addition, nine children in a children's home in Slupsk were given the USOL-D-bac virus on 16 February 1968 (Fig. 1, [12]). As stated above, no untoward post-vaccination events were observed in any of the vaccinated children or their contacts. However, in Poznán, on 14 March 1968, a four-month-old infant developed typical paralytic poliomyelitis and in mid-April and in early May two other cases occurred, one in a one-year-old child and one in an adult woman [12]. Type 3 polioviruses were found in the stools of these patients. In May 1968 six more cases were reported in the same area and from then, the epidemic spread to other parts of the country. More than half of the total of 464 paralytic cases was reported in Poznán and province and, as shown in Figure 1, the outbreak was mostly restricted to the northern and western provinces of Poland surrounding the Poznan province. The epidemic receded from September 1968 following mass vaccinations with Sabin 3 monovalent vaccine in August, with only five cases reported in October, two in November and one in December 1968. WHO collaborative studies at the time failed to identify the wild or vaccine origin of selected isolates from the epidemic (Table 2a, [13]). Isolates available from those studies were analysed in our laboratory using molecular techniques readily accessible today [14]. The complete nucleotide sequence of the USOL-D-bac strain (lot 2/66.01.12) used in the 1967-68 vaccine trials was determined and analysed to establish the predicted amino acid sequence. The genome comprises a 5' non-coding region (NCR) of 747 nucleotides, a single open reading frame of 6618 nucleotides (2206 codons), a short 3' NCR region of 71 nucleotides, and a poly(A) tract. As expected, from the three different poliovirus serotypes, the USOL-D-bac virus most closely resembled other type 3 strains, particularly through the capsid region [14].

Nucleotide sequence analysis established a close relationship between the USOL-D-bac vaccine strain and epidemic isolates (Table 2b), which contained only few mutations that could be assumed to have been acquired during replication in vaccinees, their contacts and/or patients [14]. The vaccine origin of the epidemic

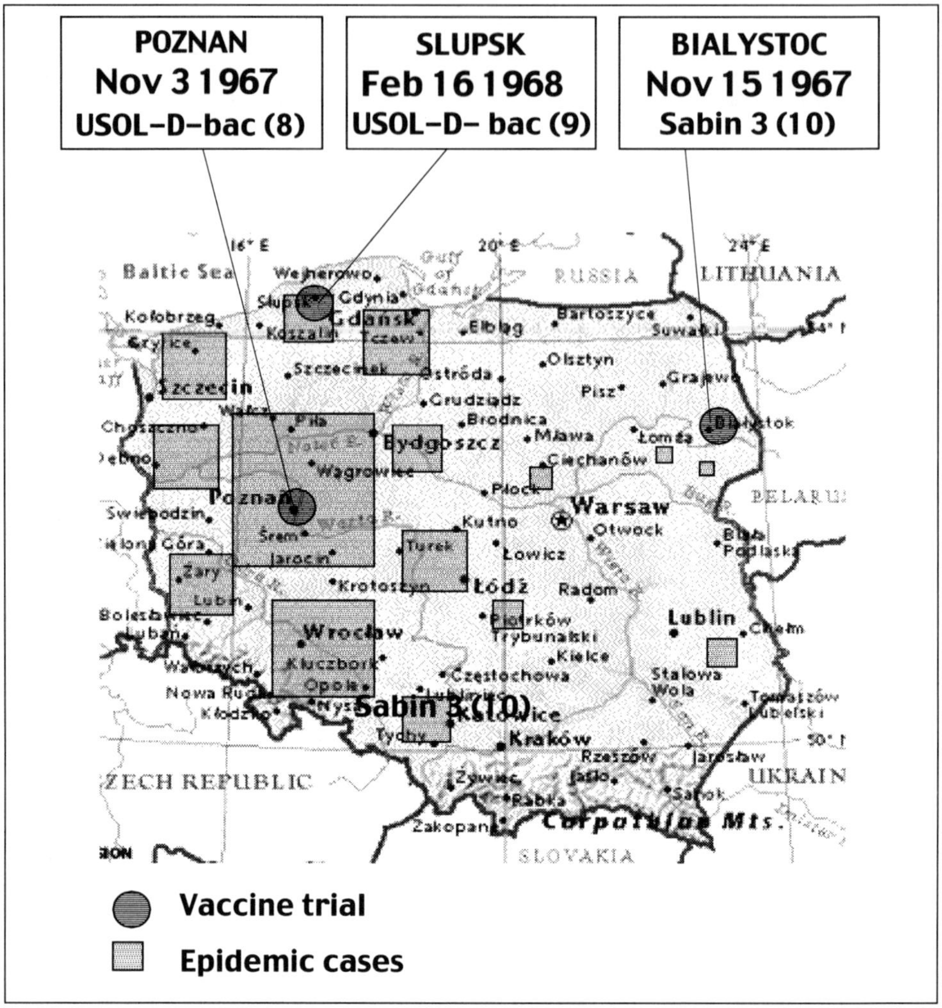

Fig. 1: Location of the vaccine trials in Poland and distribution of paralytic cases during the 1968 Polish epidemic of type 3 poliomyelitis. The number of vaccinees in each location is indicated in brackets.

was further supported by the fact that during the 1962-1967 period, not a single type 3 poliovirus strain was isolated from poliomyelitis patients or in virological surveys of healthy persons and sewage examinations carried out each year [12]. Analysis of the incorporation of nucleotide mutations at synonymous third-base codon positions, which have been shown to measure poliovirus evolution accurately, was also consistent with this hypothesis [14]. Figure 2 illustrates the comparison of the percentage of such synonymous changes in isolate 10/715 from a healthy vaccinee and two epidemic isolates (11/52 and 1/6 strains) with respect to the USOL-D-bac strain over the entire coding region, represented against the time of virus isolation. The estimated sequence evolution rate of 2.70% mutations at syn-

Table 2: Characterization of poliovirus isolates from cases of the 1968 epidemic of type 3 poliomyelitis in Poland. a) Data from WHO collaborative studies [13]. b) Nucleotide sequence analysis [14].

A						
Strain	**Origin**[a]	**Country**	**Date of isolation (days after trial)**	**Rct/40 marker**[b]	**Antigenic relationship**[c]	
					to USOL	**To Sabin 3**
USOL-D-bac	vaccine		0	–	L	D
5633/67	healthy v	Hungary	17	+		
5527/67	healthy v	Hungary	49	–		
D10/16	healthy c	Romania	52	+/–		
10/715	healthy v	Poland	66	–	D	D
5778/67	healthy v	Hungary	77	–		
11/52	case	Poland	143	+	I	D
7/61	case	Poland	168	+	I	D
4/22	case	Poland	225	+	I	D
5/91	case	Poland	227	–	I	D
1/6	case	Poland	229	+	I	D
8/01	case	Poland	232	+	I	D
20/92	case	Poland	233	+	I	D

a v: Vaccinee; c: contact.

b Calculated as [$\log_{10}$ titre at 36°C-$\log_{10}$ titre at 40°C]; +: <2.0; +/–: 2.0-5.0; –: >5.0

c Measured by the McBride neutralisation test [13]; L: Like; I: Intermediate; D: Different.

B												
Strain	**Nucleotide positions**											
	1 to 64	**65 to 747**	**748 to 1150**	**1151 to 2040**	**2041 to 2420**	**2421 to 3381**	**3382 to 4950**	**4951 to 5250**	**5251 to 6350**	**6351 to 6520**	**6521 to 7365**	**7366 to 7436**
USOL-D-bac	+[a]	+	+	+	+	+	+	+	+	+	+	+
5633/67		+		+		+		+		+		
5527/67		+		+		+		+		+		
D10/16		+		+		+		+		+		
10/715	+	+	+	+	+	+	+	+	+	+	+	+
5778/67		+		+		+		+		+		
11/52	+	+	+	+	+	+	+	+	+	+	+	+
7/61		+		+		+		+		+		
4/22		+		+		+		+		+		
5/91		+		+		+		+		+		
1/6	+	+	+	+	+	+	+	+	+	+	+	+
8/01		+		+		+		+		+		
20/92		+		+		+		+		+		
GENOMIC REGION	5'NCR		CAPSID				NON-STRUCTURAL					3'NCR

a +: indicates that the genomic fragment was sequenced and USOL-D-bac-like (>98.5% sequence identity).

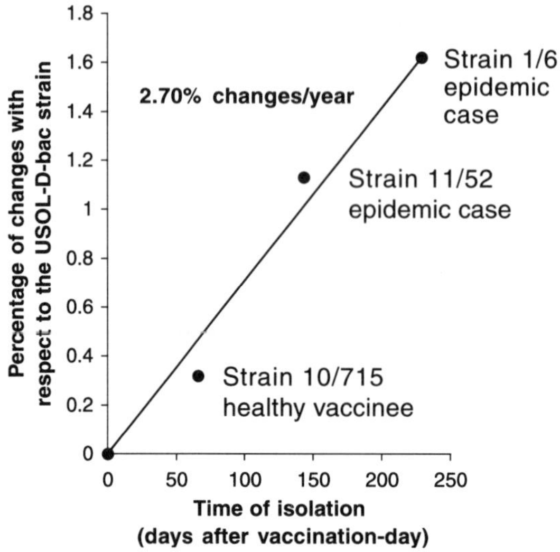

Fig. 2: Percentage of synonymous mutations at third-base codon positions over the entire coding region found in Polish poliovirus strains 10/715, 11/52 and 1/6 with respect to the USOL-D-bac strain. The sequence evolution rate calculated from the linear function is shown.

onymous third-base codon positions/year is remarkably similar to that previously calculated for wild poliovirus [15] or for Sabin-derived strains replicating for long periods in immunodeficient patients [16]. The distribution of mutations in healthy and epidemic isolates identified regions of the virus possibly involved in an increase of virus neurovirulence and/or transmissibility. Mutations were found in the 5' non-coding region and in capsid residues involved in receptor binding, virus entry and antigenic sites [14]. All epidemic strains contained a mutation at nucleotide 264 in the 5' non-coding region and amino acid changes at capsid residues VP1-7, VP1-258, VP1-294 and VP2-191. The mutations at VP1-294 (from valine to glutamic acid) and at VP2-191 (from alanine to valine) were also present in all isolates from healthy individuals indicating their possible relevance for virus growth in the gut.

The fact that USOL-D-bac vaccinees and their contacts had been shown to excrete virus more frequently, in higher titres and for longer periods than their Sabin 3 counterparts [8, 9], indicates that the excretion patterns from these individuals may have played an important role in the origin of the epidemic. In fact, two of the USOL-D-bac vaccinees in Poland were excreting poliovirus at least 80 days after vaccination, whereas Sabin 3 vaccinees did not excrete virus for more than 56 days [12].

The low immunity against type 3 poliovirus present in the Polish population at the time of the epidemic has also been suggested as a possible factor that contributed to the genesis and development of the epidemic [12, 14]. This was probably the consequence of the particular vaccine policies in Poland in the years before the epidemic, which only included type 1 and 2 components in the poliovirus live-attenuated vaccine whereas the type 3 component was given as inactivated vaccine (IPV) in conditions that only provided short-term immunity. As shown in Table 3, the significant differences between the antigenic structures of the USOL-D-bac strain and the Saukett virus, used in the inactivated type 3 poliovaccine,

Table 3: Comparison of deduced amino acid sequences at antigenic sites between USOL-d-bac-derived isolates and Saukett and Sabin type 3 vaccine strains.

Virus strain	**Antigenic site**					
	Site 1 VP1 89-100	**Site 2a VP1 217-223**	**Site 2b VP2 164-172**	**Site 3a VP1 286-290**	**Site 3b VP3 58-60, 70,71**	**Site 4 VP3 77-80**
USOL-D-bac	EVDNEQPTTRAQ	SDANDNV	TAVTSPKRE	KDGLA	ENT VR	NSLD
10/715	------------	-------	--A------	-----	--- --	---N
5633/67	------------	-------	---------	-----	--- --	----
5527/67	------------	-------	-T-------	-----	--- --	---N
D10/16	------------	-------	---------	-----	--- --	---N
5778/67	------------	-------	---------	-----	--- --	---V
11/52	------------	-------	---------	-----	--- --	----
7/61	------------	--T----	---------	-----	--- --	----
4/22	------------	--V----	---------	-----	--- --	----
5/91	------------	-------	---------	-----	--- --	----
1/6	------------	--T----	---------	-----	--- --	----
8/01	---------K--	--T----	---------	-----	--- --	----
20/92	------------	-------	---------	-----	--- --	----
Saukett[a]	------------	T-----I	---------	--N-N	-S- -T	D--Q
Sabin 3[b]	------------	T-----I	N--------	RNN-D	-S- -T	D--Q

EMBL, Accession Nos.: [a] L23846, [b] X00925.

suggest that failure to neutralise the epidemic strain specifically, as well as low immunity, may have played an important part in the emergence and establishment of the outbreak.

Conclusions

Factors such as the duration and titre of virus excretion from vaccinees and their contacts and the extent of population herd immunity, together with viral mutations acquired during multiplication in the human gut, could contribute to the establishment of vaccine-derived polio epidemics. The Sabin strains, the sole live-attenuated vaccines currently in use, may have different properties in terms of reversion to virulence and transmissibility with respect to the USOL-D-bac strain. However, the possibility of similar epidemics to that described in this report caused by Sabin-derived strains in the post-vaccination era cannot be ruled out. Vaccine-derived strains from long-term excretors could be the source of such events. This possibility has to be evaluated and considered when deciding how and when to cease polio immunisation. Studies on the prevalence of long-term excretion among the immunodeficient population and a further understanding of poliovirus transmission would be necessary before such a major decision could be taken.

REFERENCES

1 Wood DJ, Sutter RW, Dowdle WR: Stopping poliovirus vaccination after eradication. Bull World Health Org 2000;78:347-357.

2 Minor PD: The molecular biology of poliovaccines. J Gen Virol 1992;73:3065-3077.

3 Fine PE, Carneiro IA: Transmissibility and persistence of oral polio vaccine viruses: implications for the global poliomyelitis eradication initiative. Am Epidemiol 1999;150:1001-1021.

4 Racaniello VR: It is too early to stop polio vaccination. Bull World Health Org 2000;78:359-360.

5 Beale AJ, Biberi-Moroeanu S, Boulger LR, Burgasov PN, Cockburn WC, Chumakov MP, De Barbieri A, Domok I, et al: USOL-D-bac (type 3 poliovirus) vaccine studies. Bull World Health Org 1969;40:295-300.

6 Macadam AJ, Ferguson G, Stone DM, Meredith J, Almond JW, Minor PD: Rational design of a genetically-stable live-attenuated poliovirus vaccine: relevance to poliomyelitis eradication. Submitted.

7 Vonka V, Janda Z, Simon J: The properties of a new type 3 attenuated poliovirus I. Arch ges Virusforsch 1964;14:599-610.

8 Elbert LB, Chumakov MP, Ralf NM, Krutyanskaya GD, Grachyov VP, Avdeyeva LI, Dzagurov SG, Grachyova LA, Tyufanov AV, Tsypkin LB, Ravkina LI: Comparative study of two vaccine strains of type 3 poliovirus (USOL-D-bac and Leon 12a1b). Acta Virol 1967;11:89-99.

9 Vonka V, Janda Z, Simon J, Adam E: Present status of the investigation of the USOL-D-bac type 3 attenuated poliovirus. XIth Symposium of the European Association Against Poliomyelitis 1966;191-201.

10 Vonka V, Janda Z, Simon J, Adam E, Zavadova H, Starek M: Properties of a new type 3 attenuated poliovirus III. Arch ges Virusforsch 1965;15:234-243.

11 Vonka V, Janda Z, Simon J, Adam E, Zavadova H, Adamova V: The properties of a new type 3 attenuated poliovirus IV. Arch ges Virusforsch 1965;15:500-513.

12 Kostrzewski J, Kulesza A, Abgarowicz A: The epidemic of type 3 poliomyelitis in Poland in 1968. Epidem Rev (Warsz) 1970;24:89-103.

13 Melnick JL, Berencsi G, Biberi-Moroeanu S, Combiescu A A, Furesz J, Kantoch M, Kostrzewski J, Magrath DI, Perkins FT, Vonka V, Cockburn WC, Domok I, Assaad FA: WHO collaborative studies on poliovirus type 3 strains isolated during the 1968 poliomyelitis epidemic in Poland. Bull World Health Org 1972;47:287-294.

14 Martín J, Ferguson GL, Wood DJ, Minor PD: The vaccine origin of the 1968 epidemic of type 3 poliomyelitis in Poland. Submitted for publication.

15 Kew OM, Sutter RW, Nottay BK, McDonough MJ, Prevots DR, Quick L, Pallansch MA: Prolonged replication of a type 1 vaccine-derived poliovirus in an immunodeficient patient. J Clin Microbiol 1998;36:2893-2899.

16 Martín J, Dunn G, Hull R, Patel V, Minor PD: Evolution of the Sabin strain of type 3 poliovirus in an immunodeficient patient during the entire 637-day period of virus excretion. J Virol 2000;74:3001-3010.

Dr. J. Martín, Division of Virology, National Institute for Biological Standards and Control, South Mimms, Blanche Lane, Potters Bar, Herts. EN6 3QG, United Kingdom.

Brown F (ed): Progress in Polio Eradication: Vaccine Strategies for the End Game.
Dev Biol. Basel, Karger, 2001, vol 105, pp 93-98

Neurovirulence of Sabin 1-Derived Polioviruses Isolated from an Immunodeficient Patient with Prolonged Viral Excretion

T. Yoneyama[1], *H. Yoshida*[1], *H. Shimizu*[1], *K. Yoshii*[1], *N. Nagata*[2], *O. Kew*[3], *T. Miyamura*[1]

[1] Department of Virology II,
[2] Department of Safety Research on Biologics, National Institute of Infectious Diseases, Musashimurayama, Tokyo, Japan
[3] Centers for Disease Control and Prevention, Atlanta, Georgia, USA

Key words: Neurovirulence, reversion, Sabin 1 strain, transgenic mice, prolonged excretion, immunodeficient patient.

Abstract: We have analysed the neurovirulence of Sabin 1-derived isolates which persisted more than nine years in an immunodeficient patient in the U.S.A. Samples were collected from stool specimens at days 11 (St1), 23 (St2), 48 (St3), 126 (St5), and 200 (St7) after the onset of paralysis. Critical nucleotides associated with the reversion of virulence were examined. All the isolates had the substitutions at nucleotide positions 480 (G to A) in the 5'-non-coding region (NCR), 2438 (A to U) in VP3, 2795 (A to G) in VP1, and 6203 (C to U) in 3D. Serially diluted samples were injected intracerebrally to transgenic mice harbouring the human poliovirus receptor gene. Samples St2, 3, 5 and 7 showed typical virulent characters in transgenic mice, whereas the sample ST1 showed intermediate neurovirulence. It seemed that there were two variant viruses providing for a major (M) and a minor (m) populations. After disappearance of the m-variant, samples obtained at the later stages showed neurovirulence almost equivalent to that of the Mahoney strain. Thus, the Sabin 1 strain evolved towards full neuropathogenicity after long-term replication in humans by accumulating mutations. Therefore, OPV-vaccination of immunodeficient persons should be avoided.

INTRODUCTION

Orally-administered Sabin vaccine strains may change their characteristics during replication in the human intestine. This is particularly important in immunodeficient patients because poliovirus can persist longer and consequently be excreted for a longer period by such patients. During this time, different levels of mutations may accumulate. A previous report indicated that poliovirus Sabin 1 strain persisted for more than nine years in an immunodeficient patient, resulting in ~10% genomic divergence from the original vaccine strain [1]. We focused on the evolution of neuropathogenicity of excreted viruses using transgenic mice harbouring the human poliovirus receptor (PVR-Tg mice) and showed that the Sabin 1 strain could revert to a level of neurovirulence equivalent to that of the parental Mahoney strain.

Materials and Methods

Cells and viruses

HEp-2c cells were grown in monolayers in Eagle's minimum essential medium (MEM) supplemented with 10 % foetal bovine serum (FBS). Type 1 poliovirus isolates from an immunodeficient patient in the U.S.A. were passaged once in HEp-2c cells at 35°C without plaque-purification and stored at –80°C in small aliquots after determination of their titres. Those isolates were designated St1 to St7 according to order sampling for virus isolation. St1, St2, St3, St5, and St7 were collected at 11, 23, 48, 126 and 200 days after the onset of paralysis. All isolates were collected after prolonged replication in the immunodeficient patient who received his last OPV dose 6.9 years before the onset of paralysis, i.e. the initial infection started more than nine years before collection of samples by calculation of sequence evolution [1].

Nucleotide sequencing

Viral RNA was prepared from the culture supernatants by digestion with proteinase K and 0.3% sodium dodecyl sulphate followed by phenol-chloroform extraction. The nucleotide sequences were determined by dye-labelled terminator cycle sequencing using an automated DNA sequencer (ABI-Prism 310) and universal primers for polioviruses [2,3].

Assay of neurovirulence in PVR-transgenic mice

Viruses were tested for their neurovirulence in heterozygous PVR-Tg21 mice [4], which are susceptible to poliovirus infection. Groups of four- to five-week old mice were inoculated intracerebrally (i.c.) with 30μl of the virus suspensions. Ten-fold dilutions of virus stock were made in MEM containing 2% FBS. The viral dose that induced paralysis or death in 50% of mice (PD_{50}) after 14 days was calculated by the method of Karber.

Detection of virus antigen

Paralysed mice were sacrificed and their spinal cords were fixed in a solution of 10% buffered formalin. Paraffin embedded sections were examined for localization of viral antigen using hyperimmune anti-type 1 poliovirus-rabbit serum by the immunoperoxidase (avidin-biotin complex, ABC) method, and histopathological changes were visualized by haematoxylin-eosin staining.

Results

Detection of point mutations

Nucleotide substitutions considered to be critical for neurovirulence were examined [5-8]. All isolates had the nucleotide substitution (G to A) at nucleotide position 480 in the 5'-NCR (Table 1). Reversion at nucleotide position 480 is associated with increased neurovirulence, probably by restoring base pairing in a stem of domain V in the 5'-NCR. Reversions in structural proteins were found at codons VP3-225 and VP1-106, but not at codon VP1-88. In the polymerase 3D coding region a reversion at codon 3D-73 was found. Thus, all isolates had substi-

Table 1: Mutation of Sabin 1 isolates in nucleotides critical for reversion.

Isolate	Days after onset	P480	P2438	P2741	P2795	P6203
		5'-NC	VP3-225	VP1-88	VP1-106	3D-73
Sabin 1		G	A(Met)	G(Ala)	A(Thr)	C(Hys)
St1	11	A	U	G	G	U
St2	23	A	U	G	G	U
St3	48	A	U	G	G	U
St5	126	A	U	G	G	U
St7	200	A	U	G	G	U
Mahoney		A	U(Leu)	A(Thr)	G(Ala)	U(Tyr)

tutions towards reversion to the wild-type Mahoney genotype in those critical nucleotides examined, except codon VP1-88.

Neurovirulence of isolates

PVR-Tg mice have been shown to be suitable for investigating poliovirus neurovirulence [9]. PVR-Tg21, one line of PVR-Tg mice, has been introduced into safety testing of OPV preparation instead of monkeys [10], and has been used for the assay of poliovirus neurovirulence of vaccine-associated paralytic poliomyelitis (VAPP) [3,8]. Because Sabin 1-derived isolates generally showed poor or intermediate neurovirulence after viral replication in the human intestines, it was interesting to know the level of neurovirulence of those isolates collected after prolonged replication with accumulating mutations as stated above. The PD_{50}s of the isolates were compared to those of the reference strains Sabin 1 and Mahoney. The level of the neurovirulence for St1-isolate was intermediate (Table 2). Isolates at later stages were more neurovirulent, almost as neurovirulent as the Mahoney strain. It seemed that two variants consisted of major (M) and minor (m) populations in the earlier samples [1]. After disappearance of the m-variant, samples obtained at the later stages showed neurovirulence almost equivalent to the Mahoney strain. Thus, the Sabin 1 strain can change to highly neurovirulent after prolonged replication in the human intestines.

Table 2: Neurovirulence of Sabin 1 isolates in PVR-Tg21.

Isolate	[a]Dose of inoculation									[a]PD_{50}
	7.8	6.8	5.8	4.8	4.3	3.8	3.3	2.8	2.3	
Sabin 1	[b]0/5[c]	0/5								>8.3
St1		3/4	3/5	2/5						5.6
St2				5/5		0/5		1/4		4.1
St3				5/5		4/5		3/5		<2.7
St5				5/5		5/5		4/5		<2.5
St7				5/5		4/5		0/4		3.5
Mahoney					5/5		4/5		3/5	[d]<2.4

a Dose of inoculation and PD_{50} were represented in $\log_{10}$ $TCID_{50}$/mouse.
b No. of paralysed mice were represented as a numerator.
c Each group contained four or five mice.
d The data for Mahoney strain were cited in our previous paper [3].

Detection of virus antigen

To confirm that paralysis was caused by the degeneration of nerve cells after replication of the inoculated viruses, the spinal cords were examined for histopathological changes and poliovirus antigens. The mice examined showed histopathological changes characteristic of neuronal degeneration and necrosis without the inflammatory response. They were observed primarily in the anterior horns of lumbar, thoracic and cervical cords. The specific staining of poliovirus antigens was seen in the cytoplasm of degenerated and necrotic nerve cells in the lumbar and cervical anterior horns (Fig. 1).

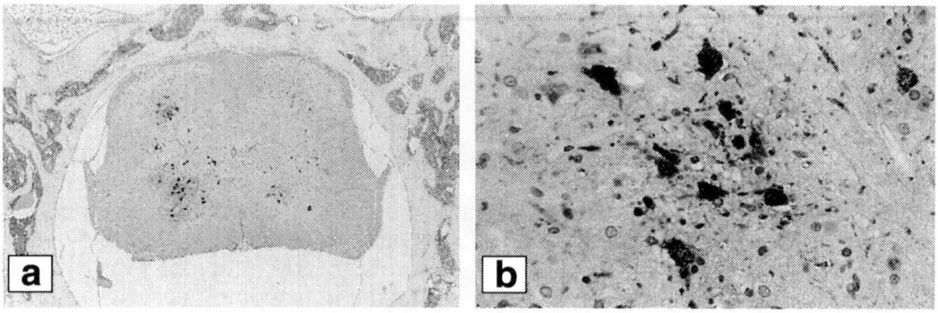

Fig. 1: The detection of poliovirus antigen in spinal cord of PVR-Tg21 mice inoculated intracerebrally with Sabin 1-derived poliovirus.
a) Lumbar spinal cord of PVR-Tg21 mouse inoculated with St7-isolate, $log_{10}4.8TCID_{50}$. The mouse showed paralysis on day 9 after inoculation and then sacrificed on the same day. Poliovirus antigens were detected in the neurons of the anterior and posterior horns (ABC method). Magnification X55.
b) Higher magnification of a part of the right anterior horn of panel (a). Poliovirus antigens are detected only in neurons. Magnification X550.

Discussion

Oral vaccine strains developed by Sabin frequently evolve towards increased neurovirulence after OPV-administration in humans and are accompanied by genomic diversity [2,3,7,8,11]. It is considered that the rare cases of VAPP are caused by such mutated vaccine-derived isolates. By normal immune defences vaccine strains were excluded within one to two months in immunocompetent persons [12]. However, in the absence of neutralizing antibodies, Sabin strains can persist for a long time and change their genomic and phenotypic characteristics after prolonged replication in the human intestines [12,13]. One case of prolonged excretion of Sabin 1 strain from an immunodeficient patient was reported recently in the U.S.A. [1] and another in Germany [14]. The isolates in the case in the U.S.A. evolved to highly neurovirulent. Association of the Sabin 1 strain with VAPP is very rare and less frequent than that of Sabin 2 or 3 [15], because the large number of genomic differences between Sabin 1 and Mahoney inhibits the shift of the Sabin strain towards Mahoney-like highly neurovirulent characteristics. Limited genomic changes of Sabin 1 strain after replication in the human intestines resulted in poor or intermediate reversion to neurovirulence [3,8].

Although there is no evidence that those excreted vaccine-derived polioviruses caused other cases of VAPP, it is possible that highly neurovirulent Sabin-derived strains could be excreted from immunodeficient persons after OPV-vaccination and might circulate in the environment for a long period. It is important to study the excretion of polioviruses and their subsequent circulation among immunodeficient persons.

Conclusion

As the diagnosis of immunodeficiency is often not established in the first year of life, some children receive OPV before this condition is recognized. Therefore, prolonged excretion of vaccine strains in immunodeficient patients presents a challenge to polio eradication. One option might be the introduction of inactivated poliovirus vaccine at the final stage of polio eradication, since it might be impossible to avoid the excretion and circulation of vaccine strains completely in the environment.

Acknowledgements

This work was supported in part by grants from the Ministry of Health and Welfare of Japan.

References

1 Kew OM, Sutter RW, Nottay BK, McDonough MJ, Prevots DR, Quick L, Pallansch MA: Prolonged replication of a type 1 vaccine-derived poliovirus in an immunodeficient patient. J Clin Microbiol 1998;36:2893-2899.

2 Furione M, Guillot S, Otelea D, Balanant J, Candrea A, Crainic R: Polioviruses with natural recombinant genomes isolated from vaccine-associated paralytic poliomyelitis. Virology 1993;196:199-208.

3 Li J, Zhang LB, Yoneyama T, Yoshida H, Shimizu H, Yoshii K, Hara M, Nomura T, Yoshikura H, Miyamura T, Hagiwara A: Genetic basis of the neurovirulence of type 1 polioviruses isolated from vaccine-associated paralytic patients. Arch Virol 1996;141:1047-1054.

4 Koike S, Taya C, Kurata T, Abe S, Ise I, Yonekawa H, Nomoto A: Transgenic mice susceptible to poliovirus. Proc Natl Acad Sci USA. 1991;88:951-955.

5 Kawamura N, Kohara M, Abe S, Komatsu T, Tago K, Arita M, Nomoto A: Determinants in the 5' noncoding region of poliovirus Sabin 1 RNA that influence the attenuation phenotype. J Virol 1989;63:1302-1309.

6 Christodoulou C, Colbere-Garapin F, Macadam A, Taffs LF, Marsden S, Minor P, Horaud F: Mapping of mutations associated with neurovirulence in monkeys infected with Sabin 1 poliovirus revertants selected at high temperature. J Virol 1990;64:4922-4929.

7 Crainic R, Furione M, Otelea D, Guillot S, Balanant J, Combiescu AA, Combiescu M, Candrea A: Natural evolution of oral vaccine poliovirus strains, in Kurstak E (ed): Measles and Poliomyelitis. Wien, Springer-Verlag, 1993, pp 371-390.

8 Georgescu MM, Balanant J, Macadam A, Otelea D, Combiescu M, Combiescu AA, Crainic R, Delpeyroux F: Evolution of the Sabin type 1 poliovirus in humans: Characterization of strains isolated from patients with vaccine-associated paralytic poliomyelitis: J Virol 1997;71:7758-7768.

9 Horie H, Koike S, Kurata T, Sato-Yoshida Y, Ise I, Ota Y, Abe S, Hioki K, Kato H, Taya C, Nomura T, Hashizume S, Yonekawa H, Nomoto A: Transgenic mice carrying the human poliovirus receptor: New animal model for study of poliovirus neurovirulence. J Virol 1994;68:681-688.

10 Abe S, Ota Y, Doi Y, Nomoto A, Nomura T, Chumakov KM, Hashizume S: Studies on neurovirulence in poliovirus-sensitive transgenic mice and cynomolgus monkeys for the different temperature-sensitive viruses derived from the Sabin type 3 virus. Virol 1995;210:160-166.

11 Georgescu MM, Delpeyroux F, Trady-Panit M, Balanant J, Combiescu M, Combiescu AA, Guillot S, Crainic R: High diversity of poliovirus strains isolated from the central nervous system from patients with vaccine-associated paralytic poliomyelitis. J Virol 1994;68:8089-8101.

12 Dowdle WR, Birmingham ME: The biologic principles of poliovirus eradication. J Infect Dis 1997;175(Suppl 1):S286-292.

13 Yoneyama T, Hagiwara A, Hara M, Shimojo H: Alteration in oligonucleotide fingerprint patterns of the viral genome in poliovirus type 2 isolated from paralytic patients. Infection and Immunity 1982;37:46-53.

14 Bellmunt A, May G, Zell R, Pring-Akerblom P, Verhagen W, Heim A: Evolution of poliovirus type 1 during 5.5 years of prolonged enteral replication in an immunodeficient patient. Virology 1999;265:178-184.

15 Shimojo H: Poliomyelitis control in Japan. Rev Infect Dis 1984;6(Suppl 2):S427-430.

Dr. T. Yoneyama, Department of Virology II, National Institute of Infectious Diseases, 4-7-1, Gakuen, Musashimurayama, Tokyo, 208-0011, Japan.

Brown F (ed): Progress in Polio Eradication: Vaccine Strategies for the End Game.
Dev Biol. Basel, Karger, 2001, vol 105, pp 99-104

Poliovirus Persistence in Human Cells in vitro

F. Colbère-Garapin, S. Jacques, A.-S. Drillet, N. Pavio, T. Couderc, B. Blondel, I. Pelletier

Unité de Neurovirologie et Régénération du Système Nerveux, Institut Pasteur, Paris, France.

Key words: poliovirus, enterovirus, picornavirus, persistent infection, poliomyelitis, receptor.

Abstract: Poliovirus (PV) can persist in vivo in the intestine of immunocompromised hosts for years. Moreover, immunocompetent individuals who have survived paralytic poliomyelitis sometimes develop the post-poliomyelitis syndrome (PPS), consisting of a variety of symptoms including new muscular atrophies. PPS may be due to PV persistence. We have developed models of PV persistence in neural cells and epidermoid cells. Cell determinants are of crucial importance for the establishment of persistent infections in human neuronal cells, whereas viral determinants play the primary role in human epidermoid HEp-2 cells. The results obtained with these in vitro models show the capacity of PV to persist and reveal a virus and cell co-evolution involving PV-receptor interactions. In addition, they suggest that several mechanisms are used by PV to establish and maintain persistent infections.

INTRODUCTION

The chronic infection of some hypogammaglobulinaemic individuals by Sabin poliovirus strains for several years following anti-polio vaccination [1] raises the question of PV persistence in the human intestine, and eventually in other organs of immunocompromised hosts. Although this phenomenon has been known for many years, it has been recognised as an obstacle to poliomyelitis and poliovirus eradication only recently. In addition, the hypothesis of PV persistence in the central nervous system as a possible cause of the post-poliomyelitis syndrome (PPS) [2] needs to be tested in several ways. Cell cultures in vitro obviously cannot be considered as perfect models of whole organisms, but they can be extremely useful for investigating the capacity of a virus to establish persistent infections and elucidating the molecular mechanisms allowing persistence. We have developed several models in cells of neuronal or epidermoid origin to improve our understanding of PV persistence in human cells [3-5]. PV mutants called PVpi are consistently selected in human neuroblastoma IMR-32 cells [4]. Our most recent results reveal virus and cell co-evolution with the involvement of PV-PV receptor (PVR) interactions during the persistent infection of IMR-32 cells. We found that mutated PVRs were expressed in PV-persistently infected IMR-32 cells, and that the miss-sense mutations mapped to PVR domain 1 [6], i.e. the domain interacting directly with PV. We have investigated whether these mutations affect PV-induced cell lysis and PV-PVR interactions.

Materials and Methods

Cells and virus

Murine thymidine kinase-negative LM cells, which have no PVR gene, LM cell derivatives (PVR-expressing clones) [6], and HEp-2 cells were grown in DMEM containing 10% newborn calf serum. The neurovirulent PV type 1 strain Mahoney (PV1/Mahoney) and Mahoney mutants Mah-KKVP1S_{95} and Mah-KKVP2Y_{142} [7] were grown on HEp-2 cells.

Resistance of cells to virus-induced lysis

PVR-expressing LM-cells (10^6) were seeded in 24-well plates and infected 18 hr later. At the time of infection, the multiplicity of infection was adjusted to 10 $TCID_{50}$ per cell. After 30 min of adsorption at 37°C, cells were washed once and 1 ml of DMEM containing 2% FCS was added to each well. After 48 h of infection, the percentage of cells surviving infection was determined as described [6].

Poliovirus conformational alteration assays

Virus was labelled with ^{35}S-methionine (ICN; 1400 Ci/mmol) and purified on a cesium chloride density gradient. Cells (10^7) were trypsinized, washed, and then incubated with ^{35}S-radiolabelled virus in a total volume of 2 ml of ice-cold DMEM-2%FCS at 4°C for 2.5 h to synchronize the infection. Alteration was initiated by adding 5 ml of DMEM-2%FCS preheated to 37°C and cells were agitated for 15 min at 37°C. Cells were then washed, pelleted and lysed as described [6]. After incubation for 20 min on ice, the cell lysates were clarified and layered on to 15 to 30% (wt/vol) sucrose gradients prepared in PBS, which were then centrifuged in a Kontron TST41.14 rotor for 2 h at 40000 rpm at 4°C .

Results

The role of PV-PVR interactions in the resistance of cells to PV-induced lysis was investigated. Murine LM cell clones expressing either the PVR form expressed in uninfected IMR-32 cells (PVR_{IMR}, with an Ala at amino acid position 67) or the PVR forms selected during the persistent infection of IMR-32 cells, were infected with the wild-type strain PV1/Mahoney, or the mutants Mah-KKVP1S_{95} and Mah-KKVP2Y_{142}. The two PV mutants harbour PVpi mutations consistently selected in cells of neuronal origin [5]. The PVR forms selected during the persistent infection of neuroblastoma cells conferred to LM cells a partial resistance to PV-induced lysis (Fig. 1). This was observed for PV1/Mahoney and the PV mutants.

PV-PVR interactions were studied in greater detail in LM cells expressing PVR_{IMR} (LM/PVR_{IMR}) and in cells expressing one of the PVR forms (PVR-Thr67) selected in persistently infected IMR-32 cells. It has been proposed that PVR-Thr67 is an allelic variant of the PVR [8]. The kinetics of adsorption of the three viruses were similar on LM/PVR_{IMR} and on LM/PVR-Thr67 (not shown). Similarly, the kinetics of elution of the three viruses were similar on both cell lines (not shown). In contrast, differences were noted when conformational modifications of the capsid

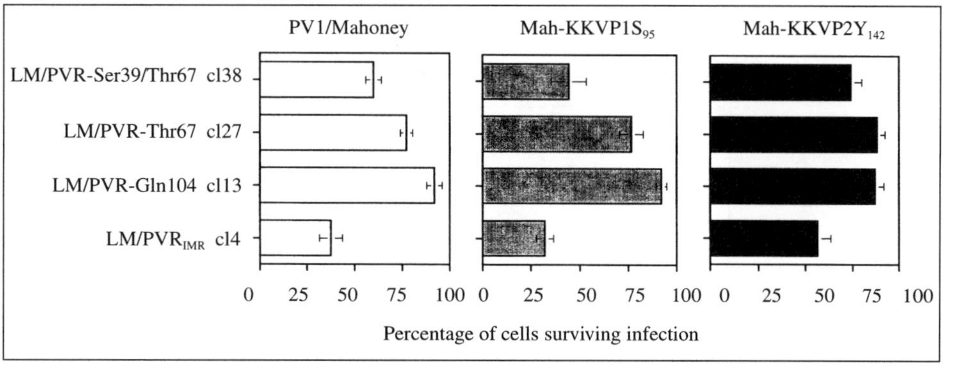

Fig. 1: Percentage of LM/PVR cells surviving after infection with PV. LM/PVR cell clones were infected at an MOI of 10 with either PV1/Mahoney, Mah-KKVP1S_{95} or Mah-KKVP2Y_{142}, and the percentage of surviving adherent cells was determined after 48 hours at 37°C. Each value is the average of four independent experiments. The standard errors of the mean are indicated.

were induced by incubating infected cells for 15 min at 37°C, after virus adsorption on to PVR-expressing cells (Fig. 2). The mutant Mah-KKVP1S_{95} seemed to form atypical 147S particles, like those that we have previously described for a type three PV [9], while Mah-KKVP2Y_{142} had a 135S/160S ratio three-fold higher than that of PV1/Mahoney, suggesting that conformational transitions are faster and/or more efficient with this mutant. In agreement with this, the results of one-step growth experiments indicated that both PV mutants had an eclipse phase more pronounced than PV1/Mahoney in LM/PVR_{IMR} and LM/PVR-Thr67 cells (Fig. 3).

Discussion

In neuronal cells in culture, most PV strains are persistent and the same viral determinants are selected in human primary foetal brain cells and neuroblastoma cells [5]. These determinants involve PV-PVR interactions and some of them modify the host tropism of PV [7]. In neuroblastoma cells, mutations are also selected in the PVR mRNA [6]. It would be interesting to know which mutations, viral or cellular, appear first, and whether the PVR mutations arise at the DNA level or by an editing mechanism. Our results indicate that the PVR mutations confer a partial resistance to lysis, not only by PV1/Mahoney but by PV mutants displaying PVpi mutations. The PVR-induced conformational transitions of Mah-KKVP1S_{95} and Mah-KKVP2Y_{142} are modified compared to those of PV1/Mahoney. Our results suggest that cells more resistant to PV-induced lysis co-evolved with PVpi capable of growing to high titres (10^6 -10^8 $TCID_{50}$/ml) in persistently infected cells [4], as observed with another picornavirus, foot-and-mouth disease virus [10].

When studying type 3 PVpi, we have found that viral determinants $VP1_{290}$ and $VP2_{13}$ affect PV-PVR interactions at the level of adsorption, elution and conformational transitions [9, 11]. They also modify the cell tropism of the virus [9]. Moreover, together they are involved in the phenotype of persistence in epidermoid HEp-2 cells [9]. In the HEp-2 cell line, during the maintenance phase of the persistent infection, the expression of the PVR is also modified [12].

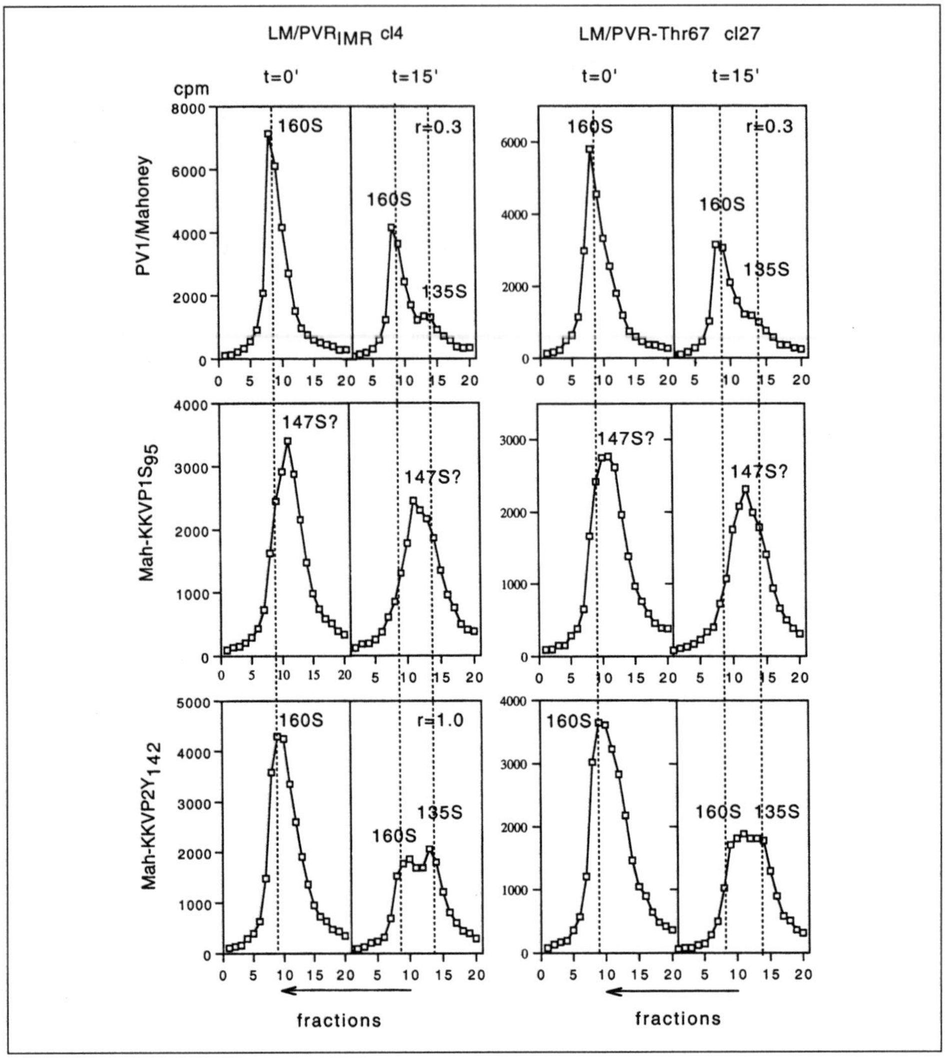

Fig. 2: PV conformational alteration assays in LM/PVR cell clones. Infection of cells with ^{35}S-radiolabelled viruses was first synchronized at 4°C for 2.5 h, then infected cells were further incubated at 4°C for 15 min (t=0') or switched to 37°C for 15 min (t=15'). The conformational modifications of the capsid following PV-PVR interactions at 37°C were analysed after sedimentation through a 15 to 30% (wt/vol) sucrose gradient (see Materials and Methods). The 135S/160S alteration ratio (r) corresponding to the area under the 135S peak divided by the area under the 160S peak is indicated.

It is remarkable that four out of 10 determinants of a type 3 PVpi are either at the same position ($VP1_{166}$) or very close ($VP1_{36}$, $VP1_{290}$, $VP2_{13}$) [9] to those found in isolates from an immunodeficient patient chronically infected for almost two years following Sabin 3 vaccination [13].

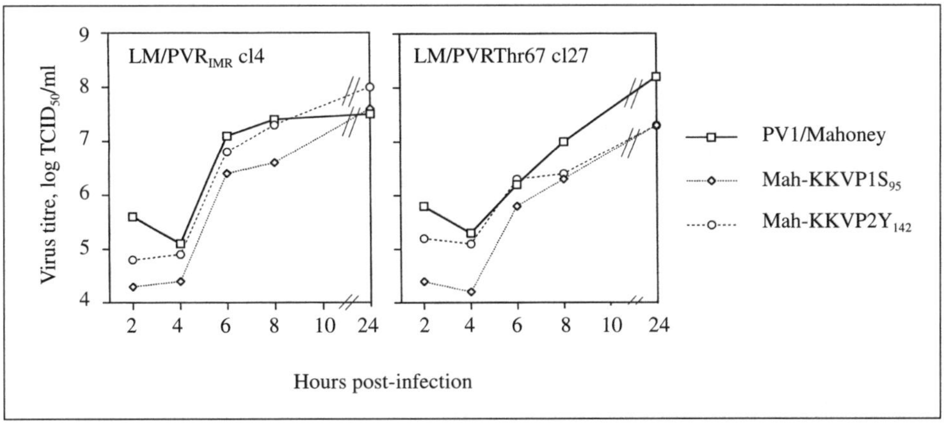

Fig. 3: Single-cycle growth curves of PV1/Mahoney, Mah-KKVP1S$_{95}$ and Mah-KKVP2Y$_{142}$ in LM/PVR$_{IMR}$ and LM/PVR-Thr67 cell clones. Cells (10^6 per well in 24-well plates) were infected at an MOI of 10. Total virus was harvested at the indicated times p.i., and titres were determined by $TCID_{50}$ assay. Each point represents the mean of four infected cultures.

Conclusions

PV easily persists in several human cell types in vitro [14]. Many of the PVpi mutations affect the host tropism [7], the cell tropism [3] and the interactions with the cell receptor. Despite common features between persistent PV infections in various human cell types, our results indicate that several mechanisms are used by PV to infect human cells persistently.

Acknowledgements

We thank Prof. Akio Nomoto and Dr. Satoshi Koike for their indispensable gift of the plasmid, pSV2-PVRa. This work was funded by the Institut Pasteur and the Association Française contre les Myopathies (contracts 6495, 6932 and 7290), and by the Direction des Recherches sur l'environnement (Recherche Environnement 6724).

References

1 Davis LE, Bodian D, Price D, Butler I, Vickers JH: Chronic progressive poliomyelitis secondary to vaccination of an immunodeficient child. N Engl J Med 1977;297:241-245.

2 Dalakas MC: New neuromuscular symptoms in patients with old poliomyelitis: a three year follow-up study. Eur Neurology 1986;25:381-387.

3 Pelletier I, Couderc T, Borzakian S, Wyckoff E, Crainic R, Ehrenfeld E, Colbère-Garapin F: Characterization of persistent poliovirus mutants selected in human neuroblastoma cells. Virology 1991;180:729-737.

4 Colbère-Garapin F, Christodoulou C, Crainic R, Pelletier I: Persistent poliovirus infection of human neuroblastoma cells. Proc Natl Acad Sci USA 1989;86:7590-7594.

5 Pavio N, Buc-Caron M-H, Colbère-Garapin F: Persistent poliovirus infection of human fetal brain cells. J Virol 1996;70:6395-6401.

6 Pavio N, Couderc T, Girard S, Sgro JY, Blondel B, Colbère-Garapin F: Expression of mutated poliovirus receptors in human neuroblastoma cells persistently infected with poliovirus. Virology 2000;274:331-342.

7 Couderc T, Guédo N, Calvez V, Pelletier I, Hogle J, Colbère-Garapin F, Blondel B: Substitutions in the capsids of poliovirus mutants selected in human neuroblastoma cells confer on the Mahoney type 1 strain a phenotype neurovirulent in mice. J Virol 1994;68:8386-8391.

8 Koike S, Ise I, Nomoto A: Functional domains of the poliovirus receptor. Proc Natl Acad Sci USA 1991;88:4104-4108.

9 Duncan G, Pelletier I, Colbère-Garapin F: Two amino acid substitutions in the type 3 poliovirus capsid contribute to the establishment of persistent infection in HEp-2c cells by modifying virus-receptor interactions. Virology 1998;241:14-29.

10 Martin-Hernandez AM, Carrillo EC, Sevilla N, Domingo E: Rapid cell variation can determine the establishment of a persistent viral infection. Proc Natl Acad Sci USA 1994;91:3705-3709.

11 Duncan G, Colbère-Garapin F: Two determinants in the capsid of a persistent type 3 poliovirus exert different effects on mutant virus uncoating. Journal of General Virology 1999;80:2601-2605.

12 Borzakian S, Couderc T, Barbier Y, Attal G, Pelletier I, Colbère-Garapin F: Persistent poliovirus infection: establishment and maintenance involve distinct mechanisms. Virology 1992;186:398-408.

13 Martin J, Dunn G, Hull R, Patel V, Minor P: Evolution of the Sabin strain of type 3 poliovirus in an immunodeficient patient during the entire 637-day period of virus excretion. J Virol 2000;74:3001-3010.

14 Pelletier I, Duncan G, Pavio N, Colbère-Garapin F: Molecular mechanisms of poliovirus persistence: key role of capsid determinants during the establishment phase. Cell Mol Life Sci 1998;54:1385-1402.

Dr. F. Colbère-Garapin, Unité de Neurovirologie et Régénération du Système nerveux, Institut Pasteur, 25, rue du Dr-Roux, F-75724 Paris Cedex 15.

Brown F (ed): Progress in Polio Eradication: Vaccine Strategies for the End Game.
Dev Biol. Basel, Karger, 2001, vol 105, pp 105-108

Rotary International: A Partner in Polio Eradication

J.L. Sever

International PolioPlus Committee, Polio Eradication Advocacy Task Force, PolioPlus Speaker's Bureau, The Rotary Foundation, Rotary International, Washington, DC, USA

Key words: Rotary International, partner, polio, eradication

Abstract: Rotary International remains committed to the goal of global eradication of polio and certification by 2005. The reports of possible sources of virulent vaccine-derived poliovirus, which may persist after the global eradication of wild poliovirus, need to be investigated rapidly. If these sources are confirmed to be significant risks to global polio eradication, methods to eliminate these sources need to be identified and implemented. Final recommendations on the stopping of vaccination need to be made by WHO.

INTRODUCTION

Rotary International is a service organization with 1.2 million members in 29,000 clubs. It was started in 1905 in Chicago, Illinois, U.S.A., and is now present in 162 countries. Rotary is an organization of business and professional persons united worldwide who provide humanitarian service, encourage high ethical standards in all vocations and help build goodwill and peace in the world. PolioPlus is Rotary's commitment to work with national and international health organizations and governments on the goal of global polio eradication and certification of eradication by the year 2005.

BACKGROUND

Rotary Clubs worldwide identify and sponsor local service activities in their own communities. Many clubs also assist other clubs in developing countries with their projects. In 1978 a new Rotary programme of Health, Hunger and Humanity (3-H) grants was started. This programme permitted the funding of larger grants using contributions from Rotarians throughout the world. The first 3-H grant was for polio vaccine for the Philippines in 1979. Other health-related grants included vaccines for measles and other diseases. Also in 1979, Rotary began to focus its vaccine efforts on polio immunization because it was needed, it was the easiest vaccine to use to introduce immunization into an unvaccinated population, and it was simple to administer by mouth.

PolioPlus – The Beginning

In 1984 Rotary convened a special advisory committee to define a major polio vaccination effort for the entire Rotary organization. That committee was called the Polio 2005 Committee. The year 2005 was selected because that will be Rotary's 100th anniversary and it was concluded that polio could be eradicated by that date. The Committee included consultants such as Dr. Albert Sabin, developer of the live oral poliovirus vaccine and Dr. Alan Hinman of the U.S. Centers for Disease Control and Prevention. From that Committee came the plan for Rotary to provide free polio vaccine for any country which needed that support. It was estimated that 100 million children in developing countries needed polio vaccine each year. Rotary would provide funds for the vaccine for five years and local Rotarians would assist with social mobilization, immunization campaigns and work with the World Health Organization (WHO) and local health authorities. It was estimated that Rotary would have to raise US$120 million to purchase the vaccine (at four cents a dose). Rotarians believed that this effort would aid in the eradication of polio. This programme was called the PolioPlus.

In 1985 Rotary embarked on a special three year PolioPlus campaign to raise US$120 million, primarily from its members to pay for the vaccine and related costs. Rotary began providing vaccine, materials for its distribution and social mobilization, and Rotarian volunteers in polio-endemic countries began assisting with polio National Immunization Days. Many of the initial efforts were directed at Latin America where the Pan American Health Organization (PAHO) was working on polio eradication in the Americas.

In 1988 Rotary completed the campaign for funds. To everyone's surprise Rotary had been able to raise not US$120 million but US$240 million for PolioPlus. At this point the WHO passed a resolution to eradicate polio worldwide and Rotary was asked to join as a partner in this effort. Rotary agreed and since that time has been working constantly with the major partners, WHO, UNICEF, the U.S. Centers for Diseases Control and Prevention and other donors and polio-endemic nations to eradicate polio.

PolioPlus Today

Rotary is a very active partner in the effort to eradicate polio and achieve certification by the year 2005. Rotary's efforts have expanded greatly. As of May 1, 2000, Rotary had committed over US$373 million for global polio eradication. By the year 2005, Rotary's contributions to the global eradication effort will be approximately half a billion dollars. In addition, millions of dollars of "in-kind" and personal contributions have been made and are being made by and through local Rotary clubs and districts for polio eradication activities. Of even greater significance has been the huge volunteer army mobilized by Rotary. Hundreds of thousands of volunteers at the local level are providing support at clinics or mobilizing their communities for immunization and polio eradication activities. More than one million Rotarians worldwide have contributed toward the success of the polio eradication effort and more than 120 nations around the world have benefited from PolioPlus grants.

Rotary's Advocacy Efforts

In 1995 the WHO reported to Rotary that there was a need for an additional $600 million of external funds to eradicate polio. To help meet this need Rotary initiated a Rotary Polio Eradication Advocacy Task Force to encourage governments in polio-free countries to contribute to the eradication of polio in endemic countries. Rotary has played a major role in decisions by donor governments to contribute over US$850 million as of June 2000 for polio eradication. Major polio-specific contributions (over US$100,000 each) have been made by the following governments: Australia, Belgium, Canada, Denmark, European Union, Finland, Germany, Italy, Japan, the Republic of Korea, the Netherlands, Norway, Portugal, Sweden, Switzerland, Taiwan, the United Kingdom and the United States of America. The private sector has given an additional US$95 million for polio eradication.

In 1999 the WHO informed Rotary that even with all present and projected donor support, including that from Rotary and the public and private sector, there was an estimated shortfall of US$300 million to eradicate polio. This is a critical problem in the effort to eradicate polio. To help meet this new need Rotary recently authorized a Rotary Polio Eradication Private Sector Initiative Task Force. This team will work with the U.N. Foundation to attempt to raise funds for this need from major corporations, foundations and wealthy individuals.

PolioPlus – Future Directions

Rotary is continuing to provide direct financial support for polio vaccines, equipment, surveillance and related activities as well as Rotary volunteers to assist with polio eradication. Rotary works with its major partners, WHO, UNICEF and U.S. Centers for Diseases and Prevention in these efforts and with other donors and local governments. Rotary is also interested in containment as part of certification. Rotary's advocacy efforts are now directed at both the public sector and the private sector to help secure the additional funds necessary to reach the goal of eradication and certification by the year 2005.

Scientific issues which require rapid investigation and resolution

There now appear to be three possible sources of virulent vaccine-derived poliovirus which may persist after the global eradication of wild poliovirus. These finding represent a significant risk to the completion of global eradication, certification and the stopping of polio vaccination. The sources include (i) the excretion of neurotropic vaccine poliovirus from patients with Vaccine-Associated paralytic Polio (VAPP); (ii) the long-term excretion of poliovirus by healthy immunodeficient patients (P. Minor at this meeting) and (iii) the transmission of virulent recombinant vaccine poliovirus over a period of years with the production of acute flaccid paralysis (M. Pallansch at this meeting). One additional study did not detect any further cases of the excretion of poliovirus by immunodeficient patients (N. Halsey at this meeting).

The possibility that virulent vaccine-derived poliovirus could continue to circulate after the eradication of wild poliovirus needs to be investigated rapidly. If these are significant risks, approaches to their control need to be implemented before polio can be considered completely eradicated and vaccination can be stopped.

Vaccination following eradication

The strategies to be used for the termination of vaccination programmes following certification of eradication need to be considered. Some of the developed countries have always used IPV and others have switched to IPV after eradication of endemic polio, but most countries use OPV. The use of IPV is considerably more expensive than OPV but eliminates the risk of VAPP. Studies are needed to determine whether the continued use of OPV after the eradication of wild poliovirus will introduce virulent vaccine-derived poliovirus, which will spread when vaccination is stopped. If this occurs, it may be necessary to switch to IPV to eliminate this risk. Recommendations on the vaccines to be used and the timing of stopping vaccination need to be made by WHO.

Prof. John L. Sever, Children's National Medical Center, 111 Michigan Avenue, N.W., Washington, DC 20010-2970, USA.

Brown F (ed): Progress in Polio Eradication: Vaccine Strategies for the End Game.
Dev Biol. Basel, Karger, 2001, vol 105, p 109

SESSION VI

Post Eradication Issues

Chairperson: *Barry Schoub*

Brown F (ed): Progress in Polio Eradication: Vaccine Strategies for the End Game.
Dev Biol. Basel, Karger, 2001, vol 105, pp 111-122

Will the Polio Niche Remain Vacant?

E. Rieder[1], *A.E. Gorbalenya*[2], *C. Xiao*[3], *Y. He*[3], *T.S. Baker*[3], *R.J. Kuhn*[3], *M.G. Rossmann*[3], *E. Wimmer*[1]

[1] Department of Molecular Genetics and Microbiology, State University of New York at Stony Brook, Stony Brook, NY, USA

[2] Advanced Biomedical Computing Ctr, SAIC/NCI-FCRDC, Frederick, MD, USA

[3] Department of Biological Sciences, Purdue University, West Lafayette, IN, USA

Key words: Poliovirus, C-cluster Coxsackie viruses, receptor interaction, receptor switching, evolution

Abstract: C-Cluster enteroviruses (C-CEVs), consisting of Coxsackie A viruses (C-CAV1, 11, 13, 15, 17, 18, 19, 20, 21, 22, 24, 24v) and polioviruses (PV1, 2, 3), have been grouped together in relation to their genomic sequences. On the basis of disease syndromes caused in humans, however, C-CAVs and PVs are vastly different: the former cause respiratory disease, just like the major receptor group rhinoviruses (magHRV), whereas PVs, on invasion of the CNS, can cause poliomyelitis. It is assumed that the difference in pathogenesis of C-CEVs is governed predominantly by cellular receptor specificity. C-CAVs use ICAM-1, just like magHRV, whereas PVs uniquely use CD155. Both ICAM-1 and CD155 are Ig-like molecules. Remarkably, based on a phylogenetic analysis of non-structural proteins, CAV 11, 13, 17 and 18 are interleaved with, rather than separated from, the three PV serotypes, e.g. PV1 is more closely related to CAV18 that to PV2. This observation suggests that PVs may have emerged from a pool of C-CAVs by evolving a unique receptor specificity. We have been studying virion structure, virion/receptor interactions, genetics, and the molecular biology of C-CEVs with the objective of identifying the molecular basis of phenotypic diversity of these viruses. Of particular interest is the prospect that C-CEVs can be genetically manipulated to switch their receptor affinity: from CD155 to ICAM-1 for PVs, or from ICAM-1 to CD155 for C-CAVs. We propose a hypothesis that in a world free of poliovirus and anti-poliovirus neutralizing antibodies C-CAVs would be given a greater chance to switch receptor specificity from ICAM-1 to CD155 and thus, to evolve gradually into a new polio-like virus.

Introduction

Picornaviridae is an ever-growing family of human and animal viruses, the members of which can cause a wide range of diseases, some fatal [1]. *Picornaviridae* have been divided into nine genera as the number of the previously recognized genera *Enterovirus, Rhinovirus, Hepatovirus, Parechovirus, Cardiovirus, Aphthovirus* has been extended recently by the three new genera *Erbovirus, Kobuvirus, and Teschovirus* [2]. A list of species and their serotypes can be found on the

Picornavirus Sequence Database (http://www.iah.bbsrc.ac.uk./virus/Picornaviridae/SequenceDatabase/Index.html).

The crystal structures of several picornavirions that are small, non-enveloped particles, have been solved [3]. In this paper, only molecular features of member viruses of the genera *Enterovirus* and *Rhinovirus* will be considered.

Briefly, the enterovirus and human rhinovirus capsids are icosahedral particles consisting of 60 identical asymmetric protomers. Each protomer is composed of a single copy each of the three non-identical, albeit structurally-related capsid proteins VP1, VP2, and VP3 (see below). Five protomers are located in a pentameric arrangement around the five-fold symmetry axis. Twelve pentamers build up the complete virus capsid. At the interface between the pentamers, two-fold and three-fold symmetry axes are located. The smallest capsid protein, VP4, is located on the inner surface of the virion. The crystal structure of PV1(Mahoney) [4] revealed remarkable similarity to that of human rhinoviruses [5] and other picornaviruses [3] (Fig. 1).

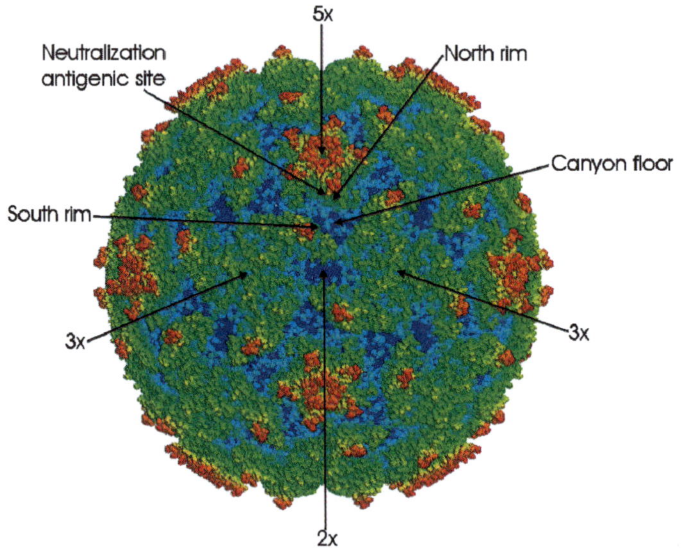

Fig. 1: **Structure of the poliovirion.** A complete capsid structure of poliovirus type 1 (Mahoney) [4] illustrated as a water-accessible molecular surface. Colours indicate the relative elevation of residues over the average diameter (red, highest, dark blue, lowest elevation). The capsid is formed by viral proteins VP1, VP2, VP3 and VP4. VP4 is buried deep inside the virus particle and is not visible from the surface. The 5X, 3X and 2X labels indicate the locations of the five-fold, the three-fold and two-fold axes of symmetry. The two-fold axis occurs at the intersection of three adjacent pentamers. The canyon's north wall, south wall, and floor are identified by arrows. The location of one (N-Ag1) of the major neutralization antigenic sites decorating the north rim of the canyon is indicated by an arrow. N-Ag2 is located at the south rim.

Although VP1, VP2 and VP3 differ in size and amino acid sequence, they have similar tertiary structures. Each capsid protein presents a common structural motif, an eight-stranded antiparallel b-barrel core. The loop extensions protruding from the surface of the virion may be well exposed. If so, they can form the four known neutralization antigenic sites, referred to here as N-Ag1, 2, 3A and 3B [6,7]. An important surface feature of the virions is a depression or 'canyon' formed at the junction of VP1 and VP3, encircling the five-fold axis. The canyon of which the "north rim" and "south rim" are decorated with components of N-Ag1 and N-Ag2, is the binding site for the cellular receptors as shown unambiguously for human rhinoviruses [8], for polioviruses [9,10] and for CAV21, a C-cluster Coxsackievirus [11; reviewed in 3].

The capsid encloses the positive-stranded RNA genome of approximately 7500 nt [12] that can be divided into three domains (Fig. 2): the 5' non-translated region (5'NTR) consisting of the cloverleaf and the internal ribosomal entry site (IRES), the long open reading frame encoding the polyprotein, and the 3'NTR, consisting of the a heteropolymeric region and poly(A). The 5' end of the genome is covalently linked to a small viral protein called VPg [13].

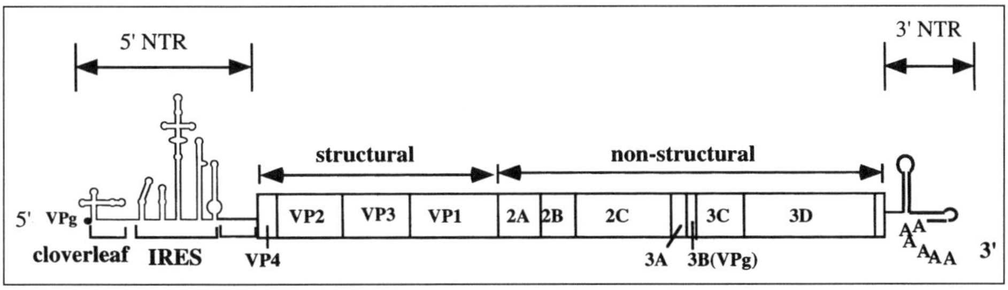

Fig. 2: **Genome organization of poliovirus**. The single-stranded genomic RNA is covalently linked to the virus-encoded VPg (3B, black dot) at the 5' end of the non-translated region (5'NTR). The 5'NTR consists of two functional domains, the cloverleaf and internal ribosomal entry site (IRES) elements. The open box depicts the polyprotein with coding regions for different viral proteins. Regions corresponding to structural (P1) and non-structural (P2, P3) protein domains are also indicated. The 3' non-translated region (3'NTR) contains an heteropolymeric region and is polyadenylylated.

The entero- and rhinoviruses cluster together form a subgroup amongst the picornaviruses (Fig. 3), implying that viruses of these genera are likely to have originated from an immediate common ancestor [1]. This close relationship is paralleled in the molecular biology of entero- and rhinoviruses that is, in broad terms, identical as member viruses of both genera produce the same set of gene products (cleavage products of the polyprotein) with similar function(s). However, exchange of gene segments from one virus to another within these genera yields, with some exceptions, lethal phenotypes. This indicates that viruses of two genera have diverged too far to retain compatibility on the genomic level. It is likely that entero-/rhinovirus chimaeras are compromised in one or more essential interactions between (i) viral proteins, (ii) viral proteins and cellular proteins, and (iii) viral proteins and the cognate genomic RNA.

Taxonomy of the Enteroviruses

Based originally on clinical manifestations in humans and in experimental animals, human enteroviruses have been divided into polioviruses (PV, 3 species),

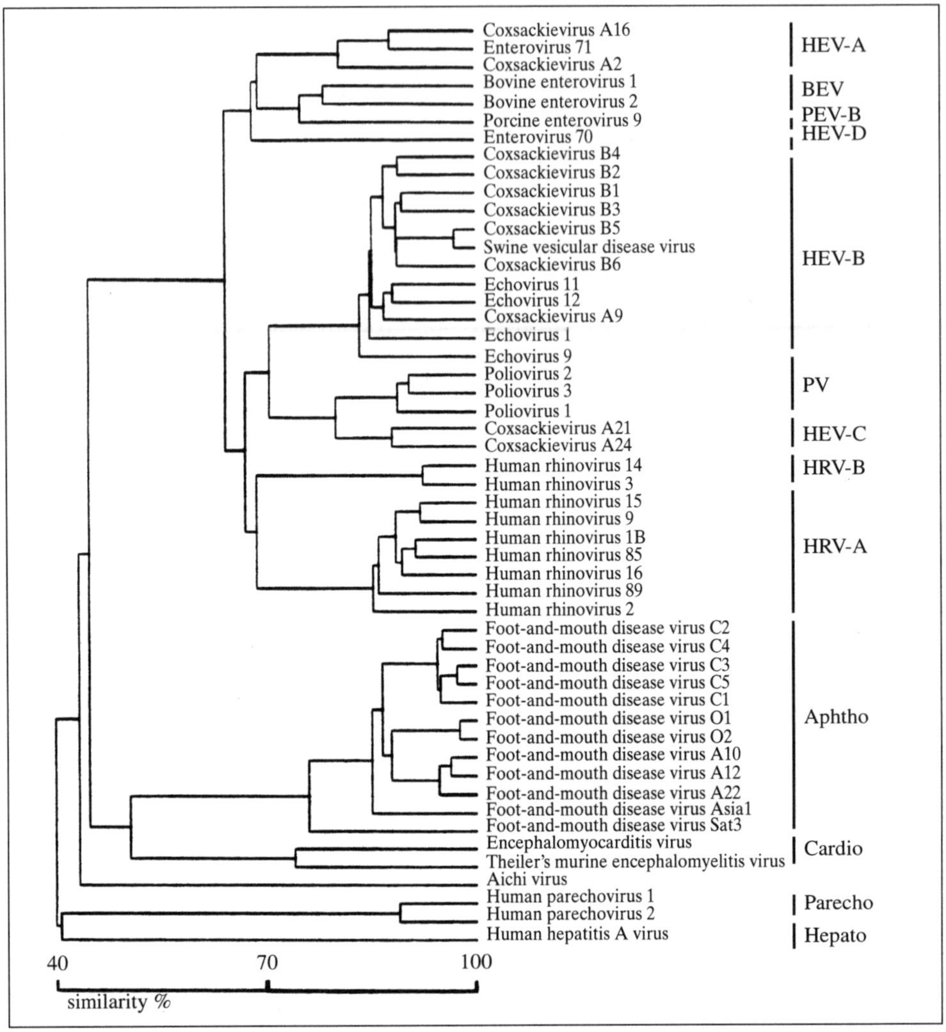

Fig. 3: **Evolutionary relationship of *Picornaviridae*.** This is a dendrogram of Picornaviridae showing amino-acid similarity in the capsid region. Sequences were aligned and the dendrogram was generated using the PILEUP Program of the Genetics computer Group software package. Reproduced from Gromeier et al [1].

Coxsackie A (CAV, 23 species) and B (CBV, 6 species) viruses, echoviruses (EV, 31 species) and enteroviruses (ENV, 4 species). Two factors have recently led to a re-evaluation of the original classification. First, different enteroviruses may cause the same disease syndromes; second, sequence analysis of enterovirus genomes has revealed unexpected kinship between viruses causing entirely different diseases. Hyypia, Hovi, Stanway and their colleagues [14] have therefore suggested the division of the human enteroviruses into the four genetic clusters A, B, C, and D [14-16] (Table 1). Additionally, some human enteroviruses were moved out of

Table 1: Characteristics of human enterovirus clusters.

Cluster	Members	5'NTR	ORF	Receptors	Pathogenesis[a]
A	CAV2,3,5,7,8, 10,12,14,16 ENV71	Ia	1	nd	paralysis in newborn mice[b], hand-foot-and-mouth disease, meningitis, paralysis
B	CBV1-6 CAV9, EV1-9,11-27,29-33[c] ENV69	Ia	2	CAR a_vb_3 CD55, a_2b_1 nd	carditis, pleurodynia, exanthema paralysis in newborn mice[b] aseptic meningitis, encephalitis,
C	PV1-3 CAV1,11,13,15,17 18,19,20,21,22,24, 24v[f]	Ib	3	CD155 ICAM-1[d]	poliomyelitis, paralysis in newborn mice[b], common cold, infantile diarrhoea acute haemorrhagic conjunctivitis[f]
D	ENV70,68[e*]	Ib, nd[*]	4	DAF	acute haemorrhagic conjunctivitis paralysis

CAV and CBV, Coxsackie A and B viruses, respectively: ENV, enterovirus; EV, echovirus; PV, poliovirus; Numbers refer to serotypes [1,13,15].

* nd, not determined.

a Common syndromes caused by one and/or other member(s) of the cluster but member viruses of other clusters may cause the same syndrome.

b Coxsackie A viruses cause flaccid paralysis, Coxsackie B viruses spastic paralysis, in newborn mice.

c For the use of receptors of different echoviruses, see [1].

d ICAM-1 is the receptor for those CAVs that have been tested in this cluster. CD55 (DAF, decay accelerating factor) may function as (non-essential) co-receptor.

e No disease syndrome has been established for EV68.

f CAV24v is a variant of CAV24 that emerged in Asia in the nineteen seventies.

the genus *Enterovirus* to form the separate, deeply rooted genera *Hepatovirus, Parechovirus,* and *Kobuvirus* [2].

Of particular interest to us are the C-CEVs consisting of the polioviruses types 1-3 and 11 Coxsackie A viruses (referred to also as Human Enteroviruses C, HE-C [2]. Dendrograms have been generated [14,16] which suggest that CAV-1, –21, and -24 may have separated first from the main C-cluster trunk, followed by the evolution of other C-CAVs which, in turn, may be the immediate ancestors of the polioviruses [1]. This scenario is evident in the tree based on sequences in the VP4-VP2 region (Fig. 4A, B). A more complex evolutionary history is apparent in a tree based on polymerase 3D sequences (Fig. 5A, B). Here, the poliovirus sequences are interleaved with, rather than separated from, the C-CAVs -11, -13, -17, -18, -20, and -20b. Hyypiä, Hovi, Stanway and their colleagues have found no evidence of recombination events in the evolution of C-CEVs which would account for the distinct grouping of these viruses in the structural and non-structural regions [14-16]. However, it should be stressed that the dendrograms have been generated on as yet limited sequence information and may need to be revised in the future as more sequences become available.

It should be noted that, until recently, each picornavirus serotype was designated as a separate species. A new definition has now been adopted as follows: "A picornavirus species is a polythetic class of phylogenetically related serotypes or strains which would normally be expected to share (i) a limited range of hosts and cellular receptors, (ii) a significant degree of compatibility in proteolytic processing, replication, encapsidation and genetic recombination, and (iii) essentially identical genome maps" [2]. The C-CEVs, therefore, contain two separate species:

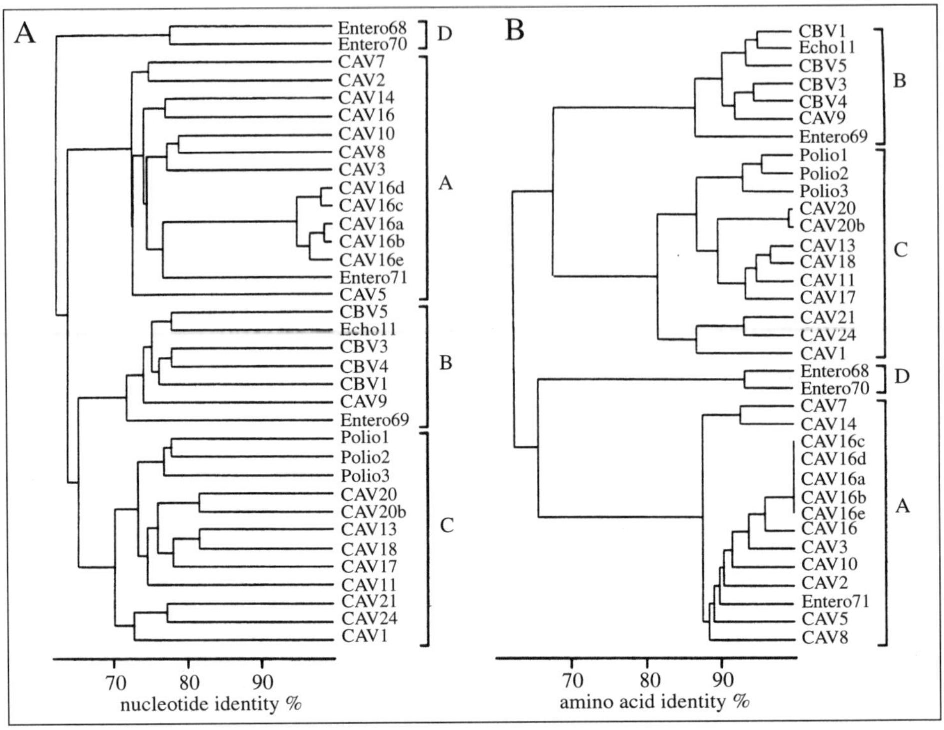

Fig. 4: **Dendrograms of enteroviruses generated using sequences from the VP4-VP2 region**. A. Nucleotide sequences (210 bp) of the indicated viruses were compared to each other. B. Amino acid sequences (70 aa) at the VP4-VP2 junction were also compared. Cluster C includes CAV1, 11, 13, 17, 18, 20, 20b, 21, and 24 which are genetically close relatives of polioviruses. Reproduced from Pulli et al [16].

the C-cluster Coxsackie A viruses (C-CAVs) and the polioviruses (PVs) which, in turn, include 11 and three serotypes, respectively.

Receptors, Virion Structure, Serotypes and Pathogenesis

Although closely related by genotype, the two species of C-cluster enteroviruses, poliovirus and C-CAV, produce very different disease syndromes in humans. Whereas poliovirus infections remain largely asymptomatic but can progress with low probability (one to two percent) to a serious neurological complication called poliomyelitis, the C-CAVs are known to cause only the common cold. The profound difference in pathogenesis is considered to be related to the different cellular receptors that these viruses are using: CD155 (also known as PVR) for PV and ICAM-1 for C-CAVs (Table 1) [1]. These receptors have distinct patterns of expression in human tissues [17-19]. However, cell-internal restriction of viral replication could also contribute to the pathogenesis of C-cluster species. For exam-

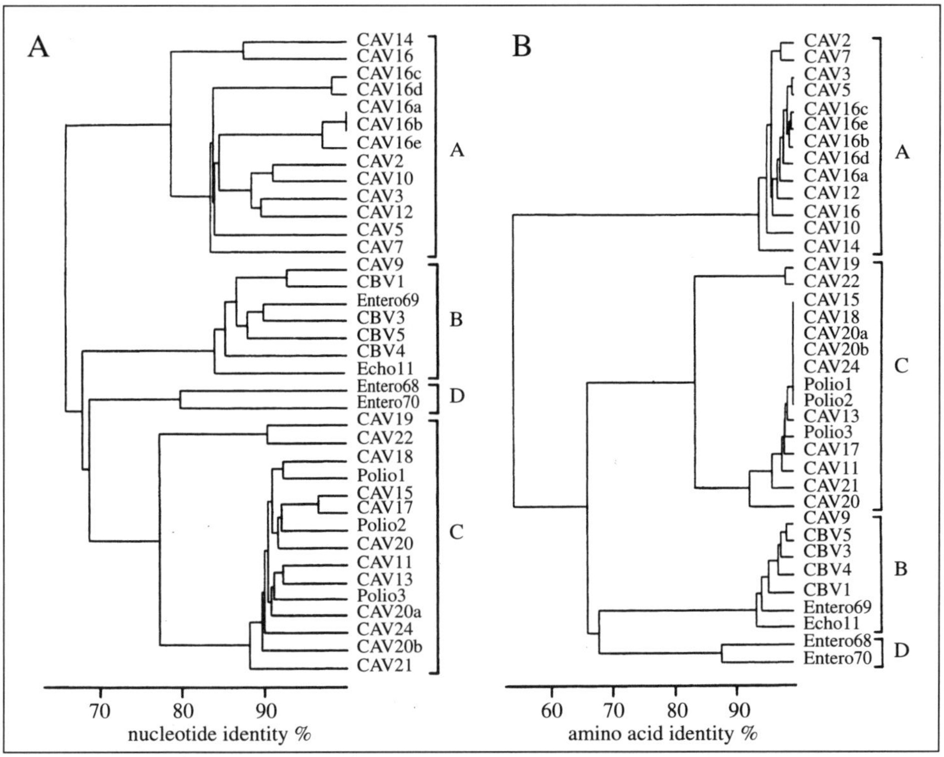

Fig. 5: **Comparison of the sequences obtained from the viral RNA polymerase (3D) coding regions**. A. Nucleotide sequences (390 bp) and, B. amino acid sequences (130 aa) were compared to each other. In this region, CAV 11, 13, 15, 17, 18, 20, 20a, 20b, and 24 group together with the polioviruses. Reproduced from Pulli et al [16].

ple, gene products or regulatory sequences (e.g. the IRES) of the viral genome may fail to function in an infected cell, thereby preventing cell destruction. IRES-driven host-range restriction has indeed been observed for PV/HRV chimaera [20,21] but not, remarkably, for a PV/C-CAV chimaera [22]. These and other observations (Rieder and Wimmer, unpublished results) demonstrate that the PVs and C-CAVs have much more in common with each other than with human rhinoviruses, despite the fact that C-CAVs and the major receptor group of human rhinoviruses (magHRVs; 92 serotypes) use the same receptor and cause the same pathology (upper respiratory disease).

Both CD155 and ICAM-1 are membrane-anchored, single-span glycoproteins belonging to the immunoglobulin super family [8,23]. CD155 and ICAM-1 have three (NH_2-V-C-C) and five (NH_2-C-C-C-C-C) extracellular domains, respectively. The N-terminal domains of the receptors serve to anchor the virion: the D1 domain (V domain) of CD155 anchors PV, the D1 domain of ICAM-1 (the N-terminal C-domain) anchors CAV21 [11] and magHRVs. In all cases, attachment occurs via the canyon [see above; 3].

Based on cryo-EM and X-ray crystallography a detailed view has emerged as to how members of the magHRVs (HRV14 and HRV16) or poliovirus type 1

(PV1) interact with their respective receptors [8-10]. ICAM-1 binds to HRV in a rather radial orientation with respect to the virion surface, interacting primarily with the canyon floor and "south wall" (considering the direction of the 5-fold axis as pointing "north"). In contrast, the interaction of the D1 domain of CD155 with the poliovirus canyon is more tangential to the surface, making extensive contact with the virion surface at the canyon rim that encompasses also N-Ag1 and N-Ag2. As mentioned above, the D1 domain of CD155 is an Ig-like V-domain that, relative to D1 of ICAM-1, has two extra b-strands (C' and C"). This difference in size by 32 residues may explain why D1 of CD155 "spills over" the canyon rim. There is also a clear difference in the orientation of the cognate receptors within the canyon. The ICAM-1 molecule leans towards the "southwest" of HRV14 or HRV16 whereas the CD155 molecules lean towards the southeast of poliovirus [3]. Interestingly, the orientation of the ICAM-1 receptor bound to CAV21 differs from that of either ICAM-1/HRV or CD155/PV [23].

Whereas the ICAM-1 has been firmly established as receptor for C-CAVs [see, for example, 24,25], it has been suggested that CD55/DAF (decay-accelerating factor) may play an (augmenting?) role as co-receptor in CAV21 infection [25]. CD55/DAF is involved in the complement cascade; it has the ability to dock several different human enteroviruses [26]. Importantly, DAF-expressing cells (lacking ICAM-1 expression) can bind CAV21 but this binding does not lead to a productive infection. It is likely, therefore, that CAV21 virions harbour two independent binding sites, one for ICAM-1, the other for DAF [24,25]. The binding site for DAF on CAV21 or for any other enterovirus, is unknown.

It remains a mystery why a virus species has adopted a certain cell surface molecule to enter a host cell. There are no discernible patterns or rules, even within a virus genus [27]. Telling examples are the HRVs of which the majority (~92) use ICAM-1 and the minority (~10) use the LDL receptor to dock on to identical host cells. ICAM-1 and LDLR are molecules that are entirely different in structure and function [28]. This receptor preference is astounding since some of the HRVs using different receptors are structurally most closely related [3]. Taken together, the above examples illustrate the remarkable plasticity of entero- and rhinoviruses and their ability to evolve new receptor specificity.

Evolution of two Receptor Specificities Amongst C-Cluster Enteroviruses

As pointed out before, it is unlikely that PVs and C-CAVs form two separate evolutionary lineages originating from a common ancestor strain [1]. Rather, the PVs may have branched off a tree previously occupied by C-CAVs. Clearly, with respect to the coding sequences of their capsid proteins, the PVs form a cluster (reflecting adaptation to their unique receptor), but even this region is more closely related to that of the C-CAVs than to capsid regions of any other enterovirus species (Fig. 3). Given the close intertwined relationship between PVs and C-CAVs in the non-structural coding sequences, it can be considered possible that the PVs evolved from the C-CAVs by receptor switching in the course of an antigenic drift. Each of the three PV serotypes may have independently emerged and adapted the new CD155 receptor [1]. If so, the binding parameters of CD155 to the three PV serotypes are likely to be different. Whereas all three serotypes interact with host cells (HeLa cells) with roughly the same binding affinity [29], profound differences in binding have indeed been observed when the three serotypes were tested with receptor mutants expressed on mouse cells [30]. Moreover, the binding phenotype to receptor mutants partially co-varied with chimaeric viruses in which neutralization antigenic sites had been exchanged [30]. These unexpected observations led to the suggestion that sequences of antigenic sites (N-Ag1 and N-Ag2) may be involved in the binding of PVs to CD155 [30], a hypothesis that has found support in the case of poliovirus type 1 [9,10] .

Birth of a New Polio-Like Virus from Benign Contemporary C-Cluster Enteroviruses by Receptor Switching: a Hypothesis

It can be envisaged that a receptor switch from ICAM-1 ⇒ CD155 of any member of the C-CAV species would give rise to a new poliovirus, provided all genetic elements of that C-CAV could function in cells known to be a target of poliovirus infection. Current studies on CAV21 and CAV24 support this assumption [22; Rieder and Wimmer, unpublished results]. On the level of the organism, both C-CAVs and PVs enter the human body via ingestion and it is possible that they reproduce at the same primary site. On the molecular level, poliovirus and C-CAV genomes have been shown to be compatible, allowing the generation of highly neurovirulent poliovirus chimaera containing a C-CAV IRES [22]. The latter observation indicates that the C-CAV IRESes have "neurovirulent" potential comparable to that of poliovirus [22]. In contrast, the HRV14 IRES, just like the HRV2 IRES, when replacing the PV IRES, has been found to function very inefficiently in neuronal cells [20,22]. Therefore, receptor switching from ICAM-1 ⇒ CD155 of a magHRV is not expected to create a neurovirulent PV-like agent.

An ICAM-1 ⇒ CD155 receptor switch would require large structural adjustments of the C-CAV virion since the docking domain of CD155 (D1, a V-domain) is larger than the docking domain of ICAM-1. The CD155 D1 may spill over the canyon rim and involve sequences at the north and south rim that are segments of N-Ags (the N-Ags of any C-CAV have not been mapped but can be assumed to be located in positions similar to that of PV). Perhaps the change of C-CAV N-Ags under the pressure of immune surveillance was the driving force of ICAM-1 ⇒ CD155 switching: surface residues at the canyon rim of a C-CAV gained affinity to CD155, thereby becoming PV-like. In other words, a C-CAV that spontaneously and/or by immune selection acquired surface sequences reminiscent of PV-like N-Ag sites also gained the propensity to adopt CD155 as receptor, thereby becoming a new species.

Obviously, the probability to the ICAM-1 ⇒ CD155 switch must involve complicated structural rearrangements because of the limited serotype diversity (only three) among the PVs. What is the probability that any of the C-CAVs will switch receptor to CD155 in the future? This depends on different factors including (i) the role that neutralization antigenic determinants of C-CAVs play in ICAM-1 binding, (ii) the size of the evolutionary space to be explored by C-CAVs in a "quest" for new receptor specificity, and (iii) the immune status of the human population.

Could global eradication of PVs increase the probability of ICAM-1 ⇒ CD155 switching by some C-CAVs?

If structural elements of N-Ags decorating the canyon rim of C-cluster enteroviruses prove to be involved in virion/receptor interaction, then a balance of antibodies against these viruses in the human population could play a decisive role in the emergence of C-cluster species with a new receptor specificity. The balance is to be drastically changed in the poliovirus-free world when anti-poliovirus antibodies are no longer present. Then, C-CAVs evolving to bind to CD155 upon a negative selection by cognate antibodies would not be cleared by anti-PV antibodies as may have happened so far [1]. We predict that C-CAVs with CD155 affinity, should they spread to the CNS, would be neurovirulent, in contrast to a virus with CD155 specificity evolved from magHRVs [20,22]. As thc pool of circulating C-CAVs will increase in an expanding world population (>60% of which will be living in mega cities), the possibility of novel polio-like viruses arising from C-CAV variants cannot be discounted.

Conclusion

We suggest that in addition to the expansive measures for the global eradication of poliovirus, strategies should be developed that aim at predicting the possible evolution of new polio-like pathogens, and prepare for their control. The results reviewed in this article may contribute to achieving this tantalizing and desirable goal [1].

Acknowledgements

The authors would like to dedicate this paper to the memory of Professor Florian Horaud.

Financial support for work described here was provided in part by NIH grants to M.G.R., R.J.K., E.W., and T.S.B., an NSF grant to T.S.B., a grant from The Brain Tumor Society to E.W., and a Purdue University reinvestment grant. The current research of A.E.G. is funded with Federal funds from the NCI and NIH under Contract No. NO1-CO-56000. The content of this publication does not necessarily reflect the views or policies of the Department of Health and Human Services, nor does mention of trade names, commercial products, or organization imply endorsement by the U.S. Government.

References

1 Gromeier M, Wimmer E, Gorbalenya AE: Genetics, pathogenesis and evolution of picornaviruses, in Domingo E, Webster RG, Holland JJ (eds): Origin and Evolution of Viruses. Academic Press,1999, pp 287-343.

2 Stanway G, Brown F, Christian P, Tapani H, Hyypia T, Knowles N, Lemon S, Minor P, Pallansch M, Palmenberg A, Skern T: Taxonomy of the picornaviridae: species designation and three new genera. Abstract. Europic 2000, Italy.

3 Rossmann MG, Bella J, Kolatkar PR, He Y, Wimmer E, Kuhn RJ, Baker TS: Cell recognition and entry by rhino- and enteroviruses. Virology 2000;269:239-247.

4 Hogle JM, Chow M, Filman DJ: The three dimensional structure of poliovirus at 2.9 A resolution. Science 1985229:1358-1365.

5 Rossman MG, Arnold E, Erikson JW, Frankenberger EA, Griflith JP, Hecht HJ, Johnson JE, Kamer G, Luo M, Mosser A, Rueckert R, Sherry B, Vriend G: Structure of a human common cold virus and functional relationship to other picornaviruses. Nature 1985;317:145-153.

6 Minor PD: Antigenic structure of picornaviruses. Cur Top Immunolog Microbiol 1990;161:121-154.

7 Pfister T, Mirzayan C, Wimmer E: Polioviruses: molecular biology, in Granoff AW, (ed): Encyclopedia of Virology. London, UK, Academic Press Ltd, 1999, vol 2, pp 1330-1348.

8 Kolatkar PR, Bella J, Olson NH, Bator CM, Baker TS, Rossmann MG: Structural studies of two rhinovirus serotypes complexed with fragments of their cellular receptor. EMBO J 1999;18:6249-6259.

9 Belnap DM, McDermott BM Jr, Filman DJ, Cheng N, Trus BL, Zuccola HJ, Racaniello VR, Hogle JM, Steven AC: Three-dimensional structure of poliovirus receptor bound to poliovirus. Proc Natl Acad Sci USA 2000;97:73-78.

10 He Y, Bowman VD, Mueller S, Bator CM, Bella J, Peng X, Baker TS, Wimmer E, Kuhn RJ, Rossmann MG: Interaction of the poliovirus receptor with poliovirus. Proc Natl Acad Sci USA 2000;97:79-84.

11 Xiao C, Bator CM, Bowman VD, Rieder, E, He Y, Hébert B, Bella J, Baker, TS, Wimmer E, Kuhn RJ, Rossmann MG: The interaction of Coxsackievirus A21 with its cellular receptor, ICAM-1. J Virol 2001;75:2444-2451.

12 Kitamura N, Semler BL, Rothberg PG, Larsen GR, Adler CJ, Dorner AJ, Emini EA, Hanecak R, Lee J, van der Werf S, Anderson CW, Wimmer E: Primary structure, gene organization and polypeptide expression of poliovirus RNA. Nature 1981;291:547-553.

13 Wimmer E, Hellen CUT, Cao XM: Genetics of poliovirus. Ann Rev Genet 1993;27:353-436.

14 Hyypia T, Hovi T, Knowles NJ, Stanway G: Classification of enteroviruses based on molecular and biological properties. J Gen Virol 1997;78:1-11.

15 Poyry T, Kinnunen L, Hyypia T, Brown B, Horsnell C, Hovi T, Stanway G: Genetics and phylogenetic clustering of enteroviruses. J Gen Virol 1996;77:1699-1717.

16 Pulli T, Koskimies P, Hyypia T: Molecular comparison of Coxsackie A virus serotypes. Virology. 1995;212:30-38.

17 Gromeier M, Solecki D, Patel DD, Wimmer E: The human poliovirus receptor/CD155 promoter directs reporter gene expression in embryonic floor plate and optic nerve of transgenic mice. Virology 2000;273:248-257.

18 Simmon DL: Functional analysis of cell adhesion molecules. Methods Mol Biol 1999;96:39-63.

19 Solecki D, Schwarz S, Wimmer E, Lipp M, Bernhardt G: 1997. The promoters for human and monkey poliovirus receptors. J. Biol Chem 1997;272:5579-5586.

20 Gromeier M, Alexander L, Wimmer E: Internal ribosomal entry site substitution eliminates neurovirulence in intergeneric poliovirus recombinants. Proc Natl Acad Sci USA 1996;93:2370-2375.

21 Gromeier M, Lachmann S, Rosenfeld MR, Gutin PH, Wimmer E: Intergeneric poliovirus recombinants for the treatment of malignant glioma (In Process Citation). Proc Natl Acad Sci USA 2000;97:6803-6808.

22 Gromeier M, Mueller S, Solecki D, Bossert B, Bernhardt G, Wimmer E: Determinants of poliovirus neurovirulence. J Neurovirol 1997;3 Suppl 1:S35-38.

23 Wimmer E, Harber JJ, Bibb JA, Gromeier M, Lu HH, Bernhardt G: Poliovirus receptors, in Wimmer E (ed): Cellular Receptors for Animal Viruses. Cold Spring Harbor, Cold Spring Harbor Laboratory, 1994; pp 101-127.

24 Shafren DR, Dorahy DJ, Greive SJ, Burns GF, Barry RD: Mouse cells expressing human intercellular adhesion molecule-1 are susceptible to infection by Coxsackievirus A21. J Virol 1997;71:785-789.

25 Shafren DR, Dorahy DJ, Ingham RA, Burns GF, Barry RD: Coxsackievirus A21 binds to decay-accelerating factor but requires intercellular adhesion molecule 1 for cell entry. J Virol 1997;71:4736-4743.

26 Evans DJ, Almond JW: Cell receptors for picornaviruses as determinants of cell tropism and pathogenesis. Trends Microbiol 1998;6:198-202.

27 Wimmer E: Introduction, in Wimmer E (ed): Cellular Receptors for Animal Viruses. Cold Spring Harbor, Cold Spring Harbor Laboratory, 1994; pp 1-13.

28 Schober D, Kronenberger P, Prchla E, Blaas D, Fuchs R: Major and minor receptor group human rhinoviruses penetrate from endosomes by different mechanisms. J Virol 1998;72:1354-1364.

29 Bibb JA, Witherell G, Bernhardt G, Wimmer E: Interaction of poliovirus with its cell surface binding site. Virology 1994;201:107-115.

30 Harber J, Bernhardt G, Lu HH, Sgro JY, Wimmer E: Serotype polymorphism of poliovirus-cellular receptor interaction: separation of events of viral attachment and uptake. Virology 1995;214:559-570.

Dr. E. Wimmer, Dept of Molecular Genetics and Microbiology, School of Medicine, State University of New York at Stony Brook, Stony Brook, NY 11794-5222, USA.

Brown F (ed): Progress in Polio Eradication: Vaccine Strategies for the End Game.
Dev Biol. Basel, Karger, 2001, vol 105, pp 123-127

The Eradication of Foot-and-Mouth Disease: a Parallel Problem

F. Brown

Plum Island Animal Disease Center, Greenport, NY, U.S.A.

Abstract: Poliomyelitis and foot-and-mouth disease (FMD) can both be prevented by vaccination. The vaccines are highly effective but they differ in that, whereas in most countries attenuated viruses have been used to control poliomyelitis, FMD vaccines are prepared from the virulent viruses. The reasons for choosing inactivated vaccines for FMD are (i) the demonstration several decades ago that a virus which was attenuated for one species could be virulent for another and (ii) the great antigenic variability of the virus. This has meant that the viruses to be used for vaccination have to "match" those occurring in the field. It also means that they should only be handled under strict conditions of containment.

An important issue therefore is whether the virus can be handled safely in an environment where the disease does not occur. A number of countries have dealt successfully with this problem for several decades. In the U.K., the virus is handled at the Government's Animal Virus Research Institute at Pirbright and the adjoining Merial facility where several million doses of vaccine are produced annually. In the U.S.A., with that country's penchant for overkill, the work is done at Plum Island, situated off the coasts of Connecticut and Long Island, New York. In addition, the Merieux Laboratory in Lyon, France, produced many million doses of vaccine for several years without endangering the local environment.

For the eradication of poliomyelitis, it will be necessary to continue vaccination for several years after the last field case of the disease is detected. To an outsider it seems logical that the vaccines should be inactivated which means that live virus is not used outside the laboratory or production facilities because of its capacity to revert to virulence. As long as live virus is present anywhere the chance of the disease re-emerging is a constant threat. This has been amply demonstrated by the outbreaks of FMD in Taiwan (1997), South Korea (2000) and Japan (2000) where the disease had not been reported for more than 60 years.

Introduction

Eradication of FMD has been achieved in several areas of the world, notably in Western Europe and South America. In addition, several countries have not had an outbreak for several decades (e.g. the U.S.A. since 1929, Canada since 1952). Dramatically, however, three countries in Asia which had been free of the disease for several decades (Taiwan, 1927; South Korea, 1936; and Japan, 1908) have had outbreaks recently. The outbreak in Taiwan in 1997 involved several million pigs and incurred the loss of lucrative export markets. The outcome of the outbreaks in South Korea and Japan is still not known.

On the positive side the success in Western Europe and several countries in South America has been achieved by the rigorous application of killed vaccines. There are two main reasons for using this kind rather than attenuated vaccines. The first is that a virus which has been attenuated for one species is not necessarily attenuated for other susceptible species. The second is the considerable antigenic variation of the virus within the seven major serotypes. This means that even within a well vaccinated population, an outbreak of the disease can occur because of the emergence of variant strains. An early example of this occurred in Europe in the mid 1960s when a virus of serotype O appeared which broke through the immunity provided by the vaccine used successfully for more than 10 years. There have been several similar instances in the interim. It is difficult to see how a suitably attenuated vaccine which is antigenically similar to a new field outbreak could be produced rapidly to meet such situations. Consequently, killed vaccines have been used almost exclusively for the past 50 years.

Thankfully, FMDV is not a hazard for humans. Of the few cases that have been reported, the symptoms were trivial [1]. It is because of the danger of handling a virus which can infect farm livestock all too readily that veterinary authorities worldwide have recognised the need for strict disease security precautions for nearly a century. Loeffler, the co-discoverer of the viral nature of the causal agent [2] was forced by pressure from the local farmers to stop his work on the disease at the University of Greisswald in Northern Germany and re-locate his laboratory to the Island of Riems in the Baltic Sea [3]. In fact, Loeffler was unlucky because it had not been recognised previously that cattle which had recovered from the disease could carry the virus for many months following the overt disease. On being returned to the farms, they infected naïve animals. At the same time it made those working with the disease aware of the importance of the carrier state.

The pertinent question in the context of this meeting is whether poliovirus can be handled safely without endangering a population in which the disease no longer occurs. I will describe the steps that have been taken to ensure that FMDV can be handled safely, making use of my long experience at the Animal Virus Research Institute in Pirbright, U.K., and at the Plum Island Animal Disease Center in the U.S.A., to describe the precautions that are taken.

I consider that there are five major requirements:

(i) the laboratory and production facility should be located in an area where there are no susceptible animals;

(ii) handling the virus should be done in laboratories maintained at a negative pressure compared to the environment, and the apparatus thoroughly disinfected before leaving the laboratory;

(iii) staff must change clothes before entering the laboratory and shower before leaving to ensure that virus is not carried to the environment;

(iv) staff must not visit farms where livestock are kept;

(v) the product, that is the vaccine, must be tested for innocuity.

Location of laboratory

The Pirbright Laboratory and the adjoining Merial Production Facility in the U.K. are located on common land on which it is forbidden to graze farm animals. Both facilities are fenced and entry is monitored. Illegal entry would be even more difficult at the U.S.A. laboratory on Plum Island.

Handling the virus under negative pressure

The evidence that the virus can be transmitted by aerosol alerted the workers for the need to operate under negative pressure, particularly when large amounts of the agent are involved. There are reports that the virus can be transmitted up to 170 miles so it is vital that it should be contained under these conditions and that the circulating air should be filtered appropriately.

Change of clothing

Since the virus can survive for considerable periods at ambient or low temperature, it is vital that it should not be carried by staff leaving the laboratory, whether on their clothes or bodies. Once regarded as irksome, but now generally accepted as sensible by personnel working with other hazardous viruses, discarding laboratory clothing and showering before re-entering the normal environment has been accepted as a routine procedure for at least 50 years by those working with FMDV.

Avoid contact with farm animals

Staff working with a virus affecting farm animals would, on balance, be expected to be interested in such animals. This would apply particularly to veterinarians. Nevertheless, on the off-chance that the virus had been carried despite the showering and change of clothing, it is sensible that contact with farm animals should be avoided. It is now generally accepted that the virus will not survive on the human body for longer than seven days, allowing appropriate guidelines to be drawn up by the laboratories involved.

Innocuity of the product

The innocuity of both the inactivated polio and FMD vaccines was a subject of considerable debate 50 years ago. Despite misgivings by several workers regarding the innocuity of the early killed poliovaccine prepared by formalin inactivation, the trials went ahead, with disastrous consequences in 1954 [4]. Some reassuring revision of the inactivating procedure was introduced, and no cases of the disease have been traced back to the killed vaccine since that time. However, doubts about the FMD vaccines produced by a similar procedure were expressed by Moosbrugger as early as 1948 [5] and subsequent work using molecular methods in the 1980s showed that most of the remaining outbreaks occurring in Western Europe at that time were caused by vaccines improperly inactivated by formaldehyde [6,7].

At this point I introduce a personal note. The doubts expressed by Moosbrugger, referred to earlier [5], were also felt by Ian Galloway, then Director of the Pirbright Laboratory. Following discussions with Galloway and Weston Hurst of Imperial Chemical Industries, Joan Crick and I [8] showed that N-acetylethyleneimine (AEI), a compound developed by that company, inactivated FMDV with first order kinetics to yield a safer highly immunogenic product. Since 1965, the Wellcome Laboratories have used AEI and its parent ethyleneimine (EI, [9]) for the preparation of billions of doses of a highly efficacious FMD vaccine, which has not been shown to possess residual infectivity.

Since it is anticipated that one of the next steps in the eradication of poliomyelitis will be an increased use of killed vaccines, it is vital that any doubts about the innocuity and immunogenicity of the product should be removed. Recent work has shown that the loss of antigenic sites can be incurred by formaldehyde inactivation. A second and possibly more serious problem is that of innocuity because FMDV and poliovirus have such similar structures that it is hard to accept that formaldehyde inactivates one virus but not the other.

To prove that a vaccine is innocuous is not easy. Work by Taylor and Bottiger and their colleagues [10, 11] in the late 1950s showed that, whereas the number of plaques obtained with poliovirus did not increase after two days incubation at 37°C, the number obtained with formalin-treated virus could be zero at two days but then start to increase for as long as 11 days. This result showed clearly that release of RNA from the virus particles is very slow after formalin treatment. Our own experiments have confirmed this because the usual methods for extracting RNA from FMDV and poliovirus particles do not release the genome from formalin-treated particles. These observations lead me to suggest that it would be worthwhile to explore imine inactivation as a method for producing poliovaccine.

The Future

One issue that has caused concern in the FMD community is the occurrence of the 'carrier' state. Animals that have been infected can carry the virus for several years. Such animals cannot be distinguished from those that have received the killed vaccine by virus neutralization tests. However, they can be distinguished from those vaccinated by a simple serological test, making use of the fact that some of the non-structural proteins are not secreted from the cells in which the virus is grown for vaccine production [12]. Consequently, the sera of vaccinated animals do not contain antibodies to these proteins.

In view of the increasing amount of information that a carrier state exists in some individuals who have received the Sabin poliovaccine, it seems important to me that a similar test should be developed to determine whether poliovirus is still extant in the environment but not causing disease by determining the serological status of selected groups. This is a vital issue in programmes to eradicate poliovirus from the environment.

References

1 Hyslop NStG: Transmission of the virus of foot-and-mouth disease between animals and man. Bull Org Mond Sante 1973; 49:577-585.

2 Loeffler F, Frosch P: Berichte der Kommission zur Erforschung der Maul-und-Klauenseuche bei dem Institut für Infektionskrankheiten in Berlin. Centralblatt Bakt 1 Abt Orig 1898;23:371-391.

3 Schiedebach H-P: The Prussian State and microbiological research - Friedrich Loeffler and his approach to the "invisible" virus. In: 100 Years of Virology ed. CH Calisher and MC Horzinek Springer 1999.

4 Nathanson N, Langmuir AD: The Cutter incident. Poliomyelitis following formaldehyde-inactivated poliovirus vaccination in the United States during the Spring of 1955. I. Background. Amer J Hyg 1963;78:16-28.

5 Moosbrugger GA: Recherches expérimentales sur la fièvre aphteuse. Schweiz Arch Tierheilk 1948;90:176-198.

6 King AMQ, Underwood BO, McCahon D, Newman JWI, Brown F: Biochemical identification of viruses causing the 1981 outbreaks of foot-and-mouth disease in the UK. Nature 1981;293:479-480.

7 Beck E, Strohmaier K: Subtyping of European foot-and-mouth disease virus strains by nucleotide sequence determination. J Virol 1987;61:1621-1629.

8 Brown F, Crick J: Application of agar gel diffusion analysis to a study of the antigenic structure of inactivated vaccines prepared from the virus of foot-and-mouth disease. J Immunol 1959;82:444-447.

9 Bahnemann HG: Binary ethyleneimine as inactivant for foot-and-mouth disease virus and its application for vaccine production. Arch Virol 1975;47:47-56.

10 Schultz P, Rightsel WA, Timm EA, Taylor FR, McLean Jr IW: Partially inactivated poliomyelitis virus: initiation of infection in tissue culture. J Immunol 1957;79:497-507.

11 Bottiger M, Lycke E, Melen B, Wrangl G: Inactivation of poliomyelitis virus by formaldehyde: incubation time in tissue culture of formalin treated virus. Arch ges Virusf 1958;8:259-266.

12 Shen F, Chen PD, Walfield AM, Ye J, House J, Brown F, Wang CY: Differentiation of convalescent animals from those vaccinated against foot-and-mouth disease. Vaccine 1999;17:3039-3049.

Prof. F. Brown, Plum Island Animal Disease Center, P.O. Box 848, Greenport, NY 11944, USA.

Brown F (ed): Progress in Polio Eradication: Vaccine Strategies for the End Game.
Dev Biol. Basel, Karger, 2001, vol 105, pp 129-147

Stopping a Polio Outbreak in the Post-Eradication Era[a]

P.E.M. Fine[1], *R.W. Sutter*[2], *W.A. Orenstein*[2]

[1] Department of Infectious and Tropical Diseases, London School of Hygiene and Tropical Medicine, London, U.K.

[2] National Immunization Program, Centers for Disease Control and Prevention, Atlanta, GA, U.S.A.

INTRODUCTION

The global Poliomyelitis Eradication Initiative is close to target. According to current predictions, wild polioviruses should cease to circulate in human populations in the year 2002, or shortly thereafter. This imminent event raises important strategic issues: (i) how best to confirm that wild virus eradication has truly occurred; (ii) how best to discontinue polio vaccination; and (iii) how best to prepare contingency plans for appropriate interventions, should wild virus reappear after its apparent eradication, or should vaccine-derived virus appear, or persist, after ceasing vaccination.

This paper is devoted to the third of these issues. It begins by describing the changing epidemiological situation associated with the final stages of the eradication programme, and discusses various outbreak scenarios that might arise. It then addresses issues surrounding intervention strategies that might be applied to control poliovirus outbreaks that might occur in the post-eradication era, and concludes with a series of recommendations.

[a] This paper was commissioned by the World Health Organization's Polio Eradication Initiative as a background document for the WHO consultation 'Polio Vaccines for the Post-Eradication and Post-Immunization Era', Geneva, Switzerland, 19-20 January 2000.

Predicting the Future

Ending the eradication programme

The "end-game" of polio eradication could unfold in various ways. The World Health Organization (WHO) will have some – but not total – control over these variations. Whatever the details, there will be three important phases

Pre-wild virus eradication

This is the current situation, with wild virus still circulating in wide areas of the world, with all countries still providing routine vaccination against poliomyelitis and all polio-endemic countries conducting supplemental immunization activities. Several features of this period are predictable:

(i) The geographical range of endemic polio will shrink. It is virtually certain that one or another South Asian or African country will be the last to remain endemic for wild polioviruses;

(ii) One by one the separate virus types should (at least appear to) cease to circulate. It is expected that type 2 will be the first to cease circulating, and type 1 the last;

(iii) Some countries will change their vaccination policies. For example, the U.S.A. discontinued the routine use of OPV vaccines from January 2000, motivated by concerns of vaccine safety rather than of efficacy;

(iv) There will be intensified vaccination efforts put into place in several areas, to ensure eradication of wild viruses (e.g. some countries will mount particularly frequent and intensive National Immunization Days [NIDs]).

Certain details of this period, which are yet unknown, may be important for determining subsequent policy:

(i) What will be the order of disappearance of wild virus types?

(ii) Where will virus persist longest, and why?

(iii) What vaccination strategies will be associated with apparent ultimate disappearance?

(iv) How will the last wild viruses be identified?

Post wild virus "eradication", vaccination still continues

After wild viruses have apparently ceased to circulate, it will be necessary to maintain intensive surveillance and vaccination activities for a period of years, before ultimately discontinuing polio vaccination altogether. Certain features of this period are predictable:

(i) It will last for several (at least three and most probably five) years, after disappearance of wild virus;

(ii) Vaccination efforts and both AFP (acute flaccid paralysis) and virus surveillance will be very intense initially, but will have a tendency to slacken with time, at least in some populations, in particular if no wild viruses are reported anywhere;

(iii) There will be much discussion of the wisdom and method of stopping vaccination altogether. Concerns about the threat of bioterrorism will undoubtedly figure in the discussion. Some sort of global policy will ultimately be recommended from WHO (which may include a massive terminal global OPV immunization day, or shifts to IPV, or coordinated shifts from trivalent to bivalent or monovalent OPV vaccines);

(iv) There will be further changes in vaccination policies in some countries, dictated by their own national advisory bodies; and some countries may elect unilaterally to discontinue vaccination, before a recommendation to do so globally. Abandonment of all vaccination at a time when OPV is still widely used elsewhere would be a bold decision, given the possibility that OPV viruses might spread into the unvaccinated population and revert to virulence.

Other features of this period are less predictable:

(i) Certain countries may persist with IPV vaccination for some time after WHO and most other countries have recommended its discontinuation;

(ii) Wild viruses may (or may not) be identified in one or another population, after their apparent absence for a period of some years. The circumstances of any such events would be important for determining future policy.

The details of how OPV vaccination is ultimately discontinued will be extremely important. In particular, the circumstances may provide a crucial test of the transmissibility of oral polio vaccine viruses (i.e. if there is a shift from trivalent to bi- or monovalent OPV vaccines, or if some countries or populations elect to discontinue vaccination altogether, while others continue to use oral vaccines).

Post ceasing vaccination

This situation is the ultimate goal of the eradication initiative. It will have certain features:

(i) There will be intensive surveillance for AFP and polioviruses for some period after ceasing vaccination. Just how long this will last, and how intensive it will be, are yet unknown.

(ii) Assuming no polioviruses are detected, there will be a gradual increase in confidence, as time goes on, that poliovirus eradication has indeed been achieved. This will reflect a declining probability that vaccine-derived viruses will reappear.

(iii) There will be a progressive decline in the prevalence of immunity in post-vaccination populations. This will reflect both the **waning of prior mucosal immunity in individuals born before ceasing vaccination** (who will become increasingly susceptible to infection, though not, or less so, to disease), and **increasing numbers of young, immunologically naïve individuals, born after ceasing vaccination** (who will be susceptible both to infection and to disease) [1,2]. This stratification means that, if virus were introduced several years after vaccination, the clinical cases would be concentrated selectively in the young, born since ceasing vaccination, whereas virus transmission could occur to some degree in all age groups because of waning mucosal immunity.

Possible post-eradication outbreak scenarios

Wild poliovirus

could "reappear" in human populations (after apparent eradication) in several ways

(i) Through persistent undetected circulation in humans:

- through long-term carriage in an immunodeficient individual;
- through persistent person-to-person transmission in the absence of detected disease, in some population or combination of populations;

(ii) Through accidental release from a "laboratory":

- from a virus research laboratory (as occurred with smallpox in Birmingham in 1978);
- from an IPV vaccine production facility;
- from some other laboratory holding or processing clinical (faecal, tissue) specimens containing undetected poliovirus;

(iii) Through intentional release ("bioterrorism" or "biological warfare"). Poliovirus is an unlikely biological weapon, as it is so indiscriminate, and would particularly affect poorer and younger rather than the high socio-economic groups and working-age populations. Its use in this way would serve little purpose beyond demonstrating a combination of stupidity and extreme anti-societal sentiment on the part of the perpetrators, who would have nothing but notoriety to gain from the act;

(iv) Through "accidental" or intentional release of a poliovirus synthesized de novo in a well equipped laboratory [3]. The possibility of such syntheses means that even the complete destruction of all polioviruses, worldwide, would not ensure the future freedom of the world from polioviruses;

(v) Through environmental persistence, e.g., in sewage, permafrost or in cadavers. By current knowledge, poliovirus is extremely unlikely to remain viable for more than a few months in any environmental setting;

(vi) Through an animal reservoir. There is at present no evidence of the existence of any such wild reservoir.

The probability of any one or more of these events happening is difficult to predict, but appears to be exceedingly small. WHO is currently undertaking studies attempting to define the risk of long-term carriage in immunodeficient individuals (carriage of vaccine-derived polioviruses [but not for wild polioviruses] for as long as ten years has now been demonstrated in three countries [4]), and is implementing various measures to reduce the risk of virus escaping from laboratories (destruction of stored viruses and potentially infectious materials, and increased containment requirements)[5].

Current experience from the polio eradication programme suggests that a genotype of poliovirus not detected for at least 12 months, under conditions of adequate surveillance, has never been detected again (personal communication, Olen Kew, CDC). Several researchers have tried to estimate the risk of continued undetected transmission, using very conservative assumptions. Eichner and Dietz [6] used computer simulation to estimate the probability of continued subclinical transmission of virus in the absence of clinical cases, under a variety of assumed conditions (e.g. 50 to 70% coverage with OPV and a case to infection ratio of 1:200, in a susceptible population of 200,000), and concluded that even after three (or five) years of no clinical cases, the probability of continued undetected circulation of virus was on the order of 5% (or 1%). These probabilities would be much less under conditions of higher OPV coverage such as are obtained in most populations today.

There will be **two important temporal trends** during the post-eradication era: the likelihood of virus reappearance will **decrease** with time; however, the seriousness of the consequences of any reappearance will **increase** with time. If wild poliovirus were to be introduced during the early post-eradication period, while vaccination is continuing, it might not even be detected, and should be relatively easily dealt with, by enhancing vaccination coverage (e.g. additional NID campaigns). But if it were to occur (long) after ceasing vaccination, the consequences would be dire, with rapid spread due to the accumulation of susceptibles and large numbers of clinical and fatal cases (there is evidence that both the clinical case to infection ratio, and the mortality rate, rise with age [7, 8]). The situation would be worsened if the response capacity were seriously hindered because the expertise and capacity to respond appropriately had waned.

Recent polio epidemics in the Netherlands, Finland, Canada and in the Amish community of the United States, demonstrate that wild polioviruses can still spread efficiently in communities whose members object to vaccination within contemporary "developed" societies with high hygiene standards.

OPV-derived virus

The possibility that vaccine-derived viruses might appear after ceasing vaccination has additional elements of uncertainty. In theory such viruses could appear or be (re)introduced through any of the circumstances listed above for wild-type viruses. In addition:

(vii) A potential source of vaccine virus will exist in unused or stored oral vaccines held in health centres, clinics and vaccine stores around the world;

(viii) Release could occur from an OPV production facility.

The ultimate transmission potential of vaccine-derived viruses in susceptible human populations is still unknown. A recent review of this subject [9] concluded that it is unlikely that OPV virus could persist by continued person-to-person transmission in the high-hygiene settings of developed countries, but that these viruses might be able to persist in poorer, less hygienic environments. The probability of such persistence will increase with time following ceasing vaccination and consequent increase in the number and proportion of susceptible individuals. Continued person-to-person transmission of these viruses might well be associated with genetic reversion towards virulence and selection towards the high transmissibility properties of the wild viruses. There appears to be at least one instance where vaccine-derived type 2 polioviruses was documented to assume wild-type characteristics (including transmissibility and neurovirulence) and caused multiple cases of paralytic disease over several years from 1988-1993 in a developing country with sub-optimal vaccination coverage. No representatives of these lineages have been detected since February 1993 [10] (personal communication: Olen Kew, CDC). A recent outbreak of type 1 vaccine-derived virus on the island of Hispaniola documents that vaccine viruses can circulate for a period of at least two years in developing countries with low vaccination coverage, and that during this period they can take on at least some of the phenotypic (transmissibility and virulence) characteristics of wild viruses [11]. An important point to appreciate is that vaccine-derived polioviruses differ from the viruses in OPV vials.

The potential for oral vaccine-derived viruses to persist in human populations is a crucially important issue, and strenuous efforts should be made to evaluate it (e.g. by controlling and monitoring the ultimate discontinuation of these vaccines).

Because of the low frequency of paralytic disease associated with vaccine polioviruses, generally estimated to be of the order of one case of vaccine-associated paralytic poliomyelitis (VAPP) per million first doses of vaccine (but probably much higher and somewhere between wild and OPV virus for vaccine-derived poliovirus), it would be difficult to detect the presence of vaccine-derived polioviruses in human populations after the ceasing vaccination. This means that many thousands – even millions – of individuals might have been infected, over very large geographical areas, before the problem was detected. This fact argues for intensive environmental surveillance (and or serosurveillance) for OPV viruses following the ceasing OPV vaccination, in particular in densely populated low-hygiene environments.

Issues Related to Outbreak Response

Outbreak control activities of vaccine-preventable diseases aim to increase immunity levels rapidly in the affected populations. Two types of vaccine are available for polio control, OPV and IPV, and there are different formulations of OPV (i.e. trivalent [tOPV] or monovalent [mOPV]). Major characteristics of these vaccines are summarized in Table 1.

The age groups to be vaccinated and the geographical focus for vaccination will depend on whether the outbreak virus is vaccine-derived or wild, on known or inferred patterns of age-specific susceptibility, and on the geographical spread of the virus as determined through disease and virus surveillance. As a general principle, vaccine should be used in a wider geographical area than already known to be

Table 1: Characteristics of different poliovirus vaccines which could be applied to control an outbreak in the post-vaccination era

	tOPV	mOPV	IPV
Immunity inducement	Slower (multiple doses required)	Faster (single dose may be sufficient)	Slower (multiple doses required)
Administration	Oral	Oral	Injection
Adverse events	VAPP	VAPP[1]	Not likely
Longer term risks	Introduction of unnecessary serotypes; Continued circulation	Continued circulation	None
Cost	Lower	Lowest	Higher

1 Risk of VAPP appears to be slightly higher, compared to tOPV, following use of type 3 mOPVs, but probably would be lower following use of type 1 mOPV.

"involved", and at a minimum should cover all children through age five years and any older cohorts born since polio vaccination was stopped. There are several important facets of outbreak control which deserve elaboration here, including: (i) delays in recognition of and response to polio cases; (ii) laboratory network needed to confirm cases; (iii) diagnostic laboratory methods; (iv) choice of vaccine for control purposes; and (v) vaccine stockpile and manufacturer capacity.

Delays and their implications

Considerable time may elapse between "introduction" of poliovirus into a population and ultimate confirmation of its presence. Several delays are involved

From introduction to first paralytic case

This delay would be dependent upon several factors: (i) the manner of "introduction" of virus into a population (the delay would be inversely proportional to the number of individuals initially infected); (ii) the rapidity of spread of infection (faster for wild than vaccine-derived viruses, inversely proportional to the prevalence of immunity in the population, and also determined by such factors as hygiene level and social mixing pattern of the population, environment and season) and (iii) the case-to-infection ratio (roughly 1/200 for wild virus; $1/10^6$ for OPV viruses; and somewhere between for vaccine-derived viruses).

There is a large number and variety of possible outbreak scenarios. In order to illustrate the numerical consequences of delays, Annex 1 shows graphically the numbers of individuals that might be infected, or diseased, over time after the introduction of a poliovirus into a population which is able to sustain its spread. The magnitude of these numbers is a function of three major factors:

(i) the average **"serial interval".** This is the **time interval between successive infections** in a chain of transmission. Annex 1 presents estimates based upon average serial intervals of either five or 10 days (the range will be from less than two days to several weeks – even years in the case of long-term chronic excreters).

(ii) the **"net (effective) reproduction number"**. This is the **average number of infection transmissions** by each infected individual. This will be highly-situation dependent, being a function of many social, hygiene and population immunity characteristics, and is illustrated in Annex 1 for a range of circumstances from one to five average transmissions per **infected** (not necessarily diseased) individual. Given the high levels of immunity prevailing in virtually all populations of the world today, this number should be, currently, appreciably below unity, for both wild and vaccine-derived viruses (and hence the declines in infection and disease incidence in these populations). It will potentially rise after ceasing vaccination, as immunity levels decline. Analysis of published data indicates that this average number of transmissions could be as high as five, for wild virus in high-hygiene situations, and as high as 15 (perhaps 20) for wild virus in low-hygiene situations **in the absence of population immunity** [9]. The number is likely to be smaller for vaccine-derived than for wild viruses.

(iii) the **population size.** Transmission will be constrained if the introduction is into a closed (e.g. island) population; but for the sake of illustration we assume in Annex 1 that the population is open (as would be the case if the population were sufficiently mobile to allow transmission over a large geographical area).

One must also consider the incubation period, from infection to clinical onset (range three to 35 days, usually seven – 14 days) in estimating the delay from introduction to first paralytic case. In Annex 1 we assume an average incubation period of 10 days.

On the basis of this background, Table 2 presents **rough** estimates of the delay that might occur, from introduction of either wild or vaccine-derived poliovirus into a population, until onset of the first paralytic case, under different conditions of population immunity (as determined by time since ceasing vaccination). This delay could be as short as a few days (if wild virus were introduced into a densely populated low hygiene environment, many years after ceasing vaccination) to as long as a year or more (if vaccine virus were introduced into a low-hygiene population just able to sustain its spread, a few years after vaccination ceased)

Delay from onset of first paralytic case to diagnostic suspicion and collection of first faecal sample

This delay will depend very much upon the population setting, the nature of the health facility to which cases are brought, the index of suspicion of the health staff and the number of cases occurring (the more cases there are, the more likely they are to attract attention). The awareness of polio among physicians and other health care professionals will be inversely related to the time since local polio elimination. It could range from less than one day (first case immediately suspected as possibly polio) to many weeks, perhaps months in the case of a vaccine-derived poliovirus outbreak.

Table 2: Estimated delay from introduction of virus into a population until the **onset** of the first paralytic case. N.B. These estimates are approximate, being dependent on a large number of variables. Importantly, if by chance the first infected individual were to experience clinical paralysis, the delay in **any** circumstance could be as short as a few days. On average, however, if the introduction were of wild virus, approximately 200 individuals would become infected before the first paralytic case[1], and many more (up to one million) if the introduction were of OPV virus.

Immunity level (time since stopping vaccination)	**Approximate delay from virus introduction into population to onset of first paralytic case**	
	Wild poliovirus	**Vaccine-derived virus**
High (one-two years since vaccination stopped)	Weeks to months	Virus unlikely to persist (no cases expected)
Moderate (three-10 years since vaccination stopped)	Several (three-10) weeks	Several months to years
Low (>10 years after vaccination stopped)	Several (>seven) days to a few (<three) weeks	Several months, possibly a year or more

[1] Average ratio for wild poliovirus type 1; for poliovirus types 2 and 3, the average ratio may be closer to one paralytic case per 1,000 or more infections among susceptible person.

Delay from clinical suspicion and stool collection to polio confirmation

In most populations of the world, confirmation of poliovirus infection requires virus identification, which in turn implies shipment of stool samples to an appropriate laboratory and appropriate cell culture isolation methods. Under current ideal conditions the isolation and serotyping requires approximately four weeks, but may take longer depending upon initial titres of virus in the specimen, presence of substances that are toxic to cultured cells, mixtures of viruses, etc.

Beyond identification of a virus as belonging to the polio family, it is essential to identify serotype (type 1, 2 or 3) and to differentiate the isolate as of wild or vaccine-derived origin. Before ceasing OPV vaccination, the isolation of vaccine-derived virus from stools raises no public health alarm beyond evidence for another VAPP or incidental virus isolation. After ceasing vaccination, however, confirmation of serotype and whether the virus is wild or vaccine-derived will be essential in order to decide upon the appropriate intervention response.

According to data from the Western Pacific Region (WPRO) of WHO, the minimum delay from stool collection to virus confirmation, including virus isolation, serotyping and intratypic differentiation has been 42 days; the longest has been many months (personal communication, Ray Sanders, WHO). The programme aims to keep this delay to below 90 days.

In the Region of the Americas, the average delay from notification to virus confirmation (as vaccine-derived) has been 74 days (range: 19-290 days) among the 27 AFP cases reported from 1992-1998 with isolation of poliovirus (personal communication, Ciro de Quadros, PAHO).

Implications

In terms of outbreak control, we are concerned with the total delay from introduction of virus until diagnostic confirmation, or until control measures could be implemented on the ground, and its implications for spread of virus. From the preceding paragraphs, we see that this total delay is likely to last for at least several weeks, and more likely for some months, under a wide variety of assumptions and circumstances.

From Annex 1, we see that many hundreds, even thousands of individuals could become infected over this interval. For example, if the net reproduction number were only 1.5, and the serial interval were five days, then 32[0], 387[2] or 4432[22] individuals would have become infected [diseased, assuming one per 200] after 30, 60 or 90 days, respectively. If the net reproductive number were two, then the cumulative numbers infected would be 127[1] after 30 days, 8191[41] after 60 days and more than half a million [2621] after 90 days. It would take twice as long to reach these numbers if the average serial interval were 10 days. Though these higher figures may be unrealistic because of their implicit assumption of a random-mixing open population (in reality one would expect the virus spread to be constrained by exhaustion of susceptibles), the spread could indeed be vast if the virus were able to invade several urban populations over this period. Given the mobility of contemporary populations, it is possible that polioviruses could spread not only between urban centres, but over a very wide geographical area, crossing national as well as continental borders, within a matter of weeks. It is clearly of great importance that all these ascertainment and confirmation delays be shortened as much as possible.

Virological considerations

Wild polioviruses types 1 and 3 are still circulating in human populations. Type 2 virus has not been detected since 1999, but we still cannot be absolutely certain of its eradication [12]. Because there is little cross-protection induced between the three wild polio virus types, all are included in the trivalent OPV or inactivated poliovirus vaccines (IPV) in current use today. They differ in certain properties: type 1 has the highest clinical attack rate of paralytic disease, followed by types 3 and then 2. There is no good evidence for differences in transmissibility between them.

If there were to be a recurrence or outbreak of either wild or vaccine-derived poliovirus, it is most likely that only a single virus type would be involved, although in theory two or even all three might appear together.

It will be necessary to determine whether any outbreak virus is wild or vaccine-derived, and by serotype, as soon as possible, as this may have an important bearing upon any intervention. Given the very different ratios of paralytic cases to infections (1/200 versus $1/10^6$), it is likely that the epidemic pattern in space and time would itself give a strong indication of whether a wild or vaccine derived virus were involved.

Laboratory network considerations

At present many laboratories work with polioviruses. Diagnostic virus isolation from stool samples is carried out in 82 national laboratories (excluding 30 provincial laboratories in China) around the world, operating generally under biosafety level 2 (BSL-2) containment. Most of these laboratories are also able to serotype polioviruses, by neutralization with type-specific antisera. Differentiation between wild and vaccine-derived viruses has additional technical requirements, and is now carried out by 14 regional laboratories located in Central African Republic, Ghana and South Africa (African Region), Egypt, Kuwait, Pakistan, Tunisia (Eastern

Mediterranean Region), Russian Federation (European Region), India, Sri Lanka, Thailand (South-East Asia Region), Australia, China (Western Pacific Region), and Brazil (American Region). In addition, six specialized laboratories located in Finland, France, Japan, the Netherlands, United Kingdom, and the United States, serve as regional reference laboratories.

Poliovirus diagnostic work will need to continue indefinitely in network laboratories, provided these laboratories do not use infectious reference poliovirus in their work. If a laboratory does detect poliovirus in a clinical sample, it would indicate that the virus is already present in the field, so it may be argued that the laboratory work at BSL-2 level should not present any undue additional risk, provided good laboratory practice is maintained. Quality control of such laboratory procedures will have to be addressed, given that it generally requires live virus. Further detailed work with poliovirus isolates should be performed only under conditions of high containment in a small number of reference laboratories.

Implications for diagnostic methods

There is potential to shorten and simplify appreciably the times required to confirm a diagnosis of poliovirus infection. In populations no longer exposed to any poliovirus vaccine, it may be possible to use **serological assays** targeting either IgG or IgM antibodies to determine whether a person who was born after ceasing vaccination has evidence of a poliovirus infection. If such assays were sufficiently robust, sensitive and specific, they could be carried out in many laboratories, with a positive serology signalling the need to collect stool for testing. Further development of such assays (none of which is yet available commercially) should have high priority on the immediate research agenda. In addition, serosurveillance of children born after ceasing vaccination may provide another means of assessing the circulation of vaccine-derived polioviruses.

It may be possible to refine methods for **direct detection of poliovirus** in stool specimens, with a potential for rapid identification of virus without need for culture isolation. If sensitivity could be improved, such assays might be able to identify viruses by serotype and as wild versus vaccine-derived using existing techniques. Even if developed, it is likely that such assays would be performed only in the reference laboratories.

Outbreak response: an argument for monovalent OPV vaccines

The only effective tools at our disposal today to combat an outbreak of polio are vaccines. Emergency measures to improve hygiene or reduce contact in high risk groups (e.g., children) may in theory help slow virus spread, but are unlikely to have much impact in controlling an outbreak. Neither immunoglobulin nor chemical antivirals are likely to be of any practical use. Because of the low case to infection ratio, cordon sanitaire or case finding and quarantine approaches are likely to be inefficient locally, though they may have a role in some circumstances on a very large geographical scale.

Combating an outbreak of wild poliovirus

It has long been accepted that wide-scale use of OPV is the preferred strategy for epidemic control of polio. There are several good reasons for this preference:

(i) the live oral vaccines induce a direct mucosal immune response, which protects better against infection than does the more strictly humoral response induced by the inactivated vaccines;

(ii) the vaccine-derived viruses are to some extent transmissible, by direct faecal-oral (predominant mode of transmission in developing countries) or by oral-oral upper respiratory spread (predominant mode of transmission in industrialized countries). Transmissibility of OPV strains varies by serotype: type 2 > 3 > 1. This has been taken as an advantage, as in effect it enhances the vaccine coverage by surreptitiously immunizing some unvaccinated individuals;

(iii) the live vaccines are more easily administered than injectable IPV, and thus can be distributed more safely and rapidly to large numbers of people than can injectable vaccines.

The argument to use OPV vaccines in outbreak situations has been accepted widely ever since their introduction, and repeatedly justified by experience (Albania, the Netherlands, Finland, Amish population, etc. [13]). Importantly, such vaccines have been employed to combat outbreaks even in populations whose fundamental preference has been for inactivated polio vaccines, as in the Netherlands and Finland. *Unless there is a major (currently unforeseen) technical innovation, there is little doubt that massive use of OPV will be the approach used to combat any outbreaks of wild poliovirus that occur.*

There are several compelling reasons to prefer monovalent OPV vaccines for outbreak control:

(i) The immune response is more rapid with monovalent than with trivalent vaccines (primarily because one dose of monovalent OPV is as immunogenic as three doses of trivalent OPV, and three doses of OPV require at least 8 weeks to administer);

(ii) The type-specific seroconversion rate is higher with monovalent than with trivalent vaccines (due to decreased inter-type competition);

(iii) Given that any outbreak is likely to involve only a single virus serotype, control with the homologous monovalent vaccine avoids seeding additional viruses into the population. Given the possibility that OPV viruses may persist, any unnecessary use of OPV in the post vaccination era should be avoided;

(iv) Monovalent vaccines are likely to be less costly per dose than trivalent vaccine.

There are certain less desirable features of the monovalent vaccines:

(i) The risk of vaccine-associated paralytic poliomyelitis (VAPP) is slighly higher with monovalent type 3 OPV, but probably lower with type 1 OPV, compared to trivalent vaccines [14];

(ii) Monovalent vials imply greater cold storage space requirements.

Combating an outbreak of vaccine-derived poliovirus

Whether vaccine-derived virus could under any circumstances persist indefinitely is not yet certain. The probability of such persistence will increase with time after ceasing vaccination as a consequence of the increase in the number of susceptibles.

There are two approaches to control a vaccine-derived virus outbreak, in terms of vaccine:

(i) **Homotypic monovalent** OPV. Obviously the use of OPV strains other than the outbreak strain would be absolutely contra-indicated, as it would make the situation worse. The use of homologous monovalent vaccines is analogous to fighting fire with fire, and the strategy implies the need to raise population immunity levels to a level equivalent to that achieved at the time of ceasing OPV vaccination (assuming that this had been sufficient to eradicate OPV at that time).

(ii) **IPV**. Experience from (the developed) countries that currently use IPV indicate that vaccine-derived viruses do not routinely continue to circulate in these populations. The relatively low levels of mucosal immunity induced by IPV thus appear to be sufficient to slow, and ultimately stop, transmission of OPV viruses, if the reproduction number is close to one. This may be the case even in low-hygiene environments, in particular shortly after ceasing vaccination. Importantly, the possible utility of such an intervention means that IPV vaccines should be available in the future.

Decisions to use one or the other approach would depend in part upon the epidemiological pattern of any vaccine-derived poliovirus outbreak. The more rapid the spread, or if there is other evidence of reversion to virulence or of a return to wild-type transmissibility, then the stronger the argument would be to use homotypic monovalent OPV.

Outbreak management

In the event of an outbreak, there will be many important operational decisions: (i) what type of vaccine to use; (ii) what should be the target population (age, geography); (iii) how many doses to administer, and according to what timetable; (iv) what other measures should be employed (i.e. enhanced case finding, virological surveillance, social mobilization, health education). Each of these issues will have major logistic implications, which will have to be dealt with on an ad hoc basis. There is much expertise in the world today in polio outbreak control. This will need to be maintained insofar as possible in the crucial years ahead. Institutions with dedicated staff and expertise will obviously be important in this regard. It will be important for such groups to devote resources to detailed planning for various outbreak scenarios that might arise in the unique epidemiological circumstances ahead.

In the longer term such expertise may be linked to, or concentrated in, organizations dedicated broadly to emergency infectious disease responses. The problems of dealing with a polio outbreak in the post-eradication era are in a sense unique, but there are analogous problems surrounding the possibility of reappearance of smallpox (or other infectious agents which may be eradicated in the future), and obvious links to "bioterrorism" and "biological warfare" control.

Vaccine stockpiles

A particularly important issue is the amount and type of polio vaccines that will need to be stockpiled for emergency use in the post-eradication era, and provisions for additional production should that be necessary.

Just what vaccines will be employed between now and the recommendation to cease polio vaccination is at present unclear, but is likely to include extensive use of both trivalent IPV and trivalent OPV. There may also be widespread use of either a bivalent (e.g. types 1 and 3) OPV vaccine (if its production and approval can be organized), or else combined use of monovalent type 1 and monovalent type 3 vaccines, or monovalent type 1 only.

Decisions concerning vaccines for the post-eradication era have major epidemiological, economic and logistic implications. We propose the following for discussion, amendment and action:

OPV

(i) emphasis should be placed upon monovalent OPV vaccines of each serotype for outbreak control in the post-eradication era;

(ii) a stockpile of at least 500 million doses[1], of high potency safety-approved product, should be maintained for each of these three vaccines. (NB this number is a "first estimate", and needs debate). Based on the "shelf life" of such product, an annual production quota should be calculated to rotate the stock;

(iii) at least 100 million doses should be maintained in e.g. 20 dose vials, ready for immediate field distribution. Facilities must be constantly in place to ensure that the remainder of the stockpiled vaccine would be available for use within five weeks of demand;

(iv) at least two manufacturers should maintain ongoing capacity to produce each of these three monovalent vaccines;

(v) these manufacturers should engage in continuous production of these vaccines, both to ensure production capability and to ensure that stockpiled vaccine is not allowed to deteriorate because of age. This is necessary given that potency testing and safety clearance of each OPV batch requires approximately 15 months;

(vi) after vaccination stops, the vaccines should be produced and stored in high security containment facilities, in roughly equal amounts, in at least four different places around the world;

1 These doses would be sufficient to vaccinate approximately three birth cohorts of the world, and would vaccinate a much greater cohort in a more defined geographical area.

(vii) the vaccines should be "owned" by the World Health Organization. A protocol for their release needs to be prepared which may require approval from WHO's Director-General;

(viii) the World Health Assembly should approve the plan for a future vaccine stockpile. Any future change in this protocol would also require approval by the World Health Assembly;

(ix) though individual nations may elect to produce and stockpile additional OPV for their own purposes after OPV vaccination stops, this vaccine must be produced and stored under WHO-approved high containment conditions.

IPV

Whether or not there will be any role for IPV vaccine in the post-eradication era is at present unclear. If it is deemed necessary, for example, to ensure the disappearance of OPV vaccine derived viruses in some environment, then it too must be stockpiled for potential emergency use in the future. We thus propose:

(i) A global stockpile of trivalent IPV vaccine should be maintained, if it is deemed necessary, to ensure disappearance of OPV vaccine-derived viruses from some environments.

(ii) It would be desirable that future IPV be produced only with non-wild-type strains.

(iii) Details of the production, stockpiling and access requirements for IPV vaccines should be agreed by the World Health Assembly before the WHO recommendation to discontinue all polio vaccination.

Recommendations

Given that we are entering a period of unique epidemiological uncertainty, expert groups should formulate predictions, and their underlying arguments, explicitly, and these should be openly evaluated against what actually transpires.

The recommendations below are intended for a hypothetical scenario of a world that has stopped polio vaccination. At this point, it is uncertain which option for stopping vaccination will be employed, if any.

Policy

(i) active surveillance of paralytic polio, including maintenance of the global polio laboratory network, should be maintained as a high priority before and for at least five years after ceasing polio vaccination. After that period, surveillance for poliomyelitis cases should continue indefinitely;

(ii) strenuous efforts should be made to minimize delays from clinical onset of polio to final virological confirmation, serotyping and intratypic differentiation (i.e., distinction between wild and vaccine-derived virus);

(iii) after stopping use of OPV, all poliovirus work, except primary isolation and serotyping, should be restricted to a few laboratories working under high-level containment (safe means must be found for quality control of laboratories undertaking primary isolation);

(iv) a stockpile of at least 500 million doses of each of the three types of monovalent OPV vaccine should be maintained in case of an outbreak of polio after ceasing vaccination. At least 100 million doses should constantly be available in 20-dose vials for immediate shipment;

(v) OPV vaccine manufacturer capacity must be maintained for global use in two laboratories. This production should be continuous, to ensure maintenance of production capability;

(vi) the need for IPV vaccines in the post-eradication era should be reassessed after ceasing OPV vaccination, in particular with regard to their use in eradicating the circulation of vaccine-derived viruses;

(vii) poliovirus vaccines stockpiled for global use should be owned and controlled by the WHO, who should be formally responsible for their release in any particular situation;

(viii) the WHO should ensure that the capacity for planning and overseeing the control of poliovirus outbreaks be maintained in the post-eradication era;

(ix) the WHO should develop a model protocol for responding to the occurrence of cases of polio or poliovirus infections. As part of the certification process of polio eradication, countries should adopt these protocols to local conditions. It is likely that outbreak response should involve the vaccination of at least all children under five years of age, and all individuals born since ceasing vaccination in the populations concerned, which would extend appreciably beyond areas already known to be infected.

Research

(i) Research on more rapid diagnostic tools to confirm poliovirus infection (e.g. serology or direct PCR) deserves high priority;

(ii) Methods for enhancing the sensitivity of environmental surveillance for polioviruses (e.g. through sampling sewage) remain important, and their further development deserves high priority. Such technology may be invaluable in monitoring the disappearance of OPV viruses after ceasing OPV vaccination, and in ascertaining the extent of spread of polioviruses should they reappear in the post-eradication and post-vaccination era;

(iii) Research on the transmissibility of vaccine-derived polioviruses is of high priority. Special studies should be mounted to coincide with the ceasing vaccination in order to monitor any persistence of OPV.

ANNEX

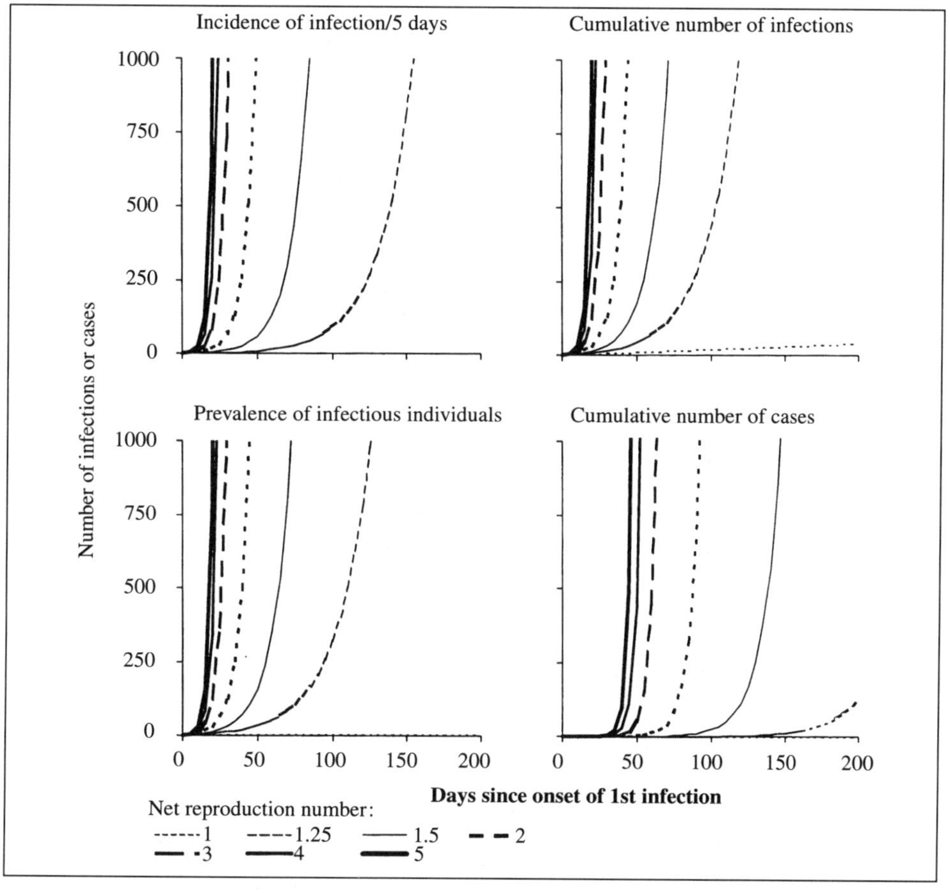

Predicted incidence and cumulative incidence of polio virus infections, prevalence of infectious individuals and the cumulative number of paralytic cases expected at different time intervals after the introduction of polio virus into a population, for different values for the net reproduction number. Calculations assume a single infected individual at the outset, that individuals remain infectious for 28 days, and that one in every 200 infected individuals suffers paralytic disease after an incubation period of 10 days. The serial interval (average time interval between onset of infection of successive cases in a chain of transmission) is assumed to be five days.

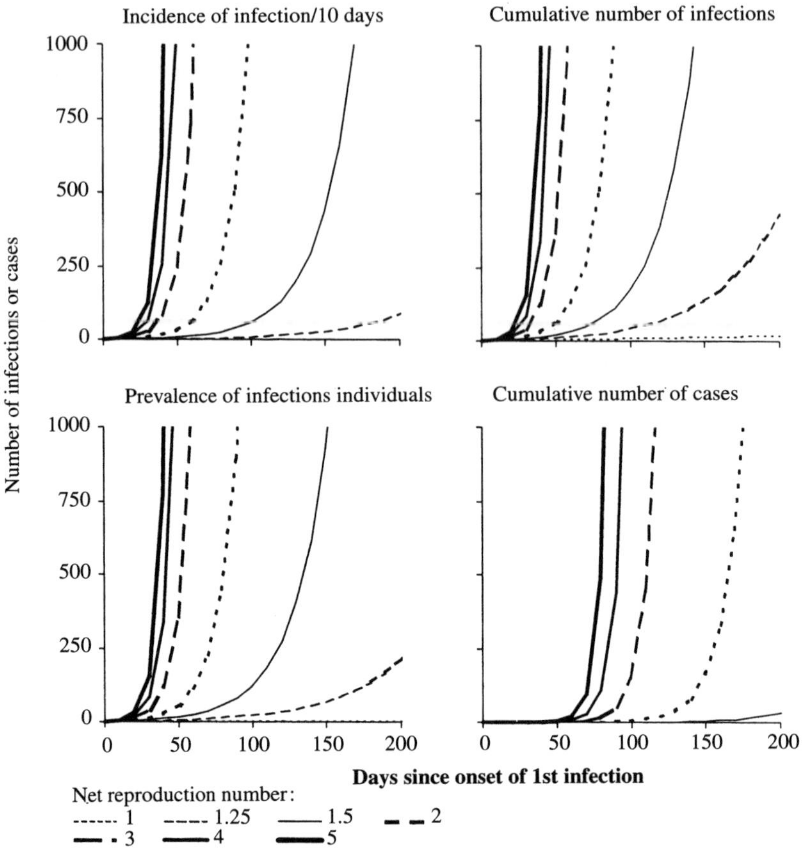

Predicted incidence and cumulative incidence of polio virus infections, prevalence of infectious individuals and the cumulative number of paralytic cases expected at different time intervals after the introduction of polio virus into a population, for different values for the net reproduction number. Calculations assume a single infected individual at the outset, that individuals remain infectious for 28 days, and that one in every 200 infected individuals suffers paralytic disease after an incubation period of 10 days. The serial interval (average time interval between onset of infection of successive cases in a chain of transmission) is assumed to be 10 days.

Acknowledgements

The authors thank Dr E Vynnycky for important contributions to the text and Annex of this document, respectively, and Drs S Cochi, C de Quadros, W Dowdle. O Kew, M Pallansch, P Patriarca, and R Sanders for helpful comments. PEMF's contribution was supported in part by WHO.

References

1 Sutter RW, Patriarca PA: Inactivated and live, attenuated poliovirus vaccines: mucosal immunity, in Kurstak E (ed): Measles and Poliomyelitis. Vaccines, Immunization, and Control. Wien, Austria, Springer Verlag, 1993:22:279-294.

2 Nishio O, Ishihara Y, Sakae K, Nonmura Y, Kuno A, Yasukawa S, Inoue H, Miyamura K, Kono R: The trend of acquired immunity with live poliovirus vaccine and the effect of revaccination: Followup of vaccinees for 10 years. J Biol Stand 1984;12:1-10.

3 Racaniello VR, Baltimore D: Cloned poliovirus complementary DNA is infectious in mammalian cells. Science 1981;214:916-919.

4 Wood D, Sutter RW, Dowdle W: Stopping vaccination following poliomyelitis eradication: Issues and challenges. Bull WHO 2000;78:347-357.

5 Vaccines and Biologicals Department. WHO Global Plan of Action for Laboratory Containment of Wild Polioviruses. Geneva, Switzerland: World Health Organization, WHO/V&B/99,32.

6 Eichner M, Dietz K: Eradication of poliomyelitis: when can one be sure that polio virus transmission has been terminated. Am J Epidemiol 1996;143:816-822.

7 Prevots DR, Ciofi degli Atti ML, Sallabanda A, Diamante E, Aylward RB, Kakariqqi E, Fiore L, Ylli A, van der Avoort H, Sutter RW, Tozzi AE, Panei P, Schineia N, Genovese D, Oblapenko G, Greco D, Wassilak SGF: Outbreak of paralytic poliomyelitis in Albania, 1996: High attack rate among adults and apparent interruption of transmission following nationwide mass vaccination. Clin Infect Dis 1998;26:419-425.

8 Sabin AB: Paralytic consequences of poliomyelitis infection in different parts of the world and in different population groups. Am J Public Health 1951;41:1215-1230.

9 Fine PEM, Carneiro IAM: Transmissibility and persistence of oral polio vaccine viruses. Implications for the global poliomyelitis eradication initiative. Am J Epidemiol 1999;150:1001-1021.

10 CDC. Circulation of a Type 2 vaccine derived poliovirus - Egypt, 1982-1993. MMWR 2001;50:41-42, 51.

11 CDC. Public Health Dispatch: Outbreak of Poliomyelitis - Dominican Republic and Haiti, 2000-2001. MMWR 2001;50:147-148.

12 CDC. Apparent global interruption of wild poliovirus type 2 transmission. MMWR 2001;50:222-224.

13 Patriarca PA, Sutter RW, Oostvogel PM: Outbreaks of paralytic poliomyelitis, 1976-1995. J Infect Dis 1997;175(suppl1):S165-172.

14 Domok I: Experience associated with the use of live poliovirus vaccine in Hungary, 1959-1982. Rev Infect Dis 1984;6(suppl2):S413-418.

Dr. P.E.M. Fine, London School of Hygiene and Tropical Medicine, Keppel Street, London WC1E 7HT, U.K.

Brown F (ed): Progress in Polio Eradication: Vaccine Strategies for the End Game.
Dev Biol. Basel, Karger, 2001, vol 105, pp 149-150

ROUNDTABLE DISCUSSION

What are the Gaps in our Scientific Knowledge Relevant to Stopping Polio Immunisation?

D. Wood

National Institute for Biological Standards and Control, Potters Bar, U.K.

The roundtable identified a number of important gaps in our current knowledge. These included the following:

(i) The frequency and duration of long-term carriage in a variety of different country settings. Related to this were the risks that long-term excretors would pose for reintroduction of polioviruses into future unimmunised communities. It was suggested that mathematical modelling be applied to evaluate different scenarios, ranging from the known situation of the presence of a single long-term excretor in a population to the hypothetical situation of hundreds of long-term excretors. Development of such models would be considerably aided by more knowledge of the natural history of long-term polio excretion such as the sites and titres of shed viruses and the transmissibility of such viruses to family members. Environmental studies around identified long-term excretors would also be very informative.

(ii) More studies are urgently needed to supplement studies in progress of polio infections in HIV-infected persons. This should include studies of the natural history of polio in HIV-infected persons such as whether they excrete poliovirus for longer or at higher titres than usual.

(iii) The risk of OPV-derived viruses establishing wild type transmissibility. In this context the excellent studies from Cuba which suggest this will not occur need to be extended to other countries, particularly with lower hygiene/ higher density settings. In addition, the search for viruses similar to the recombinant Sabin 2 strains from Egypt that showed wild-type characteristics needs to be extended. A number of studies of OPV circulation in countries that switch to IPV would also help in this context.

(iv) There are important gaps in our knowledge about new vaccines or re-formulations of the current trivalent OPV. In particular it was pointed out that licences for monovalent OPV may have lapsed in many countries and if mOPV was to be stockpiled for potential emergency use, this needed to be reviewed quickly and, if necessary, dialogue initiated with regulatory authorities on how to expedite re-licencing.

(v) Work was needed to establish a mechanism, which included appropriate verification, for recall of unused OPV after OPV immunisation stops. These stocks were likely to be much more widely distributed than laboratory stocks of wild poliovirus; hence the logistics of such an exercise were likely to be an order of magnitude more complex.

(vi) Improved methods to detect silent circulation of polioviruses in a population are required, including efforts to exclude the hypothetical occurrence of cryptic excretion of poliovirus that may not be detected by conventional virus culture methods. Furthermore it was suggested that the independent global certification commission criterion for certification that requires the absence of wild poliovirus circulation for three years in the presence of good quality surveillance might not be achievable in all countries, especially in Africa. Alternative criteria may need to be considered in case this concern becomes a reality.

(vii) A gap in funding to support this research and the continued use of vaccines was identified, should stopping immunisation need to be delayed much beyond the projected timescale. This will need vigorous advocacy to rectify.

(viii) Manufacturers needed clear guidance on the types and quantities of vaccine needed in the period between certification and cessation of immunisation and in the stockpiles that will be needed in the post-immunisation era. The mechanisms for achieving a co-ordinated cessation of immunisation, especially for OPV, need to be determined.

(ix) As well as the virological and epidemiological considerations, it was also suggested that attention be given to the socio-economic and political dimensions of when and how to stop immunisation.

Dr. D. Wood, N.I.B.S.C., Blanche Lame, South Mimms, Potters Bar, Herts EN6 3QG, U.K.

Brown F (ed): Progress in Polio Eradication: Vaccine Strategies for the End Game.
Dev Biol. Basel, Karger, 2001, vol 105, p 151

SESSION VII

Possible Strategies for Stopping Immunisation

Chairperson: *Sir Joe Smith*

Brown F (ed): Progress in Polio Eradication: Vaccine Strategies for the End Game.
Dev Biol. Basel, Karger, 2001, vol 105, pp 153-158

Possible Global Strategies for Stopping Polio Vaccination and How They Could be Harmonized

S.L. Cochi, R.W. Sutter, R.B. Aylward

Centers for Disease Control and Prevention, National Immunization Program, Vaccine-Preventable Disease Eradication Division, Atlanta, GA, USA

Global Polio Eradication Initiative, Department of Vaccines & Biologicals, Geneva, Switzerland

Abstract: One of the challenges of the polio eradication initiative over the next few years will be the formulation of an optimal strategy for stopping poliovirus vaccination after global certification of polio eradication has been accomplished. This strategy must maximize the benefits and minimize the risks. A number of strategies are currently under consideration, including: (i) synchronized global discontinuation of use of oral poliovirus vaccine (OPV); (ii) regional or subregional coordinated OPV discontinuation; and (iii) moving from trivalent to bivalent or monovalent OPV. Other options include moving from OPV to global use of IPV for an interim period before cessation of IPV use (to eliminate circulation of vaccine-derived poliovirus, if necessary) or development of new OPV strains that are not transmissible. Each of these strategies is associated with specific advantages (financial benefits for OPV discontinuation) and disadvantages (cost of switch to IPV) and inherent uncertainties (risk of continued poliovirus circulation in certain populations or prolonged virus replication in immunodeficient persons). An ambitious research agenda addresses the remaining questions and issues. Nevertheless, several generalities are already clear. Unprecedented collaboration between countries, regions, and indeed the entire world will be required to implement a global OPV discontinuation strategy. Regulatory approval will be needed for an interim bivalent OPV or for monovalent OPV in many countries. Manufacturers will need sufficient lead time to produce sufficient quantities of IPV. Finally, the financial implications for any of these strategies need to be considered. Whatever strategy is followed it will be necessary to stockpile supplies of a poliovirus-containing vaccine (most probably all three types of monovalent OPV), and to develop contingency plans to respond should an outbreak of polio occur after stopping vaccination.

Introduction

Global progress towards polio eradication continues to proceed rapidly such that the initiative remains on target for the complete eradication of naturally occurring polio within the next two years, and global certification by the year 2005 [1]. The anticipated time frame for interrupting poliovirus transmission, and for certification, containment, and cessation of OPV administration is outlined in Figure 1.

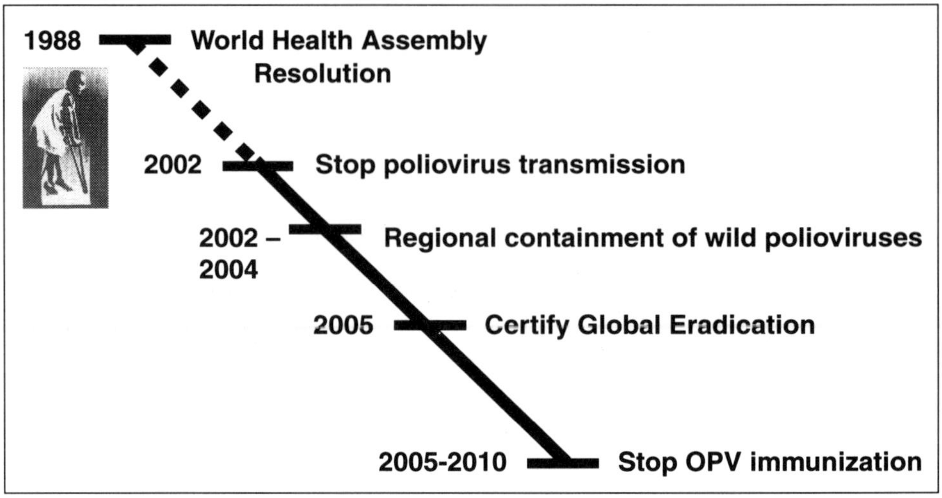

Fig. 1: Polio eradication timeline.

No country can stop polio immunization safely until wild polioviruses have been eradicated globally. One of the challenges of the polio eradication initiative over the next few years will be the formulation of an optimal strategy to stop poliovirus vaccination after global certification of eradication has been accomplished. This strategy must both maximize the benefits and minimize the risks.

The rapid progress being achieved towards the global eradication of wild polioviruses makes it imperative that WHO be prepared to recommend a strategy for stopping immunization when global eradication is imminent. This will permit the strategy to be implemented as quickly as possible after eradication is certified globally and maximize its benefits. Since 1997, increasing attention has been focused on potential strategies for stopping immunization once eradication has been achieved [2-5].

The single issue that dominates the debate on strategies for stopping immunization is whether vaccine-derived poliovirus strains (VDPV) will continue to circulate after the use of OPV is discontinued [2-5]. Should this occur, vaccine-derived strains could, theoretically, revert to fully neurovirulent strains. Persistent circulation could occur if VDPV excreted by the last cohorts of vaccinees established chains of transmission in new cohorts of non-OPV vaccinated individuals. Alternatively, VDPV from persistently infected, immunocompromised individuals could potentially spread to and circulate in the general population [6-8].

Strategies for Stopping Immunization

If evidence does not indicate a risk of continued circulation of VDPV strains, then what are the options for discontinuing OPV vaccination? This issue was discussed at length in 1998 at a WHO-sponsored meeting on the scientific basis for stopping polio immunization [4]. It was concluded that «OPV vaccination should stop and IPV vaccination can stop when there is:

1. eradication of wild-type polioviruses;
2. laboratory containment of stocks; and
3. evidence that VDPV will circulate for only a limited period.»

Thus, any scenario for stopping vaccination must be preceded by a process in which each country and region is certified as polio-free (Fig. 2). The most important criterion for certification of a country, a region, or indeed the world, is the absence of polio virus isolation for at least three years in the presence of excellent surveillance [9].

While it is not possible at present to recommend a definitive strategy for stopping immunization, only a limited number of possible strategies can be envisaged (Fig. 3) [2-5]. Each of the possible strategies has vaccine supply and quality issues which must be addressed, so the options must continue to be assessed on a continuing basis. Besides the option of «no change» (i.e., continuation of universal childhood vaccination with OPV), these options include the following:

(i) coordinated cessation of OPV simultaneously worldwide, or country-by-country;

(ii) global use of IPV for a limited interim period or indefinitely;

(iii) sequential removal of one or two of the Sabin strains from OPV or use of monovalent OPV; or

(iv) development and use of new vaccines, either live or inactivated, for an interim period.

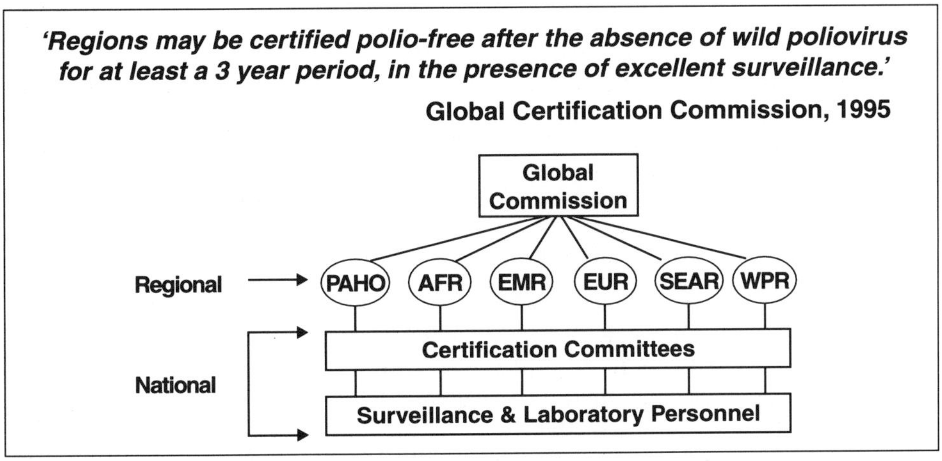

Fig. 2: Containment and certification.

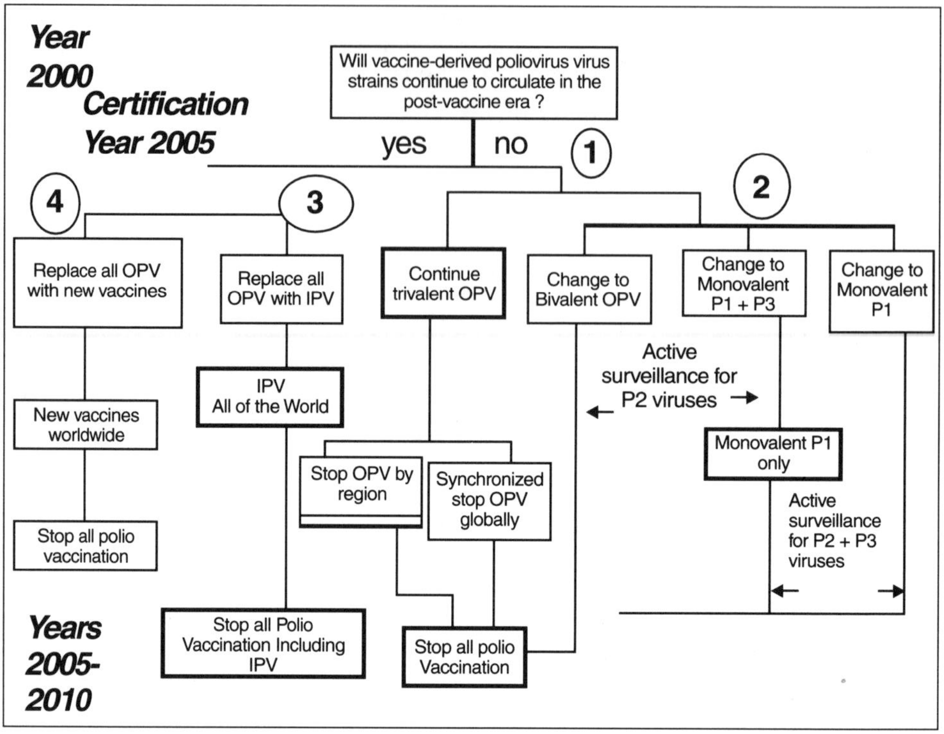

Fig. 3: A decision tree for stopping polio vaccination.

The simplest and least costly strategy would be simply to stop immunization with OPV. While each of the above options requires further evaluation, the discontinuation of OPV in a synchronised effort worldwide remains the most plausible strategy. Ideally, cessation would be coordinated between countries to reduce the chances of cross border transmission of VDPV. A final series of mass campaigns may be necessary to maximize population immunity before stopping vaccination.

Another approach would be to stop administration of the three Sabin types sequentially. Because type 2 wild virus disappears quickly with effective implementation of immunization programmes, it would probably be the first vaccine strain removed. This option has the potential advantage of allowing monitoring of the effect of stopping vaccination against one serotype (type 2) following its apparent eradication-essentially serving as a preliminary «trial» of stopping vaccination altogether. Either a bivalent type 1 and 3 vaccine or monovalent vaccines could be used. For a bivalent vaccine, however, safety and efficacy trials would be required to gain regulatory approval, which pose substantial difficulties in gaining such approval [10-11]. If both wild types 1 and 3 have been eradicated, then monovalent type 1 vaccine could be considered, which has an historical record for both routine use and outbreak control, so regulatory concerns may be fewer. It is important to note that all these strategy options are only interim solutions, and require selection of a final strategy downstream.

If VDPV do circulate persistently, the IPV could be used for an interim period of, as yet, undefined length [4,11]. However, the effectiveness and feasibility of this strategy must be validated. This would also be the most costly strategy. The immunogenicity of IPV in developing countries cannot be inferred from studies in industrialized countries. One recent study of IPV administered in developing countries using WHO's current infant immunization schedule (6, 10 and 14 weeks of age) demonstrated a suboptimal serological response. Low routine immunization coverage in populations at the highest risk for persistent circulation may also limit the effectiveness of an IPV strategy. If implemented, IPV could be administered efficiently in a combination product with DTP and, possibly, other antigens. Vaccine manufacturers have indicated that five to seven years would be required to establish a global IPV production capacity. Manufacturers would also need to be assured that they would recover their investment before expanding their facilities. To evaluate an IPV strategy, it would be useful to monitor the disappearance of VDPV in polio-free countries changing from OPV to IPV.

New vaccine strains for either OPV or IPV vaccine might be useful in the final stages of vaccination [12]. However, there would be a lengthy and costly process to gain regulatory approval. An exception may be the production of IPV from Sabin strains, with which three manufacturers have reported previous experience. Such a vaccine would simplify future containment requirements during vaccine manufacture and increase the safety margin in case of inadvertent release. Continued research on candidate new vaccines should continue, but an aggressive approach will be required from researchers, industry and regulatory authorities for any candidate vaccines to reach clinical trials.

Summary and Conclusions

Manufacturing and regulatory issues need to be resolved regarding a decision to undertake any of the following vaccination strategies: (i) bivalent OPV; (ii) large-scale use of monovalent OPV; (iii) global IPV use, which does not appear feasible at present; and (iv) use of new vaccine strains for either OPV or IPV.

Progress toward polio eradication has come so far that we are fortunate now, at this stage of the eradication initiative, to be able to consider and seek consensus on how to stop vaccination. An important theme underlying all such considerations is that global and regional certification procedures, laboratory virus containment issues, and strategy decisions about stopping polio vaccination are interrelated, requiring close coordination of the respective plans of action that address these issues.

The decision-making process for stopping polio vaccination will be greatly assisted by identifying relevant research questions and aggressively implementing a research agenda to address them [5]. Before determining how to stop polio vaccination, further scientific study is needed of: (i) the persistence of VDPV in immunodeficient persons and in under-immunized populations; and (ii) the potential, if any, for spread of virus from immunodeficient individuals to the non-immune general population.

Whatever strategy is used it will be necessary to stockpile supplies of both OPV and (possibly) IPV, and to develop contingency plans to respond should an outbreak of polio occur after vaccination is stopped.

References

1 Centers for Disease Control and Prevention. Progress toward global eradication of poliomyelitis, 1999. MMWR 2000;49:349-354.

2 Cochi SL, Sutter RW, Kew OM, Pallansch MA, Dowdle WA: Decision tree for stopping polio immunization. Presented at the Technical Consultation on the Global Eradication of Poliomyelitis, Geneva, 28-29 April, 1997.

3 Cochi SL, Sutter RW, Kew OM, Pallansch MA, Dowdle WR: Possible strategies for stopping polio immunization. Meeting on the scientific basis for stopping immunization against poliomyelitis, Geneva, 23-25 March 1998. (unpublished WHO document WHO/EPI/POLIO/SIM.98/WP1.2).

4 Expanded Programme on Immunization, Global Programme for Vaccines and Immunization. Global eradication of poliomyelitis: "Report of the Meeting on the Scientific Basis for Stopping Immunization Against Poliomyelitis", Geneva, 23-25 March 1998. (unpublished WHO/EPI/GEN/98.12).

5 Wood DJ, Sutter RW, Dowdle WR: Stopping poliovirus vaccination after eradication: issues and challenges. Bull WHO 2000;78:347-357.

6 Davis LE, Bodian D, Price D, Butler IJ, Vickers JH: Chronic progressive poliomyelitis secondary to vaccination of an immunodeficient child. N Engl J Med 1977;297:241-245.

7 Hara M, Saito Y, Komatsu T, Kodama H, Abo W, Chiba S, Nakao T: Antigenic analysis of polioviruses isolated from a child with agammaglobulinemia after Sabin vaccine administration. Microb Immunol 1981;25:905-913.

8 Kew OM, Sutter RW, Nottay BK, McDonough MJ, Prevots DR, Quick L, Pallansch MA: Prolonged replication of a type 1 vaccine-derived poliovirus in an immunodeficient patient. J Clin Microbiol 1998;36:2893-2899.

9 Global Programme for Vaccines and Immunization. "Report of the First Meeting of the Global Commission for the Certification of the Eradication of Poliomyelitis". Geneva, World Health Organization, 1995 (unpublished WHO document WHO/EPI/GEN/95.6).

10 Milstien J: Manufacturing and regulatory considerations for a "2-less OPV" or a "global IPV" strategy. Presented at the Technical Consultation on the Global Eradication of Poliomyelitis, Geneva, 28-29 April, 1997.

11 Milstien J: Feasibility of a global IPV strategy and sequential removal of Sabin strains. Meeting on the scientific basis for stopping immunization against poliomyelitis, Geneva, 23-25 March 1998. (unpublished WHO document WHO/EPI/POLIO/SIM.98/WP6.1).

12 Department of Vaccines and Biologicals. "Report of the Meeting on New Polio Vaccines for the Post-Eradication Era". Geneva, World Health Organization, 2000 (in press).

Dr. S.L. Cochi, Centers for Disease Control and Prevention, National Immunization Program, Mailstop E-05, 1600 Clifton Road, NE, Atlanta, GA 30333, USA.

Brown F (ed): Progress in Polio Eradication: Vaccine Strategies for the End Game.
Dev Biol. Basel, Karger, 2001, vol 105, p 159

Roundtable Discussion

Possible Strategies for Stopping Immunisation

D.J. Wood

The discussants agreed that at the moment it was not possible to recommend a single strategy of when and how to stop immunisation. At present the thinking in policy development needs to remain flexible and irrevocable steps should not yet be taken. However, this makes it difficult for manufacturers to predict what to do. A decision therefore must be taken soon. The discussants recognised that some countries may wish to buy time to see if long-term excretors will be a problem in the post-OPV era and may unilaterally elect to continue to use IPV after a co-ordinated cessation of OPV. Strategies are urgently needed to contain the spread, if any, of virus from long-term excretors to provide an alternative course of action. These new strategies should be built into the current options being considered for stopping immunisation. The occurrence of a few long-term excretors may not preclude global cessation of OPV nor require the global use of IPV.

An important consideration is the need to build political consensus on how to stop OPV immunisation. This may be difficult to achieve, and therefore deserves special attention. Particular difficulties were envisaged if some countries unilaterally elect to continue with IPV after cessation of OPV is recommended globally. The global use of IPV for an interim period after global OPV cessation was strongly advocated by some discussants, but strongly opposed by others and remains the most controversial of the potential strategies. There was general agreement that introduction of a new live attenuated vaccine was extremely unlikely at this stage but research, including limited clinical evaluation, should continue so we know as much as possible about the various candidates before studies of poliovirus vaccines become impossible.

Dr. D. Wood, N.I.B.S.C., Blanche Lane, South Mimms, Potters Bar, Herts EN6 3QG, U.K.

Brown F (ed): Progress in Polio Eradication: Vaccine Strategies for the End Game.
Dev Biol. Basel, Karger, 2001, vol 105, p 161

SESSION VIII

What Vaccines Could be Used Post Eradication if They Were Needed

Chairperson: *John Petricciani*

Brown F (ed): Progress in Polio Eradication: Vaccine Strategies for the End Game.
Dev Biol. Basel, Karger, 2001, vol 105, pp 163-169

Progress with Inactivated Poliovirus Vaccines Derived from the Sabin Strains

Y. Doi, S. Abe, H. Yamamoto, H. Horie, H. Ohyama, K. Satoh, Y. Tano, Y. Ota, M. Miyazawa, K. Wakabayashi, S. Hashizume

Japan Poliomyelitis Research Institute, 5-34-4, Kumegawa-cho, Higashimurayama-shi, Tokyo, Japan

Key words: IPV, inactivated poliovirus vaccine, D-antigen, Sabin strains

Abstract: To produce a safe and effective inactivated poliovirus vaccine (IPV), we have developed S-IPV using Vero cells infected with the Sabin strains in a semi-production scale. All production steps including virus culture on microcarrier beads were highly reproducible. Mean recovery percents of infectious viruses or D-antigens during all processes for concentration, purification and inactivation were 30-50% in the three types. The S-IPV potency was adjusted for D-antigen content as determined by in-house ELISA and was comparable to WHO reference IPV derived from the virulent strains in immunogenicity tests in rats. Antibody development in more than 30 seronegative infant volunteers after two shots of S-IPV at four-week interval were 100% without notable adverse reactions. The mean antibody titres ($\log_2$) to Sabin 1, 2 and 3 viruses were 11.1, 8.3 and 8.9, respectively. The antibodies neutralized the Mahoney, MEF-1, and Saukett virulent strains with slightly inferior titres to those of the Sabin strains. D-antigens for each type of S-IPV were stable at 4°C without any significant decrease over more than two years.

Introduction

There is an international consensus that each country has to provide immunization against poliovirus until there are no cases of wild poliovirus-induced paralysis in the world [1]. It is also known that vaccine-associated paralytic polio (VAPP) is unavoidable while we use OPV, although VAPP is very rare. VAPP is a burden not only to the patients but also to manufacturers and to the governments that must provide immunization against polio with OPV in countries where wild polioviruses have already been eradicated. We have been developing a safe polio vaccine derived from the Sabin strains to contribute toward elimination of VAPP and eradication of polio.

Materials and Methods

Cells and viruses

Manufacturer's working cell bank (MWCB) at the 134-passage level was established from an ampoule of Vero cells purchased from ATCC at the 124-passage level. The cells from the MWCB at the 140-passage level, which should be used for virus culture, and the 150-passage level, passed all the tests for WHO requirements [2].

Seed viruses, Sabin type 1 (LSc, 2ab), type 2 (P712, Ch, 2ab) and type 3 (Leon, $12a_1b$) that have been used for OPV production, were used for virus culture.

Vaccine preparation

Vero cells for virus culture were prepared on microcarrier beads (Cytodex 1, Pharmacia Biotech, Sweden) in a 14LCelligen Plus glass vessel (New Brunswick Scientific, USA). Pooled virus fluid was concentrated and purified mainly by the method of van Wezel et al [3]. The virus fluid was concentrated by ultrafiltration (Pall Filtron, USA), and then further concentrated by ultracentrifugation at 100,000g for four hours and the pellet was resuspended in 0.1M PB (phosphate-buffered solution). The highly concentrated virus fluid was subjected to filtration through a DEAE Sepharose CL-6B column (Pharmacia Biotech, Sweden) and eluted with 0.1M PB. Fractions that had absorption ratios at 260nm/280nm greater than 1.5 were pooled as purified virus fluid. Before inactivation, the purified virus fluid was diluted about 10 times with M-199 (Earle's base solution without Ca, Mg, PO_4 and phenol red, Dainihon Seiyaku Co. Japan), glycine added to 0.5%, and then filtered through a 0.2μm pore filter. Each filtered virus fluid was inactivated with 0.025% formalin for 12 days at 37°C. Test samples taken from all production steps were assayed in accordance with WHO requirements [4]. Some S-IPV lots were blended with each type of monovalent IPV to make an expected D-antigen content, diluting with M-199 as mentioned above. As a preservative, 2-phenoxethanol was added to 0.5% and the pH adjusted to 7.1-7.3. The inactivated virus fluid was filtered through a 0.45μm pore filter and distributed in siliconized glass vials.

D-antigen titration

D-antigens were quantified with an in-house sandwich ELISA. Poliovirus type and D-antigen specific mouse monoclonal antibodies for each type were used as capture antibody, and type-specific neutralizing rabbit antisera were used as detector antibodies. In-house reference D-antigens for each type of Sabin strain were determined with reference to WHO S-IPV (91/672 supplied courtesy of Dr D.J.Wood, NIBSC) [5] by ELISA. D-antigen titres of test samples were then measured against in-house reference D-antigens by parallel line assay.

Potency tests in rats

Immunogenicity of vaccines was measured by the method of Steenis et al [6]. Briefly, undiluted and three-fold dilutions of test vaccine were diluted 1:2 and injected once intramuscularly with 0.5mL of the vaccine to the left and right legs of 10-12 Wistar rats per vaccine dilution. After three weeks, blood samples were collected from each rat. For a two-injection test in rats, a vaccine containing the same antigen dose was injected three weeks after the first injection, and blood was collected two weeks after the second inoculation. All sera from the rats were tested for neutralizing antibody.

Neutralization test

Neutralizing antibody titration for rat and human sera was performed by the micromethod using HEp-2C cells. Serial two-fold dilutions for each sample were made in duplicate wells starting from a 1:4 dilution, and were challenged with viral 32-320 $CCID_{50}$ for each type of Sabin or virulent strain. Serum and virus mixtures were incubated at 36°C for three hours and kept at 4°C overnight. Antibody titres were expressed as the highest dilution of 50% CPE suppression in $\log_2$.

Clinical tests in adult and infant volunteers

Phase 1 clinical tests were performed in accordance with GCP requirements of Japan. Phase 2/3 clinical tests have been proceeding under the new GCP of Japan. In phase 1 clinical test, 10 healthy male adult volunteers without a history of polio vaccination were inoculated with S-IPV. As a control group, five healthy adults were immunized following the same schedule, but were inoculated with M-199 without antigens. For the 2/3 phase clinical test, healthy infant volunteers from 14 different hospitals with no history of polio vaccination were added to the trial.

Results

Vaccine preparation

In our experience the burst size of infectious virus from an infected Vero cell is about one half compared to that of primary monkey kidney cells. But this weakness is compensated for by using Vero cells in a tight monolayer on micro-beads in the microcarrier system – Celligen Plus. Virus titres of each type of single harvest were 10 9.2-9.4 $CCID_{50}$/mL.

Mean recovery of infectious virus by ultrafiltration was 60-80%. Virus recovery from ultracentrifugation to DEAE chromatography was 50-75%, and D-antigen recovery between pre- and post-inactivation was 70-80%. Total recovery from crude virus to the end of inactivation was around 30-50%.

Table 1 shows the purity of virus in fluid during the production processes. The final product of trivalent S-IPV, 0.5mL per human dose, has acceptable purity by WHO IPV requirements [4].

Table 1: Purity of virus fluid during production process.

Production process	Volume	Protein (mg/mL)	Cellular DNA (ng/mL)	Bovine albumin (mg/mL)
Crude virus fluid	600	100-300	100-1000	40
Pooled virus fluid (0.2 mm filtrate)	600	100-300	<0.04	n.t.
Concentrated by ultra filt.	20	300-900	n.t.	500
Concentrated by u.c.f.g.	1	n.t.	n.t.	74
Gel filtrate	1	250-800	n.t.	<0.001
Monovalent S-IPV	10	25-80	<0.04	<0.001
Trivalent S-IPV	50-120	0.6-16	<0.04	<0.001

n.t. = not tested.

To make S-IPV with immunogenicity comparable to WHO V-IPV (91/547, D-antigen content for types 1, 2 and 3 are 40, 10 and 30 units, respectively) [7], some S-IPV lots composed of different D-antigen contents were given once to rats. Figure 1 shows the mean neutralizing antibody titres of 10-12 rats and seroconversion rates for the rats. Type 1 S-IPV showed superior immunogenicity to type 1 V-IPV, and type 2 S-IPV; WHO S-IPV (91/672) [5], showed poorer immunogenicity than type 2 V-IPV (WHO 91/574). Type 3 S-IPV showed slightly inferior (1:1.5) immunogenicity to type 3 V-IPV. From these experiments, D-antigen contents in S-IPV were tentatively set at 30 units/0.5mL/dose for types 1 and 2, and 50 units for type 3.

Stability of S-IPV

Stability of D-antigens in S-IPV at different temperatures was tested at –20°, 4°, 25° and 36°C. D-antigens for each type of S-IPV were very stable at 4°C, showing no decrease over two years. At 25°C, D-antigen content gradually

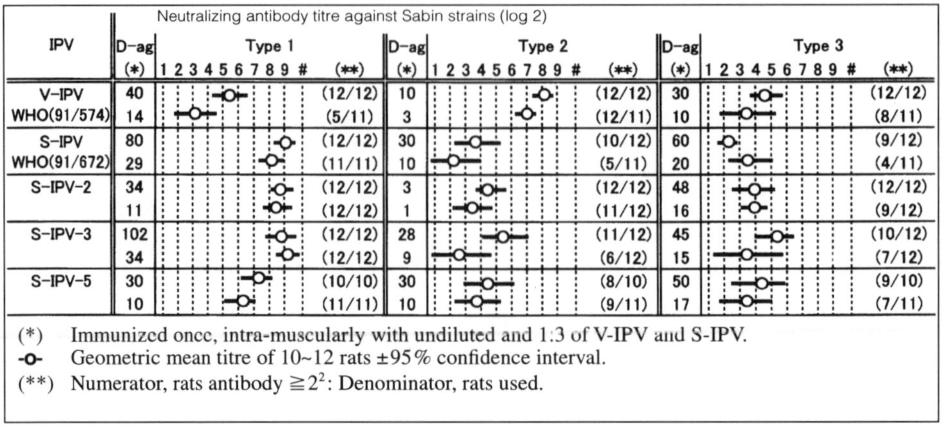

Fig. 1: Antibody development in rats inoculated with different D-antigen contents of V-IPV and S-IPV.

decreased, but the half-life was not less than 12 months. Storage at –20°C was not suitable for S-IPV, and stability was worse at 37°C.

Neutralizing antibody development in human volunteers

The products of S-IPV-5 comprising 30, 30 and 50 D-antigen units for types 1, 2 and 3 were given twice, 0.5mL each subcutaneously to adults, and serum samples were collected on the days of the first and second immunizations and two weeks after the second immunization. Neutralizing antibody titres per person against Sabin and virulent strains are shown in Figure 2. Seroconversion or booster effects of S-IPV were evident and the antibodies also neutralized the virulent strains.

The immunization schedule for the infant volunteers was as follows. The lot of S-IPV-11 composed of a similar D-antigen content to S-IPV-5 was given twice, 0.5mL each, subcutaneously at four week intervals. Two weeks after the second S-IPV inoculation, a dose of conventional OPV was administered orally. Serum samples were collected from each infant on the days of the first S-IPV inoculation, two weeks after the second S-IPV, and six weeks after OPV administration. All sero-negative infants developed higher antibody levels (Table 2), and types 1 and 3 antibodies seemed to plateau after two immunizations with S-IPV. Infant neutralizing antibodies also showed potent neutralizing activity against virulent strains although the titres were 1/3.9, 1/2.3 and 1/1.3 times lower than those to the Sabin strains for types 1, 2 and 3 respectively.

Discussion and Conclusions

We have noticed that some inactivated antigens from the purified Sabin strains adsorbs to glass. To prevent loss of antigens during the production processes, plastic containers have been used. Siliconized glass vials were used as containers for these clinical S-IPV studies. To prevent the adsorption, Kersten et al [8] tried a number of excipients such as Tween 80, albumin, and amino acids. They con-

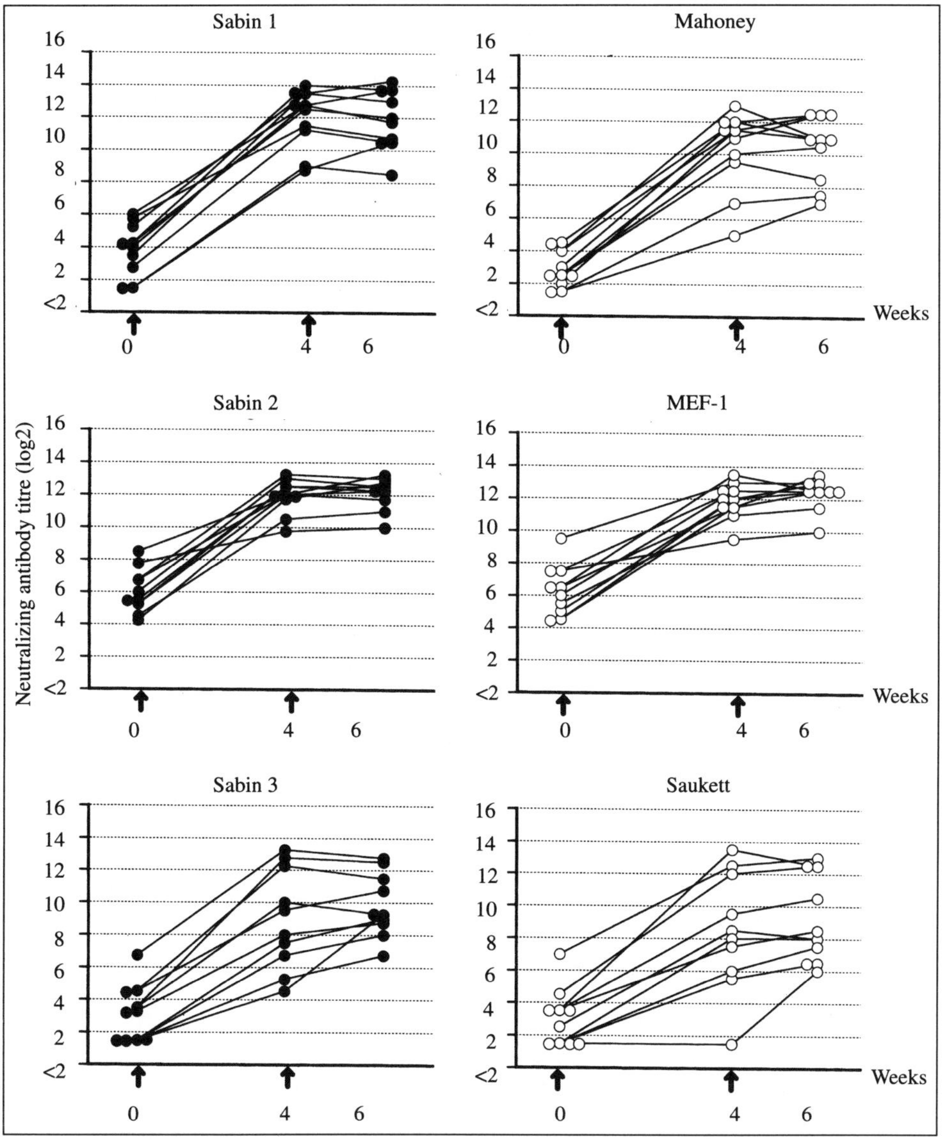

Fig. 2: Seroconversion of adult volunteers after one and two inoculations with S-IPV.
↑ S-IPV-5 ※ inoculation, 0.5 ml s.c.
※ (D-antigen content of types 1,2,3 : 30,30,50)

cluded that siliconized vials could completely prevent the adsorption. Now we are making stability tests in plastic containers for future products.

Our previous studies on S-IPV [9] show that the immunogenic potency of S-IPV as well as V-IPV can be expressed by AELV (antigenic extinction limiting

Table 2: Neutralizing antibody development in sero negative infant volunteers immunized with S-IPV and OPV.

Vaccination	Mean antibody titre against Sabin strain (log 2)		
	Type 1	Type 2	Type 3
Two doses of S-IPV[*1]	n=39 11.1±0.4[*2]	n=31 8.2±0.7	n=42 8.9±0.6
Two doses of S-IPV[*1] and 1 dose of OPV	n=26 9.9±0.4	n=20 10.1±0.7	n=28 8.8±0.9

[*1] D-antigen contents of types 1,2,3: 30,30,50.

[*2] 95 % confidence interval.

value) by immunizing guinea pigs with a few serial 10-fold dilutions of the IPV injected twice subcutaneously, at two weeks interval. This time we only tried the rat potency test (cf. WHO collaborative study [6]).

Figure 3 shows antibody development of eight or nine rats immunized with different D-antigen doses for each type of S-IPV. After the first immunization with type 2 or type 3 containing 24 and 72 D units respectively, the rats showed very poor sero-conversion, but their antibodies rose very well after the second immunization, even when immunized with lower D units. From the very good immunogenicity of S-IPV-5 and S-IPV-11 in human volunteers, we believe that two-shot immunization in rats reflects a suitable potency for human use.

There are no noticeable adverse reactions to S-IPV inoculation in adult and infant volunteers. It seems that S-IPV may be a promising candidate poliovirus vaccine to realize the WHO's Global Plan of Action for Laboratory Containment of Wild and Virulent Polioviruses.

References

1 Meeting on the scientific basis for stopping immunization against poliomyelitis. WHO/EPI/POLIO/SIM.98.WP5.3.

2 Requirements for the use of animal cells as in vitro substrates for the production of biologicals. Tech Rept Series 1998;878:19-56.

3 Wezel van AL, Steenis van G, Hannik CA, Cohn H: New approach to the production of concentrated and purified inactivated polio and rabies tissue culture vaccines, in Regamey RH (ed): Vaccinations in the Developing Countries. Dev Biol Stand. Basel, Karger, 1978, vol 41, pp 159-168.

4 Requirements for poliomyelitis vaccine (inactivated). WHO Tech Rept Seri 1982;673:40-77.

5 Wood DJ, Heath AB, Sawyer LA: A WHO collaborative study on assays of the antigenic content of inactivated poliovirus vaccines. Biologicals 1995;23:83-94.

6 Steenis van G, Wezel van AL, Sekhuis VM: Potency testing of killed polio vaccine in rats, in Hennessen W, van Wezel AL (eds): Reassessment of Inactivated Poliomyelitis Vaccine. Dev Biol Stand. Basel, Karger, 1981, vol 47, pp 119-128.

7 Wood DJ, Heath AB, Kersten GFA, Hazendonk T, Lantinga M, Beuvery EC: A new WHO international reference reagent for use in potency assays of inactivated poliomyelitis vaccine. Biologicals 1997;25:59-64.

8 Kersten G, Hazendonk T, Beuvery C: Antigenic and immunogenic properties of inactivated polio vaccine made from Sabin strains. Vaccine 1999;17:2059-2066.

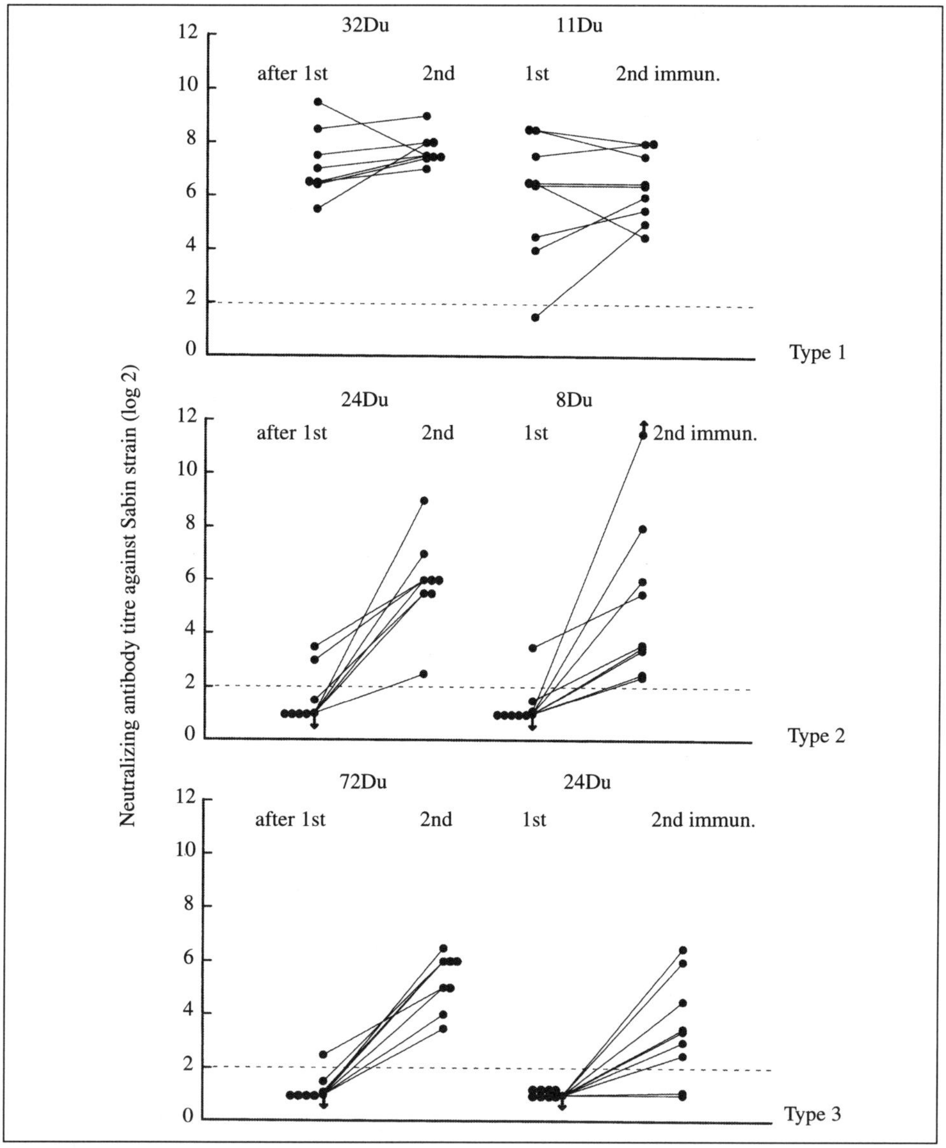

Fig. 3: Neutralizing antibody development in rats after one and two immunizations with S-IPV.

9 Abe S, Yamaki A, Doi Y, Yoshioka I: Effect of Arildon on the immunogenicity of formalin-inactivated polioviruses. Japan J Med Sci Biol 1987;21:1-13.

10 Wood DJ, Heath AB: A WHO collaborative study of immunogenicity assays of inactivated poliovirus vaccines. Biologicals 1995;23:301-311.

Dr. Y. Doi, Japan Poliomyelitis Research Institute, 5-34-4, Kumegawa-cho, Higashimurayama-shi, Tokyo 189-0003, Japan

Brown F (ed): Progress in Polio Eradication: Vaccine Strategies for the End Game.
Dev Biol. Basel, Karger, 2001, vol 105, pp 171-177

Inactivated Vaccines Based on Alternatives to Wild-Type Seed Virus

K. Chumakov[1], E. Dragunsky[1], A. Ivshina[1], J. Enterline[1], V. Wells[1], T. Nomura[2], M. Gromeier[3], E. Wimmer[3]

[1] Center for Biologics Evaluation and Research, FDA, USA
[2] Central Institute for Experimental Animals, Japan
[3] Department Microbiology, State University of New York, Stony Brook, USA

Worldwide eradication of poliomyelitis has entered its final phases, but continues to present substantial new challenges. The possibility of stopping immunization against poliomyelitis and the ways to achieve this goal are still being debated. The prevailing opinion is that before all immunization can stop, there should be an interim period when inactivated poliovirus vaccine must be used instead of live OPV. Such transition would stop circulation of all polioviruses including vaccine ones, and the careful monitoring of the epidemiological situation while affording adequate protection of the human population. In developed countries where poliomyelitis has been eradicated, the switch to IPV is already taking place. In the future, if and when routine immunization stops, there may be a need for maintaining an emergency stockpile of polio vaccines, which will require at least some limited production and use of IPV. Since current IPV is produced from virulent strains of poliovirus, vaccine production will become a major reservoir of wild-type poliovirus requiring top containment measures. Manufacture of IPV from apathogenic strains would avoid the potential danger of re-introduction of poliovirus into communities. There are two ways to address this issue. First, wild-type polioviruses used as substrates for IPV production can be genetically modified to eliminate their pathogenicity. Second, IPV can be made from attenuated Sabin strains. We have studied recombinant poliovirus strains having the 5'-UTR of rhinovirus 2 and a coding region of poliovirus and found that they retained their capacity to grow to high titres while possessing substantially reduced neurovirulence. When tested in monkeys, rhino-poliovirus chimaeras had neurovirulence comparable to that of Sabin strains. The paralytic dose on intraspinal inoculation of Tg-PVR 21 transgenic mice was about 100-fold higher than that of Sabin strains. In addition, unlike mice inoculated with the wild-type polioviruses, mice inoculated with the chimaeras exhibited only transient paralysis and survived. This shows that it is possible to create highly attenuated and vigorously replicating poliovirus strains that can be used for IPV manufacture. Both new engineered strains and Sabin strains have their advantages and disadvantages as substrates for vaccine production. Sabin strains have a well-established safety record in humans, but their immunogenicity needs further study. On the other hand, the capsid structure and antigenicity of genetically engineered strains are identical to those of wild-type strains, but their safety in humans remains unknown. Urgency of the transition to apathogenic strains for IPV production calls for a coordinated international study for evaluating the merits of both approaches.

Introduction

World-wide eradication of poliomyelitis is an unprecedented public health endeavour not only because of its scale measured by the number of countries, people, and resources involved, but also because of the number of serious and unique challenges that have to be met. It became especially clear as we approached final phases of the effort, and suddenly faced realities of the post-eradication, polio-free world which appears to be within reach, but the ways to achieve it are still unclear. It is critically important for the success of the entire effort that these final steps be taken in a considered, responsible, and scientifically sound manner to prevent any possible set-back, both in the short term, and in the distant future. It is especially important since the success of the polio eradication initiative can open doors to similar campaigns to eradicate other diseases. In contrast, its failure will result in a loss of confidence of the general public in the ability of scientific and public health communities to deliver, which ultimately will make progress of vaccinology more difficult. Thus the final steps of the eradication programme should be planned very carefully, and we should go an extra mile to ensure its ultimate and lasting succes. We must avoid controversial decisions and pursuit of short-term savings by taking shortcuts based on unfounded optimism.

What are these challenges? Perhaps the two biggest questions are whether after stopping poliovirus circulation in nature it would be safe to stop vaccination, and if so, what is the sequence of steps that should be made to ensure that such transition does not result in re-emergence of the disease. While there are a number of theoretical considerations and mathematical models that suggest that it may be safe to stop all vaccination and that re-introduction of poliovirus into circulation (from any of the number of potential sources) can be readily detected and taken care of [1,2], there is no tangible proof at this point that this can de done. Only the future course of events will show whether this is true, and we have only one chance to check this. Discussion of the reliability of poliovirus containment, impact of long-term excretion of poliovirus by some individuals [3], re-emergence by natural evolution or possibility of a malevolent release of the virus goes beyond the scope of this paper and is covered by others at this forum. These issues, however, call for gradualism in our approach to transition into a post-vaccination period, and suggest that the prudent strategy must envision an interim transition period of continued vaccination. Stopping all immunization immediately will inevitably destroy infrastructure and result in a loss of essential expertise necessary for the production and control of poliovirus vaccines, which can become a serious problem in case there is a need to replenish the emergency vaccine stockpile or to resume immunization. Vigorous and extensive monitoring of the environment should be performed during the cooling-off period, while the outstanding scientific issues need to be resolved to determine when and if ultimate cessation of vaccination will become possible. In the meantime at least limited routine immunization in developed countries and in high-risk areas throughout the world should continue.

But even this conservative approach has challenges of its own. Two vaccines that were instrumental in eradicating poliomyelitis are no longer acceptable for the post-eradication period. Some features of the vaccines that were advantageous in the early phases of eradication have become liabilities. For instance, the ability of Oral Poliovirus Vaccine (OPV) to spread and vaccinate contacts was helpful initially, but it is hardly acceptable now because of the possibility of reversions and emergence of "runaway" strains. While risk-benefit ratio was strongly in favour of this vaccine when wild-type polio was a real threat, even the extremely low rate of vaccine-associated paralysis is no longer acceptable when OPV becomes the major source of paralytic poliomyelitis. These considerations have led most industrial countries to switch to Inactivated Poliovirus Vaccine (IPV), but it has problems of its own. Besides a somewhat narrower range of protection, its major disadvantage is that currently it is being produced from virulent wild-type strains. There are documented cases of unintended re-introduction of wild-type strain from a production facility into the community [4], leaving us to wonder what could have happen if the population was not universally immune to poliovirus.

Therefore new vaccines are needed for the interim period between completion of polio eradication and stopping immunization. The best solution would be to use genetically stable strains for OPV production, so that the new vaccine inherits the efficacy and low cost of the current OPV, but will not cause vaccine-associated paralytic poliomyelitis (VAPP). There is a number of improved vaccine strains that have been proposed for this purpose, and bringing them to large-scale clinical trials must definitely be a high priority. One significant obstacle may the scale of these trials. Since the incidence of VAPP after Sabin OPV administration is of the order of one case per million doses, many millions of individuals will need to be immunized to establish unambiguously that the improved strains are safer.

Another possibility is to use avirulent strains for production of IPV, so that even if the virus accidentally escapes from production facility, this will not result in an outbreak of paralytic poliomyelitis. One obvious choice would be Sabin strains, while other possibilities include a number of genetically engineered attenuated strains. Considering the short window of opportunity available for development and evaluation of new poliovirus vaccines, all realistic options should be explored in a concerted effort of polio virologists, vaccine industry, and regulators. This is why we performed this pilot neurovirulence safety to determine whether the new recombinant poliovirus strains can be considered as substrates for IPV production.

Materials and Methods

Derivation of recombinant strains containing the 5'-UTR of rhinovirus 14 and coding region of Mahoney poliovirus type 1 (RIPO) or attenuated Sabin type 1 strain (RIPOS) were described before [6]. RL-

3 strain is a recombinant with the 5'-UTR from rhinovirus 2, and the coding region from the Leon/37 strain of type 3 poliovirus. The virus strains were grown in Vero cells, and infectious titre determined by the end-point dilution method in HEp-2c cells [5]. Neurovirulence tests in monkeys were performed according to the WHO procedure [5] with 14 Rhesus monkeys for type 1, and 24 monkeys for type 3 poliovirus. In each experiment an equal group of monkeys was inoculated with the respective reference strain (Sabin strain, U.S. Reference NC-4 for type 1, and NC-2 for type 3). Neurovirulence test in Tg-PVR21 transgenic mice was performed by intraspinal inoculation of mice with varying doses of poliovirus, and subsequent observation for clinical signs for 14 days.

Results

Initial studies of chimaeras between the 5'-UTR of rhinovirus 2 and a coding region of wild-type Mahoney strain of poliovirus indicated that the strain may have a markedly decreased tropism towards neuronal cells. Peripheral inoculation of the strain into transgenic mice showed that it is highly attenuated [6]. To assess the degree of attenuation of the strain in comparison with Sabin strains, we tested RIPO in a standard WHO monkey neurovirulence test concurrently with the U.S. National neurovirulence reference (NA-4). 14 monkeys were inoculated with 100 TCID50 of each virus, and after 17 days of clinical observation sacrificed for histological examination of their spinal cord and brain. Some monkeys developed partial paralysis, and the number of paralysed monkeys in the group inoculated with RIPO was similar to that in the control group inoculated with Sabin strain. The mean histological lesion score for these groups is presented in Table 1. It is clear from these results that neurovirulence of RIPO is no higher than that of the Sabin strain.

Table 1: Monkey neurovirulence test (WHO) of rhino-poliovirus chimera.

Strain	Number of monkeys	Lesion score
Sabin (NA-4)	14	0.87±0.38
RIPO	14	0.92±0.42

Another new method for evaluating poliovirus neurovirulence is a test in Tg-PVR21 transgenic mice expressing human poliovirus receptor (CD155). The test, developed in our laboratory [7,8] allows accurate and sensitive discrimination of vaccine samples with low levels of neurovirulence. We inoculated groups of 10 mice with varying doses of RIPO, Sabin strain, and wild-type Mahoney strain. The results show that wild-type Mahoney strain possesses the highest neurovirulence with both PD50 and LD50 of about 100 TCID50 (Fig.1). The Sabin strain is about 100 times less virulent, with both LD50 and PD50 equal to 10^4 TCID50. In contrast to the wild-type and Sabin strains, both RIPO and RIPOS had PD50 and LD50 values not only much higher than for the Sabin strain, but they were also significantly different, and a substantial fraction of paralysed mice survived and recovered from partial paralysis. This result demonstrates that RIPO and RIPOS have significantly lower neurovirulence for transgenic mice than the Sabin strain.

We also evaluated a similar recombinant construct between rhinovirus 2 and wild-type Leon/37 poliovirus of type 3. The results on Figure 2 show that it is also

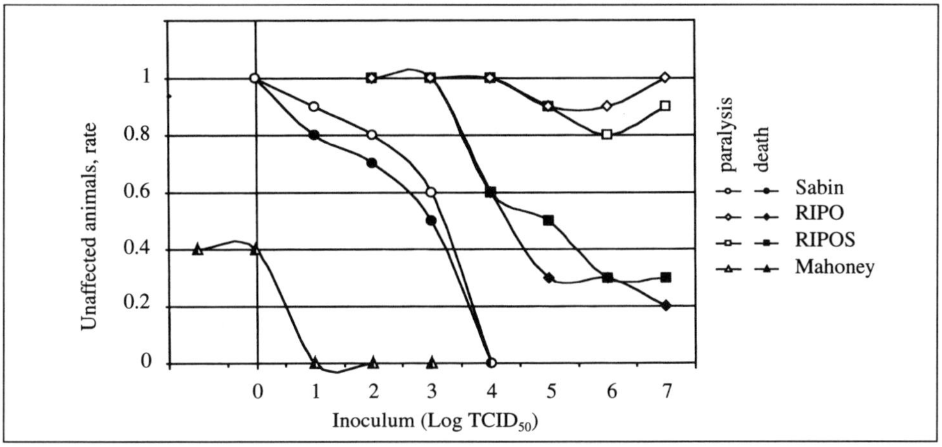

Fig. 1.

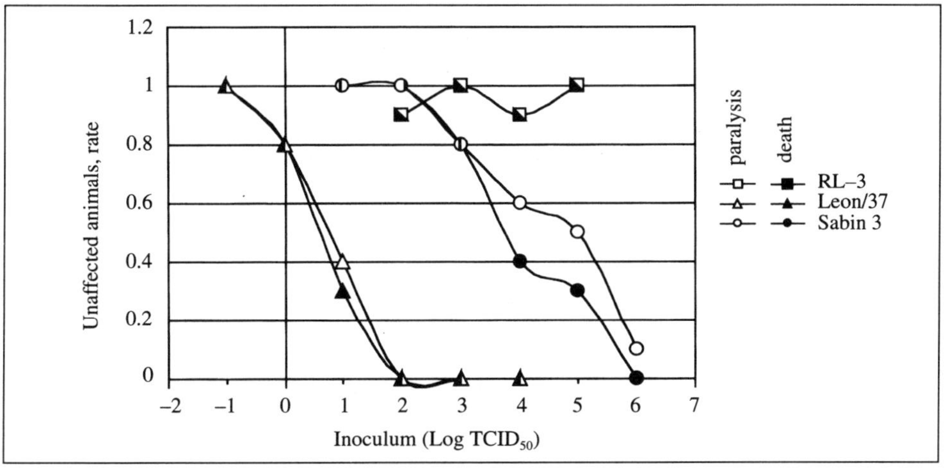

Fig. 2.

highly attenuated and, as with type 1 strains, some of the paralysed mice survive and recover.

Discussion

There are a number of additional requirements that strains appropriate for manufacture of IPV in the post-eradication era should meet in addition to the ones that apply to the current strains. The most important one is the absence of pathogenicity for humans and genetic stability of this property upon replication both in vitro and in vivo. Experiments in vitro showed that human neuroblastoma cells are much more resistant 60 rhino-poliovirus chimaeras, suggesting that the strains should possess lower neurovirulence. The experiments in Rhesus monkeys and transgenic mice reported in this paper confirm that the level of attenuation provided by substitution of 5'UTR is comparable to that of the Sabin strain. The next step in evaluating the safety of these strains should be a study in higher primates, and then in human volunteers. These studies are also important because of another potential use of these recombinant strains to treat human gliomas, as was recently proposed [9]. Before this can be done, however, it would be important to assess the genetic stability of these strains in cell cultures to determine whether their attenuated phenotype can be reversed.

In general, the new strains suitable for IPV production in the post-eradication period should probably conform to safety standards currently applied to OPV. Evaluation of the strains involves not only neurovirulence tests, but also studies of transmissibility of the virus, and must at some point involve at least some limited field trials of the live virus in human populations. This makes the entire effort more difficult, and raises some ethical issues. Many of the additional studies could be avoided if the Sabin strains could be used as substrates for IPV production. There is ample evidence for the safety of Sabin strains. First, it is not clear that Sabin strains can establish sustainable chains of transmission in communities. Second, the rate of VAPP associated with Sabin strains is negligibly low even upon mass administration of the live virus. Since the human population will not be exposed to the live virus unless there is a manufacturing accident (which can be easily detected by ongoing monitoring), the possibility of VAPP can be largely discounted.

There are some perceived problems with the Sabin strains as substrates for IPV production. Several groups tried to produce IPV from Sabin strains, but abandoned the effort because of the lower immunogenicity of the resulting vaccine compared to the conventional IPV. It is not clear however, that all options were explored to make an adequate product from the Sabin strains. There are several possible reasons why IPV made from Sabin strains possess lower potency. First, the lower stability of Sabin strain capsids was shown, potentially leading to partial destruction of D-antigen upon treatment with formaldehyde. There are a number of alternative inactivating agents that rapidly inactivate infectivity while leaving protein capsids intact, and their use for IPV production can be explored [10-13]. Another possible reason why previous attempts to make Sabin-based IPV have failed is the slight differences in antigenic properties between wild-type and Sabin strains. Potentially this can be overcome by changing formulation of IPV to increase the amount of antigen. There are a number of other ways IPV made from Sabin strains can be improved to increase its potency and efficacy, which can be explored.

There is an additional benefit to using the same strain for both OPV and IPV production. One of the outstanding logistical issues of the polio eradication campaign is creation of a sufficient stockpile of OPV. Such a stockpile may be needed for an emergency response in case poliovirus is re-introduced into the population. There are both scientific issues (e.g. monovalent vs. polyvalent OPV), as well as logistical and financial ones (e.g. how many doses are needed, how to finance its creation and maintenance). One more issue to be considered is that stopping routine vaccine manufacture will result in the loss of production capacity and expertise needed for manufacture and control. Since the length of time the stockpile may be needed cannot be determined at present (and there is a possibility that it may be needed indefinitely), the best solution should be based on a stable self-sustaining arrangement. For instance, if after the shelf-life of OPV stockpile expires, the bulk can be re-processed for IPV that can be sold to be used in countries that will elect to continue using IPV, and in high-risk situations (health workers, urban areas in under-developed countries, major metropolitan areas with high mobility of population that are also plausible targets for bio-terrorism, etc.).

Considering that the creation of a new generation of poliovirus vaccines is a high priority world-health issue, and the short timeframe that is still available to make the switch, the most efficient way to do this would be to organize an international collaboration with participation of manufacturers and regulatory authorities from different countries. This will shorten the time needed for development and approval of this product, and is more likely to result in finding the optimal solution.

References

1 Dowdle WR, Birmingham ME: The biologic principles of poliovirus eradication. J Infect Dis 1997;175:S286-292.

2 Wood DJ, Sutter RW, Dowdle WR: Stopping poliovirus vaccination after eradication: issues and challenges. Bull World Health Organ 2000,78:347-357.

3 Kew OM, Sutter RW, Nottay BK, McDonough MJ, Prevots DR, Quick L, Pallansch MA: Prolonged replication of a type 1 vaccine-derived poliovirus in an immunodeficient patient. J Clin Microbiol. 1998;36:2893-2899.

4 Mulders MN, Reimerink JH, Koopmans MP, van Loon AM, van der Avoort HG: Genetic analysis of wild-type poliovirus importation into The Netherlands (1979-1995). J Infect Dis 1997;176:617-624.

5 Requirements for poliomyelitis vaccine (oral): WHO Technical Report, WHO 1990, vol Ser 800, pp 30-65.

6 Gromeier M, Alexander L, Wimmer E: Internal ribosomal entry site substitution eliminates neurovirulence in intergeneric poliovirus recombinants. Proc Natl Acad Sci USA 1996;93:2370-2375.

7 Dragunsky E, Taffs R, Chernokhvostova Y, Nomura T, Hioki K, Gardner D, Norwood L, Levenbook I: A poliovirus-susceptible transgenic mouse model as a possible replacement for the monkey neurovirulence test of oral poliovirus vaccine. Biologicals 1996;24:77-86.

8 Dragunsky E, Chernokhvostova Y, Taffs R, Chumakov K, Gardner D, Asher D, Nomura T, Hioki K, Levenbook I: TgPVR21 mice for testing type-3 oral poliovirus vaccines: role of clinical observation and histological examination. Vaccine 1997:15:1863-1866.

9 Gromeier M, Lachmann S, Rosenfeld MR, Gutin PH, Wimmer E: Intergeneric poliovirus recombinants for the treatment of malignant glioma. Proc Natl Acad Sci USA 2000;97:6803-6808.

10 Jiang SD, Pye D, Cox JC: Inactivation of poliovirus with beta-propiolactone. J Biol Stand 1986;14:103-109.

11 Budowsky EI, Zalesskaya MA, Nepomnyashchaya NM, Kosyanovsky RG: Principles of selective inactivation of the virual genome: Dependence of the rate of viral RNA modification on the number of protonizable groups in ethyleneimine oligomers. Vaccine Research 1996;5:29-39.

12 Burrage T, Kramer E, Brown F: Structural differences between foot-and-mouth disease and poliomyelitis viruses influence their inactivation by aziridines. Vaccine 2000;18:2454-2461.

13 Burrage T, Kramer E, Brown F: Inactivation of viruses by aziridines, in Brown F, Vyas G (eds): Advances in Transfusion Safety. Dev Biol. Basel, Karger, 2000, vol 102, pp 131-139.

Dr. K. Chumakov, Centers for Biologics Evaluation and Research, FDA, Division of Viral Products,
1401 Rockville Pike, HEM 255, Rockville, MD 20852, USA.

Brown F (ed): Progress in Polio Eradication: Vaccine Strategies for the End Game.
Dev Biol. Basel, Karger, 2001, vol 105, pp 179-187

Live-Attenuated Strains of Improved Genetic Stability

A.J. Macadam[1], G. Ferguson[1], D.M. Stone[2], J. Meredith[2], J.W. Almond[2], P.D. Minor[1]

[1] National Institute for Biological Standards and Control, Potters Bar, U.K.
[2] University of Reading, Reading, U.K.

Key words: Poliovirus, vaccines, genetic stability, attenuation, 5' noncoding

Abstract: The current live-attenuated vaccine strains of poliovirus are genetically unstable and capable of rapid evolution in human hosts, resulting in reversion to neurovirulence and, occasionally, disease. They can also be shed by recipients for a considerable time after vaccination. This raises questions about how and when to stop vaccination after wild-type viruses have been eliminated. Persistence of vaccine revertant viruses in the population would present a risk to new cohorts of unvaccinated children and threaten the success of the eradication programme. A number of Sabin vaccine strain derivatives have been described that are, in theory, genetically more stable than the present vaccines and therefore less likely to revert to virulence. The approaches used in their derivation are outlined here and data presented for two strains showing a significant improvement in genetic stability. These strains were designed according to our understanding of the molecular basis of attenuation and incorporate changes in the sequence of an RNA structural domain that plays a key role in attenuation. They may also be less transmissible than the current type 3 vaccine strain and are potentially useful in the strategically difficult final stages of poliomyelitis eradication.

INTRODUCTION

In 1991, at a meeting co-sponsored by the IABS and WHO amongst others, a document was presented summarising discussions at the WHO on the potential use of new poliovaccines [1]. These discussions were held in response to progress in understanding the molecular biology and mechanisms of attenuation of Sabin's live vaccines which suggested possible approaches to overcoming some of the limitations of existing strains. The climate of opinion in which these recommendations were made was quite different from the present one as we approach the final eradication of wild poliomyelitis, but much of the document is still highly relevant. The primary research objectives identified were enhanced immunogenicity of OPV in developing countries, improved thermostability and greater genetic stability in order to decrease rates of vaccine-associated disease. The first two have been addressed by repeated mass vaccination campaigns and implementation of an efficient cold-chain. The third objective can be considered even more relevant today as we near a time when the only poliomyelitis will be vaccine-derived. The genetic instability of the Sabin strains is well documented and can be explained in terms of the small number of point mutations that give rise to attenuation phenotypes and the selection pressure against them on growth in the human gut.

Criteria for selection and characterisation of candidate vaccine strains were laid down at the 1991 meeting [1]:

(i) candidate strains should be derived from the attenuated Sabin strains;

(ii) strains should have comparable or better attenuation phenotypes than existing strains, ideally without compromising growth properties in non-neural tissues;

(iii) strains should have more stable attenuation phenotypes during passage in cell culture systems, preferably under strongly selective conditions;

(iv) stability should be measured by molecular methods as well as at the phenotypic level by monkey neurovirulence tests and rct assay;

(v) preferably, stability should be assessed in appropriate animal models such as enteric infection of chimpanzees;

(vi) consistency in production must be established;

(vii) the extent and duration of excretion in human vaccinees and their contacts, and the properties of excreted viruses should be assessed;

(viii) the sequences on which attenuation is dependent and the attenuation phenotypes should be maintained in excreted strains for longer periods than those of Sabin strains;

(ix) human trials should move sequentially from highly immune adults to progressively more susceptible individuals.

Leaving aside the questions of whether new strains are needed and the practicability of their assessment, these criteria are still broadly applicable.

Candidate Strains

A number of strains have been described that potentially have more stable attenuation phenotypes than the Sabin strains (Table 1). Different approaches have been taken and in many cases the potentially useful properties have been discovered serendipitously during studies designed to understand the structure-function relationship of the 5' noncoding region (ncr), the site of major attenuating mutations in all three Sabin strains. A common theme is that of deletion or substitution of (large) stretches of nucleotides in the 5' ncr. Two groups (A and F [2,7]) specifically set out to construct safer vaccine candidates designed on the basis of an understanding of the molecular mechanisms of attenuation of Sabin's live vaccines. All strains are based on Sabin strains or their parents in which case the approach used could be transferred to a Sabin genetic background. All are as atten-

Table 1: New vaccines candidates.

	Description	Reference
A	Capsid protein recombinants between Sabin 1 and Sabin 2 or Sabin 3	2
B	5'ncr deletion mutant of Sabin 3	3
C	5'ncr deletion mutants of Mahoney / Sabin 1	4
D	5'ncr deletion mutants of Mahoney	5
E	5'ncr recombinants between Mahoney / Sabin 1 and HRV2	6
F	5'ncr point mutants of Sabin 3	7

uated as, or more attenuated than, the parental strain when tested in monkeys and/or (transgenic) mice. There are good reasons to believe attenuation phenotypes of these strains might be more genetically stable than those of the parental strains although this has not been formally tested except for candidate B [3] which has undergone a limited human trial and candidate F for which data are presented below. Three other approaches will be described briefly.

The approach taken by Nomoto and colleagues (Fig. 1a [2]) was founded on the superior safety record of Sabin 1 compared to the other two vaccine strains. Sabin 1 associated cases of paralysis are extremely rare and this may be due in part to the stability of the attenuating residue at nucleotide 480 in the 5'ncr which reverts less rapidly than analogous mutations in the 5'ncrs of Sabin 2 and Sabin 3 during growth in the human gut. The capsid proteins of Sabin 1 were replaced by those of the other two vaccine strains, thus transferring antigenic properties and presumably determinants of attenuation, which have been identified in the capsid proteins of all serotypes [8]. The new type 2 strain was approximately as attenuated as Sabin 2 and the type 3 strain was more attenuated than Sabin 3. Clinical trial lots of these strains were prepared but the genetic stability of the attenuation phenotypes has not been assessed.

The Nomoto and Agol groups found that deletions of approximately 150 nucleotides at the 3' end of the Sabin 1 or Mahoney 5'ncr, downstream of the IRES, resulted in attenuation [4, 5]. Attenuation correlated with replacement of the cryptic AUG, which is part of an essential OAT (oligopyrimidine/AUG tandem) motif, with the initiator codon (Fig. 1b, [5]). An AUG at this position is required for ribosomal entry but when that AUG was the initiator codon the resultant virus was attenuated. The mechanism of attenuation operating in viruses Mah(L)/74 and Mah(L)/90 is not known but the deletions had no effect on virus yields in HeLa cells and SK-N-MC human neuroblastoma cells nor on template activity in Krebs-2 cell extracts, in contrast to effects of attenuating mutations in the 5'ncrs of the Sabin strains. The effect on growth may thus be confined to neurones in the CNS. Attenuation phenotypes of these viruses are theoretically more genetically stable than those of the Sabin strains because of the requirement for complex rearrangements rather than simple point mutations to restore wild type OAT configurations, although this has not been experimentally tested.

Wimmer and colleagues replaced the entire Mahoney IRES with that of human rhinovirus 2 (HRV2, Fig. 1c) and found that the resultant construct, PV1(RIPO), was attenuated in monkeys and TgPVR mice [6]. A second construct containing the Sabin 1 capsid proteins, PV1(RIPOS), was also attenuated. Growth of

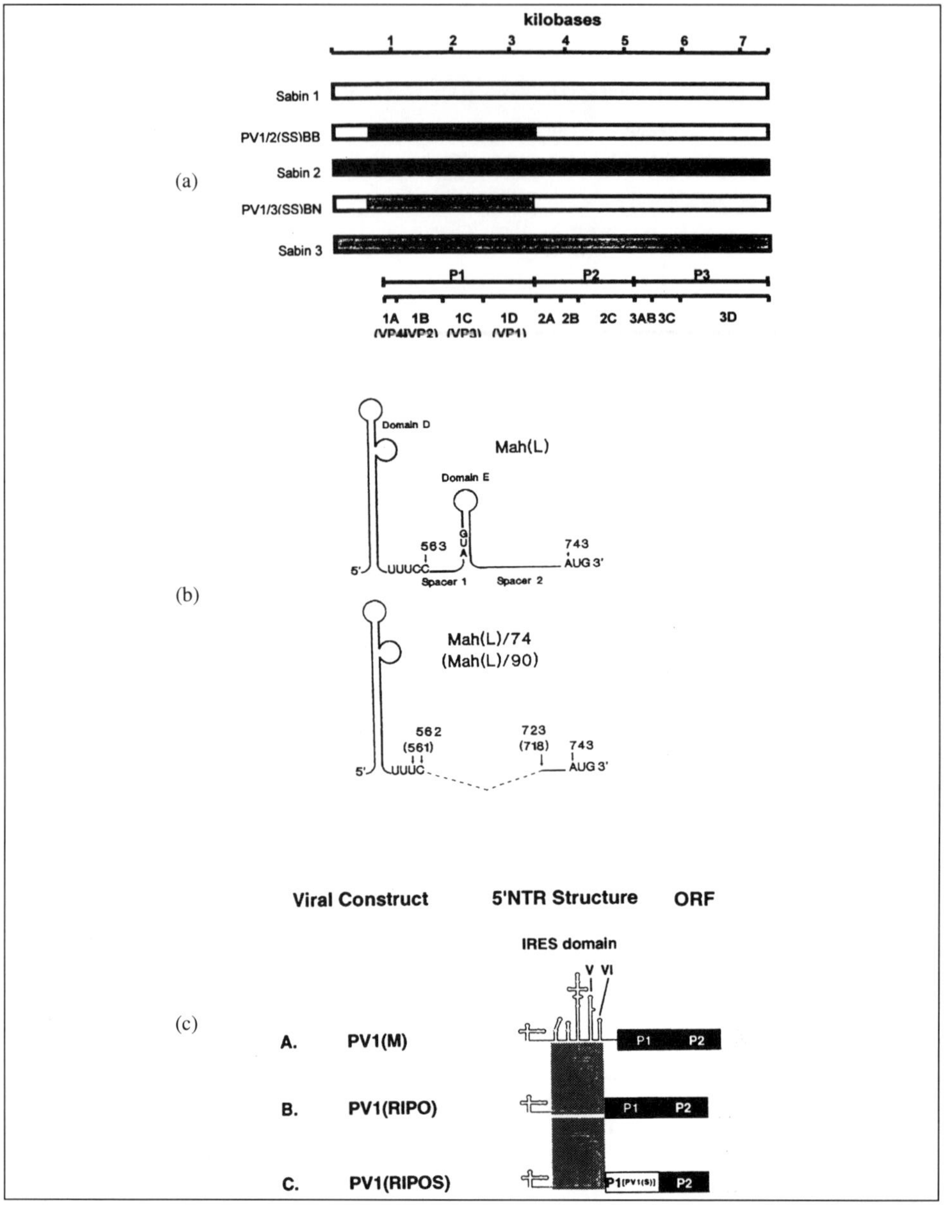

Fig. 1: Approaches to construction of new strains. (a) Genome structures of capsid protein recombinants. Light grey, black and dark grey boxes represent sequences of Sabin 1, Sabin 2 and Sabin 3 genomes respectively (adapted from [2]). (b) Schematic representation of a distal portion of the 5'ncr of wild-type poliovirus [Mah(L)] and deletion mutants. Domains D and E are also known as domains V and VI. Dotted lines represent deletions in mutants Mah(L)/74 and Mah(L)/90 (adapted from [5]). (c) PV1/HRV2 chimeras featuring heterologous IRESes derived from PV1/Mahoney (unshaded) and HRV2 (grey shading). All viruses had the wt PV1(M) cloverleaf (5'ncr domain I) and ORF except PV1(RIPOS) which had a capsid protein coding region derived from PV1/Sabin. (adapted from [6]).

PV1(RIPO) was indistinguishable from that of PV1(M) in HEp2C cells but was abrogated in SK-N-MC human neuroblastoma cells. In contrast to PV1(M), PV1(RIPO) failed to replicate in TgPVR mouse spinal cords and caused no detectable histological damage following i.c. inoculation, but replicated to wild-type levels in muscle following i.m. inoculation. The mechanism of attenuation is not known but the viral determinants reside in stem-loops V and VI (Fig. 1c). The important regions are poorly conserved between poliovirus and HRV2 but the residues involved in attenuation have not yet been identified, so it is difficult to estimate how many mutations would be required for reversion to virulence. Stability on passage under selective conditions has not been assessed.

Genetically Stabilised Type 3 Strains

Each Sabin strain has an important attenuating mutation domain V of the 5'ncr [8]. The least stable of these is in the type 3 strain. Viruses from all vaccinees that excrete type 3 virus for longer than five days post-vaccination have reverted this attenuating mutation [9]. Furthermore, somewhere between a half and two-thirds of vaccine-associated cases in immunocompetents are thought to be caused by Sabin 3 revertants and all viruses from these cases have reverted the 5'ncr mutation. The attenuating residue in question is 472U in domain V of the 5'ncr (Fig. 2). Revertants have a C at this position like the wild parent Leon. The evidence that

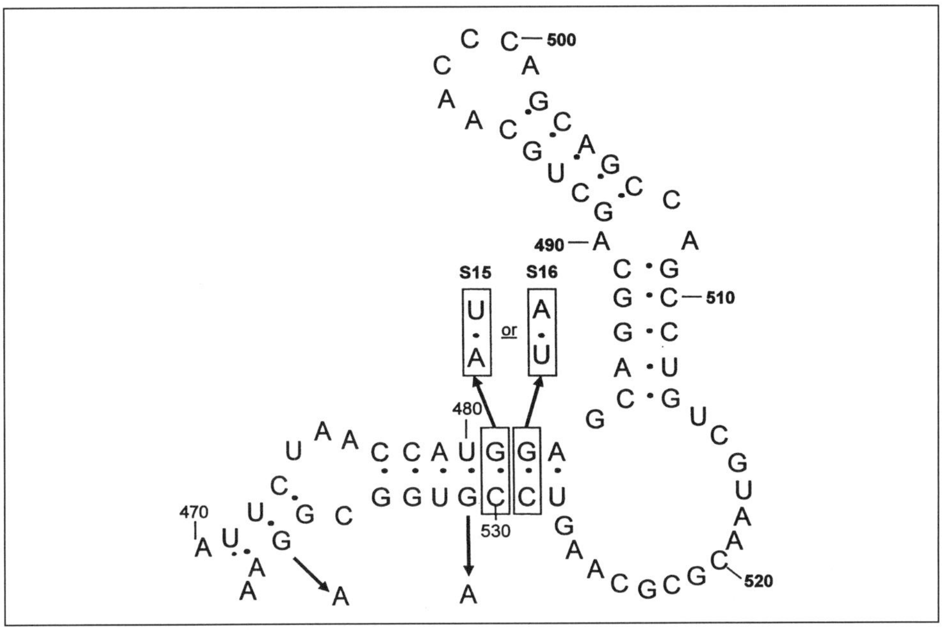

Fig. 2: Predicted RNA secondary structure of domain V (nucleotides 471-538) of the type 3 vaccine strain, Sabin 3 (adapted from [13]), showing mutations introduced into 5'ncrs of strains S15 and S16. Both strains had G→A substitutions at positions 537 and 531 converting U-G to U-A base-pairs. In strain S15 the G-C base-pair at 481/530 was substituted for a U-A base-pair and in strain S16 the G-C base-pair at 482/529 was substituted for an A-U base-pair.

472U attenuates by weakening the base-pair at 472/537 from CG to UG is well documented [10]. We proposed that it is the structural stability of the whole domain that is important, irrespective of the actual sequence [11] and reasoned that if all UG and mismatch base-pairs were removed from domain V and other positions were changed to adjust the overall thermodynamic stability of this domain to that of the vaccine strain, we would have an attenuated but genetically stable strain. If the structural prediction was correct there would be no single mutation that could increase the thermodynamic stability of domain V. Increase of structural stability would require two mutations, the first of which would disrupt whichever base-pair it participated in and therefore be selected against.

A number of strains were constructed but only results with two of them, S15 and S16, will be described here. Both strains have G→A substitutions at positions 537 and 531, converting U-G to U-A base-pairs. In strain S15 the G-C base-pair at 481/530 is substituted for a U-A base-pair and in strain S16 the G-C base-pair at 482/529 is substituted for an A-U base-pair (Fig. 2). Thus strains S15 and S16 differ from Sabin 3 at four positions in the 5'ncr and nowhere else and all base-pairs in domain V are Watson-Crick.

The viruses satisfied the first two of the selection criteria above in that they were derived from, and of comparable attenuation to, Sabin 3. In neurovirulence tests in monkeys no animals were paralysed by any of the viruses and mean histological lesion scores were similar (Table 2). The genetic stability of the attenuation phenotypes was assessed during passage in tissue-culture systems that were expected to mimic the strong selection against 472U in the human gut. Stability was monitored by molecular methods and phenotypic assays, particularly monkey neurovirulence tests.

Table 2: Neurovirulence before and after passage in L20B and Vero cells.

Virus	Unpassaged		L20B Passage 5		Vero Passage 10	
	Clinical[a]	MLS[b]	Clinical	MLS	Clinical	MLS
Sabin 3 (S3)	0/10	0.62	1/4	1.92	4/5	1.95
Strain S15	0/4	0.61	0/4	0.53	0/5	1.41
Strain S16	0/4	0.42	0/4	0.68	0/5	0.88
S3/472C	0/4	1.58				
S3/2034C	1/8	1.45				
S3/472C/2034C	3/4	2.07				

[a] Number of paralysed animals/total number.
[b] Mean (histological) lesion score.

On passage of Sabin 3 in L20B cells at 37° C it was found that nucleotide 472U reverted rapidly to C. These cells are mouse L cells expressing human poliovirus receptor cDNA. By the second passage nearly half of the Sabin 3 virus population had a C at nucleotide 472 and by the 5th passage nearly 85% had a C at this position (Fig. 3a). No nucleotide changes were found in domain V of either S15 or S16 in any passage isolate (Fig. 3a) nor in the entire 5'ncr of 5th passage isolates. No mutations were detected in the capsid proteins of any of the three strains. Thus under stringent selective conditions the sequences responsible for attenuation of S15 and S16 were completely stable.

Reversion at nucleotide 472 was also selected, more slowly, in Vero cells (derived from African Green monkey kidney) at 37°C so that by the 10th passage over 60% of the Sabin 3 virus population had a C at nucleotide 472 (Fig. 3b). During this period no mutations were introduced into domain V regions of strains S15 or S16 which again appeared genetically stable (Fig. 3b).

The second major attenuating mutation in Sabin 3 is at nucleotide 2034, resulting in a Phe at VP3-91 in the capsid proteins [8]. This residue is also the major determinant of temperature-sensitivity (ts) in Sabin 3. Both ts and neurovirulence phenotypes are reverted simultaneously by second-site mutations in the capsid proteins selected in vivo or in vitro [12]. Vero passage 10 isolates of Sabin 3, S15 and S16 each had a single, different, point mutation in the capsid proteins which resulted in a coding change. These changes were all selected at similar rates during

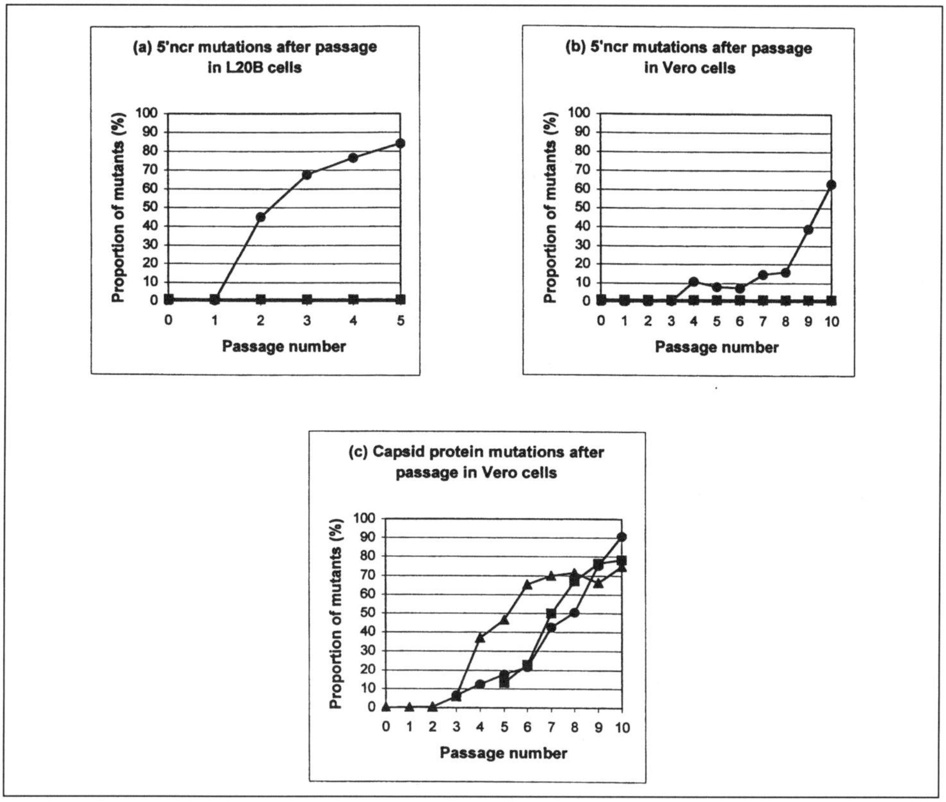

Fig. 3: Genetic stability of Sabin 3 (S3), S15 and S16 after passage in different cell lines. S3, S15 and S16 were passaged (a) five times in L20B cells or (b, c)10 times in Vero cells at 37°C using a multiplicity of infection of 10. Nucleotide changes were monitored by sequencing. Proportions of S3 virus populations with 472C (a,b) and of all virus populations with capsid protein mutations (c) were measured by PCR and restriction endonuclease digestion (MAPREC) [14]. Symbols: 2, Sabin 3; 4, S15; 8, S16.

passage in Vero cells (Fig. 3c). Selection mirrored loss of the ts phenotype in HEp2C cells (not shown) and consequently partial reversion to virulence.

Table 2 shows paralysis rates and mean histological lesion scores for viruses before and after passage in L20B and Vero cells. Also shown are phenotypes of site-directed mutants of Sabin 3 with reversions at 472, 2034 or both positions. After five passages in L20B cells Sabin 3 showed a marked increase in virulence in terms of both clinical and histological lesion scores, appearing slightly more virulent than a site-directed mutant of Sabin 3 with a C at 472, consistent with sequence data in Fig.3a. Strains S15 and S16 were approximately as attenuated as the parental viruses and the vaccine strain. No animals were paralysed by either virus. The mean lesion for S15 decreased slightly and that of S16 increased slightly although differences were not significant. This means that under conditions which rapidly selected neurovirulent variants of Sabin 3 the phenotypes of strains S15 and S16, as well as their 5'ncr sequences, were stable.

After 10 passages in Vero cells Sabin 3 was virulent. The virus caused paralysis in four our of five animals within five days and gave a high lesion score. Its phenotype was similar to that of a site-directed mutant of Sabin 3 with a C at 472 and a C at 2034, consistent with the nucleotide sequence data above. Neither S15 nor S16 caused any paralysis although both displayed increases in histological lesion scores, S15 more than S16. These were consistent with the partial reversion of the attenuating mutation in the capsid proteins indicated by data in Figure 3c. Neither was any more virulent than a site-directed mutant of Sabin 3 with a C at 2034. Again it appeared that attenuation due to domain V was completely stable.

By changing just four nucleotides in part of the 5'ncr viruses were constructed that were not only theoretically more stable than Sabin 3 but under stringent selection pressures proved to be completely stable in the 5'ncr. This was achieved while maintaining the attenuation levels of Sabin 3 and using the same mechanisms of attenuation, involving weakening the RNA secondary structure of domain V. These strains may also be less transmissible than Sabin 3. The type 3 vaccine strain does not "take", or establish itself, very efficiently and is eliminated from the human gut within five days unless mutants with a C at 472 arise [9]. Take rates for excreted Sabin 3-derived strains will be substantially higher than that of the vaccine since these viruses all have a C at nucleotide 472 already. But take rates for S15- or S16-derived strains in secondary hosts, because or their genetic stability, are likely to be similar to those of the original strains. Limited transmission of Sabin strains is considered an advantage in mass vaccination campaigns but may be a disadvantage when it comes to stopping vaccination.

Conclusions

There are two major questions concerning the use of new live-attenuated poliovaccines: will they be needed/useful, and can the ethical/regulatory obstacles be surmounted? It is often said that changing the poliovaccine strains would be impossible because clinical trials would require immunisation of millions of susceptible infants to establish superior safety. Ultimately that is probably true but it should not be used as a reason to abandon all research in this area. There are limited human trials that can be conducted to establish immunogenicity and genetic stability using small numbers of individuals, a framework for which was established by the WHO in 1991 [1]. If safe, genetically-stable vaccines were available on the shelf they would be the live vaccines of choice in a number of potential situations: (i) if it were considered too risky to stop vaccination in view of inadequate surveillance or containment or knowledge of the extent of persistent virus excretion. At this stage safer vaccines would have ethical value; (ii) if a sequential approach to cessation of vaccination were adopted since the regulatory issues would not be affected by including a new type 3 strain into the bivalent preparation; (iii) as part of an outbreak response in the post-vaccination era when genetically stabilised strains would have the advantage of increased safety for vaccine recipients and contacts and, potentially, a decreased likelihood of re-emergence of poliomyelitis after vaccination is stopped for the second time.

References

1 Ghendon Y: WHO recommendation on potential use of new poliomyelitis vaccines, in Brown F, Lewis BP (eds): Poliovirus Attenuation: Molecular Mechanisms and Practical Aspects. Dev Biol Stand. Basel, Karger, 1993, vol 78, pp 133-139.

2 Kohara M, Abe S, Yoshioka I, Nomoto A: Development of candidates for new type 2 and type 3 oral poliovirus vaccines, in Brown F, Lewis BP (eds): Poliovirus Attenuation: Molecular Mechanisms and Practical Aspects. Dev Biol Stand. Basel, Karger, 1993, vol 78, pp 141-148.

3 Ubertini TR, Cioni C, Perini L, Gagnoni S: Non-neurovirulent, genetically stable clone of poliovirus (Sabin type III strain). Vaccine 1988;6:481-482.

4 Iizuka N, Kohara M, Hagino-Yagamishi K, Abe S, Komatsu T, Tago K, Arita M, Nomoto A: Construction of less neurovirulent polioviruses by introducing deletions into th 5' noncoding sequence of the genome. J Virol 1989;63:5354-5363.

5 Slobodskaya OR, Gmyl AP, Maslova SV, Tolskaya EA, Viktorova EG, Agol VI: Poliovirus neurovirulence correlates with the presence of a cryptic AUG upstream of the initiator codon. Virology 1996;221:141-150.

6 Gromeier M, Bossert B, Arita M, Nomoto A, Wimmer E: Dual stem loops within the poliovirus internal ribosomal entry site control neurovirulence. J Virol 1999;73:958-964.

7 Macadam AJ, Ferguson G, Stone DM, Meredith J, Almond JW, Minor PD: Rational design of a genetically-stable live-attenuated poliovirus vaccine: relevance to poliomyelitis eradication. J Virol (submitted).

8 Minor PD: The molecular biology of poliovaccines: J Gen Virol 1992;73:3065-3077.

9 Dunn G, Begg NT, Cammack N, Minor PD: Virus excretion and mutation by infants following primary vaccination with live oral poliovaccine from two sources. J Med Virol 1990;32:92-95.

10 Macadam AJ, Stone DM, Almond JW, Minor PD: The 5' noncoding region and virulence of poliovirus vaccine strains. Trends Microbiol 1994;2:449-454.

11 Almond JW, Stone D, Burke K, Skinner MA, Macadam AJ, Wood D, Ferguson M, Minor PD: Approaches to the construction of new candidate poliovirus type 3 vaccine strains. Dev Biol Stand 1993;78:161-170.

12 Macadam AJ, Arnold C, Howlett J, John A, Marsden S, Taffs F, Reeve P, Hamada N, Wareham K, Almond JW, Cammack N, Minor PD: Reversion of the attenuated and temperature-sensitive phenotypes of the Sabin type 3 strain of poliovirus in vaccinees. Virology 1989;172:408-414.

13 Skinner MA, Racaniello VR, Dunn G, Cooper J, Minor PD, Almond JW: New model for the secondary structure of the 5' non-coding RNA of poliovirus is supported by biochemical and genetic data that also show that RNA secondary structure is important in neurovirulence. J Mol Biol 1989;207:379-392.

14 Chumakov KM, Powers LB, Noonan KE, Roninson IB, Levenbook IS: Correlation between amount of virus with altered nucleotide sequence and the monkey test for acceptability of oral poliovirus vaccine. Proc Natl Acad Sci USA 1991;88:199-203.

Dr. A.J. Macadam, N.I.B.S.C., Blanche Lane, South Mimms, Potters Bar, Herts EN6 3QG, U.K.

Brown F (ed): Progress in Polio Eradication: Vaccine Strategies for the End Game.
Dev Biol. Basel, Karger, 2001, vol 105, pp 189-194

Vaccines Based on Recombinant Antigen Strategies

P. Minor

National Institute for Biological Standards and Control, Potters Bar, Herts, U.K.

INTRODUCTION

There are two highly effective and extremely safe vaccines against poliovirus which have been used successfully for over 40 years. The characteristics of inactivated polio vaccine (IPV) were established in the 1950s where the effect on the incidence of poliomyelitis was rapidly evident, and many countries in Europe, as well as the U.S.A., have altered their national vaccination policy to the use of IPV away from oral poliovaccine (OPV). Scandinavian countries and the Netherlands predominantly used IPV from the outset and have eradicated poliomyelitis, although it has been suggested that this may have been made easier by their high standards of hygiene or other epidemiological factors [1].

In most of the world eradication has depended on the use of oral poliovaccine (OPV) to interrupt transmission. OPV is associated with a very low level of vaccine-associated paralysis, estimated at one per 530,000 first time recipients or one per 1.2 million vaccinees overall [2]. This is a tiny rate of adverse reactions for a medical intervention, and is extremely difficult to measure in any circumstances other than complete national immunisation over a period of years.

With this background the development of vaccines based on the recombinant technologies available becomes extremely difficult, primarily because of the need to demonstrate safety and efficacy comparable to that of the existing vaccines, which is likely to be nearly impossible. A second problem arises from the nature of poliovirus as an antigen. Certain recombinant produced vaccines are either in widespread use, as for the hepatitis B vaccine produced by expression of the surface antigen in yeast, or theoretically possible, as for sub-unit influenza vaccines containing the surface glycoproteins. In these instances the protein immunogen alone is able to generate a protective immune response. This does not appear to be the case to an equal degree for poliovirus where the capsid has a complex quaternary structure.

The advantages of vaccines produced by recombinant technology would be the elimination of the need to grow infectious virus or to give infectious virus to the population at large. After eradication of wild-type poliovirus, these are likely to be the chief routes by which individuals could become infected and poliomyelitis re-emerge.

Antigenic Structure of Poliovirus

Polio occurs in three serotypes such that immunity to one serotype does not protect against the other two, and smaller antigenic differences exist between strains within a serotype. However, a preparation of a particular strain also contains two distinct antigenic forms of particles, originally designated D and C antigen [3] based on their sedimentation in an ultracentrifugation step gradient, D being denser than C. It was shown that serum from acute phase cases of poliomyelitis reacted predominantly with C antigen, while serum from convalescent cases, where recovery was underway, reacted with D antigen; the D antigen fraction also contained most of the virus infectivity and is now known to represent intact mature virus particles, while the C antigen fraction contains empty capsids. Because antibodies to D antigen neutralise virus infectivity it has been considered that inactivated vaccines should be standardised in terms of their D antigen content. The difference between the two antigenic forms is attributable to a major conformational rearrangement which can be induced by relatively mild treatments including heating at 56°C, adsorption to surfaces or UV treatment [4]. A recombinant antigen would have to be able to induce antibody reacting with D antigen to be able to protect against infection.

The antigenic structure of poliovirus of all three serotypes has been studied intensively over the years [5] and four main targets of antibodies identified as independent antigenic sites, chiefly by the isolation of mutants resistant to neutralisation by monoclonal antibodies. The independent sites are formed by amino acids which cluster in the structure of the virus [6,7]. Site 1 is composed of three loops from the viral protein VP1 located around the pentameric apex of the virus particle, of which one, designated the B-C loop, [6] is the most significant. Site 2 is composed of a sequence from VP2 which clusters with a shorter sequence from VP1. Site 3 includes short exposed sequences from VP3 and VP1, and site 4 involves sequences of VP3 on adjacent pentameric subunits of the virus. Neutralising monoclonal antibodies against site 1 can react with both D and C antigen, or with D antigen alone; the epitopes recognised are chiefly located on the exposed B-C loop. A monoclonal antibody reacting exclusively with C antigen has been shown to recognise the same loop in a different conformation [8]. Similarly, neutralising antibodies directed against site 2 may react with both D and C antigen. Neutralising antibodies against sites 3 and 4 react exclusively with D antigen because of the short contiguous sequences recognised.

The conformations of the antigenic sites recognised by neutralising antibodies are therefore fragile and depend to a large extent on the complex quaternary structure of the infectious virus. Except for site 1 they are composed of elements from different capsid proteins, although some sequences are more exposed than others. This poses a major challenge to the development of recombinant based antigens which would have to imitate the structure found on the infectious virus in order to induce antibodies against it.

Use of the Single Purified Capsid Proteins as Immunogens

Proteins purified from the virus particles of certain picornaviruses have been shown to induce neutralising antibody. The VP1 protein from foot and mouth disease virus has been consistently reported to induce neutralising antibody [9] and, when expressed in a bacterial system, could be shown to induce a protective response experimentally [10]. Capsid protein VP2 of Coxsackie virus B was reported to induce high levels of neutralising antibodies [11].

The data for poliovirus are less consistent, some reporting that no protein is effective, others that VP1 or all proteins can induce a neutralising response [9,12,13]. The preparation of the protein from the virus has been considered crucial [14] although the complex intertwining of the proteins in the virus particle requires that they be extensively denatured before purification, so losing their structure which may be difficult to regenerate. Purification of proteins from virus fixed with formalin was also reported to give material inducing a neutralising response [15]. This underlines the need to imitate the structures on the virion, and suggests that expression of a single protein is unlikely to be effective. The levels of antibodies induced by purified poliovirus proteins have in general been low and inconsistent and expression of a single protein is most unlikely to provide a satisfactory vaccine.

Peptide Based Vaccines

Peptides based on the amino acid sequence of sections of the foot-and-mouth disease capsid protein VP1 have been potent inducers of protective immune responses, particularly when expressed as part of a protein with a strong ability to induce a T cell response, such as the hepatitis B core antigen [16]. Similar studies with poliovirus peptide sequences have been less striking in the responses induced, although credible antibody levels can be induced [17,18]. In general the responses are only induced where the sites react with D and C antigen specific antibodies, and may be more flexible in their conformation. Where the antibodies react with linear peptides in ELISA systems, as for the foot-and-mouth disease virus peptides, they induce the strongest responses, and the sequences can be shown to be disordered in the structure. Conversely it might be expected that a peptide which takes up a particular conformation by virtue of its amino acid sequence, such as one with several proline residues, could also be effective in imitating the conformation of the same sequence on the virus.

The need for accurate imitation of the native conformation and the difficulty in doing so have been demonstrated by the preparation of chimaeric polioviruses, constructed by exchanging antigenic sequences between serotypes in cDNA clones. The viruses recovered would be, for example, largely serotype 1, but with elements of antigenic site 1 replaced by the corresponding sequence of type 3. The viruses can express dual antigenicity [19,20], although usually imperfectly [21,22], and usually only where the replaced site is a long contiguous sequence or can be imitated by peptides. Even where peptides are presented in the context of a structurally closely analogous virus, where the conformation should be most appropriate, therefore, they are not particularly effective, if judged as alternatives to the existing vaccines.

Generation of Virus Like Particles (VLPs)

As the conformation of the proteins is crucially dependent on the intact virus structure, a way in which they could be expressed accurately would be to generate virus-like particles in which all the proteins are present but the genomic RNA is excluded. Poliovirus proteins are translated from a single open reading frame into a polyprotein which is processed by virus-encoded proteases to give the functional polypeptides. Two protease activities are recognised, one of which (P2A) cleaves the capsid proteins en bloc from the non-structural proteins while the other (P3C or P3CD) performs the remaining cleavages, including those generating the individual capsid proteins. The formation of virus-like particles is therefore likely to require the expression of the capsid proteins, P3CD and, depending on the construct, P2A as well. When constructs were made including these three elements in vaccinia virus, they were ineffective because P2A is involved in shutting off the cap-dependent translation of host RNAs, and therefore also affected vaccinia virus replication. An alternative was to express the capsid proteins alone in vaccinia virus with P3CD, so obviating the need for P2A. This approach has not been vigorously pursued for generating VLPs. Another alternative is to use the baculovirus system with expression under the control of the polyhedrin gene promoter. This has the potential advantage that expression levels of proteins can be extremely high in this system. As polyhedrin is a late protein the replication of the baculovirus can be completed before cap-dependent translation is shut off. It would also be possible to manipulate the system to obviate the need for P2A, although this has not been reported. Urakawa et al [23] reported the construction of a baculovirus containing the entire coding region of the type 3 poliovirus strain Leon, lacking only the 5' non-coding region and therefore unable to replicate. Virus-like particles were produced, although in relatively low amounts for this expression system, and shown to induce neutralising antibodies in mice. The particles had the morphology of empty capsids. It is expected that they would express D antigenicity, but be very fragile and likely to convert to C antigen.

DNA Vaccines

When DNA encoding an antigen of interest is placed in expression plasmids under the control of a eukaryotic promoter, such as the CMV IE gene promoter, it is able to induce immune responses on inoculation into experimental animals. This procedure has been described for a variety of immunogens, including proteins from influenza and hepatitis B viruses and the malaria parasite. So far as is known it has not been attempted for poliovirus, but it is possible that constructs capable of producing VLPs in vitro could also do so in vivo, in which case the immune response generated might be significant as the VLPs would be made in situ. There are several clinical trials of DNA vaccines in humans in progress at the time of writing, although none with polio constructs so far as is known.

Conclusions

The advantages of poliovaccines prepared by expression would be mainly that they would remove the need for infectious virus in production or immunisation. The complex structure of the virion makes this a difficult problem, and while neutralising antibodies have been induced by isolated proteins or peptides the results have not been reliable or convincing enough to make them the basis for development of a new vaccine type. It is possible that the expression of virus-like particles would give a more effective product, and this, together with DNA vaccines, are worth further exploration.

References

1 Sabin AB: Paralytic poliomyelitis: old dogmas and new perspectives. Rev Inf Dis 1981;3:543-564.

2 Nkowane BU, Wassilak SG, Oversteen WA, Bart KJ, Schonberger LB, Hinman, AR, Kew OM: Vaccine associated paralytic poliomyelitis in the United States: 1973 through 1984. Journal of the American Medical Association 1987;257:1385-1390.

3 Mayer MM, Rapp HJ, Roizman B, Klein SW, Cowan KM, Lukens D, Schwerk CE, Schaffer FL, Charney J: The purification of poliomyelitis viruses studied by complement fixation. J Immunol 1957;78:435-455.

4 Le Bouvier GL: The modification of poliovirus antigens by heat and ultraviolet light. Lancet 1955;ii:1013-1016.

5 Minor PD: Antigenic structure of picornaviruses, in Racaniello VR (ed): Picornaviruses: Current Topics in Microbiology Immunology, Springer-Verlag, 1990;16:122-154.

6 Hogle JM, Chow M, Filman DJ: Three dimensional structure of poliovirus at 2-9Å resolution. Science 1985;229:1358-1365.

7 Filman DJ, Syed R, Chow M, Macadam AJ, Minor PD, Hogle JM: Structural factors that control conformation transition and serotype specificity in type 3 poliovirus. EMBO J 1989;8:1567-1579.

8 Ferguson M, Minor PD: Differences in conformation of type 3 poliovirus antigenic sites on non-infectious empty particles and infectious virus. J Gen Virol 1990;71:1271-1274.

9 Meloen RH, Rowland DJ, Brown F: Comparison of the antibodies elicited by the individual structural polypeptides of foot-and-mouth disease and polioviruses. J Gen Virol 1979;45:761-763.

10 Klied DG, Yansura D, Small B, Dowbenko D, Moore DM, Grubman MJ, McKercher PD, Morgan DO, Robertson BH, Bachrach HL: Cloned viral protein vaccine for foot and mouth disease: responses in cattle and swine. Science 1981;214:1125-1129.

11 Beatrice ST, Katze MG, Zajac BA, Crowe RL: Induction of neutralizing antibodies by the coxsackievirus B9 virion polypeptide, VP2. Virology 1980;104:426-438.

12 Chow M, Baltimore D: Isolated capsid protein VP1 induces a neutralising response in rats. Proc Nat Acad Sci USA 1982;79:7508-7512.

13 Emini EA, Dorner AJ, Dorner LF, Jameson BA, Wimmer E: Identification of a poliovirus neutralisation epitope through use of neutralising antiserum raised against a purified viral structural protein. Virology 1983;124:144-151.

14 Dernick R, Heukeshjoven J, Hilbrig M: Induction of neutralising antibodies by all three structural poliovirus polypeptides. Virology 1983;130:243-246.

15 Van der Marel P, Hazendonk TG, Henneke MAC, van Wezel AL: Induction of neutralising antibodies by poliovirus capsid polypeptides VP1, IP2 and VP3. Vaccine 1983;117-22.

16 Clarke BE, Newton SE, Carroll AR, Francis MJ, Appleyard G, Syned AD, Highfield PE, Rowlands DJ, Brown F: Improved immunogenicity of a peptide epitope after fusion to hepatitis B core protein. Nature 1987;330:381-384.

17 Emini, EA, Jameson BA, Wimmer E: Priming for and induction of antipoliovirus neutralising antibodies by synthetic peptides. Nature 1983;304:699-703.

18 Ferguson M, Evans DMA, Magrath, DI, Minor PD, Almond JW, Schild GC: Induction of broadly reactive type specific neutralising antibody to poliovirus type 3 by synthetic peptides. Virology 1985;143:505-515.

19 Burke K, Dunn G, Ferguson M, Minor PD, Almond JW: Antigenic chimaeras of poliovirus: potential novel vaccines against picornaviral infections. Nature 1988;332:81-82.

20 Murray MG, Kuhn RJ, Arita M, Kawamura N, Nomoto A, Wimmer E: Poliovirus type 1/type 3 antigenicity brid virus constructed in vitro elicits type 1 and type 3 neutralising antibodies in rabbits and monkeys. Proc Natl Acad Sci USA 1988;85:3203-3207.

21 Minor PD, Ferguson M, Katrak K, Wood D, John A, Howlett J, Dunn G, Burke K, Almond JW: Antigenic structure of chimeras of type 1 and type 3 poliovirus involving antigenic site 1. J Gen Virol 1990;71:2543-2551.

22 Minor PD, Ferguson M, Katrak K, Wood D, John A, Howlett J, Dunn G, Burke K, Almond JW: Antigenic structure of chimeras of type 1 and type 3 polioviruses involving antigenic sites 2, 3 and 4. J Gen Virol 1991;72:2475-2481.

23 Urakawa T, Ferguson M, Minor PD, Cooper J, Sullivan M, Almond JW, Bishop DHL: Synthesis of immunogenic but non-infectious poliovirus particles in insect cells by a baculovirus expression vector. J Gen Virol 1989;70:1453-1463.

Dr. P.D. Minor, N.I.B.S.C., Blanche Lane, South Mimms, Potters Bar, Herts EN6 3QG, U.K.

Brown F (ed): Progress in Polio Eradication: Vaccine Strategies for the End Game.
Dev Biol. Basel, Karger, 2001, vol 105, p 195

Poster Session II

Brown F (ed): Progress in Polio Eradication: Vaccine Strategies for the End Game.
Dev Biol. Basel, Karger, 2001, vol 105, pp 197-208

Anomalous Observations on IPV and OPV Vaccination

T.J. John

Kerala State Institute of Virology and Infectious Diseases, Alapuzha, Kerala, India.

Abstract: Anomalies of vaccine performance are events or observations that go counter to the current **paradigms** on the properties of a vaccine. In the current paradigm, inactivated poliovirus vaccine (IPV) induces serum immunity to protect the individual from poliomyelitis, but not mucosal immunity to prevent subsequent wild poliovirus infection. Therefore, it is believed not to be suitable to interrupt virus transmission in polio-endemic tropical and developing countries, where poliovirus transmission is thought to be predominantly faecal-oral, unlike in countries with excellent sanitation, where it is predominantly respiratory. Oral poliovirus vaccine (OPV), because it is believed to mimic natural (wild) poliovirus infection and to induce serum and mucosal immunity, is considered ideal to interrupt virus transmission in countries with poor sanitation and endemic polio. Moreover, the vaccine viruses are shed in the stools and it is presumed to spread faeco-orally to unvaccinated children in the vicinity, thus increasing its effectiveness in the community. These paradigms on both vaccines may be seen in standard textbooks of virology and paediatrics. In reality, IPV induces very high mucosal immunity in a monkey model, lasting at least 12 months and providing complete protection against oral challenge with wild virus. In field trials, IPV has been found to have very high vaccine efficacy (VE) and to retard significantly wild-virus transmission in communities. OPV, requiring five to seven doses for individual protection, does not seem to induce effective mucosal immunity. Hence, 10-15 doses of OPV and near 100% vaccination coverage are necessary for interruption of virus transmission in countries with poor sanitation. In the monkey model, wild poliovirus infection did not offer any mucosal protection against a second infection, indicating that live virus infection is not the best way to induce mucosal immunity (unless repeated several times). The immunity induced by OPV has two arms, individual protection (by serum immunity) and mucosal protection from later infection by wild virus; these are dichotomous, as evidenced further by protected children participating in wild virus transmission in breakthrough outbreaks in communities well vaccinated with OPV.

There is no evidence that polioviruses, wild or vaccine, spread faeco-orally to any meaningful extent. The median age of polio in India, in the pre-vaccine era, and even in recent years was 12-18 months. No other faeco-oral infection has such a low median age. Measles virus transmission is respiratory, and the median age of measles is over two years. Wild virus is shed faecally, but by the age when faecal microbes infect children, most of them are already immune to disease caused by polioviruses. As for vaccine viruses, even when heavy inocula are fed repeatedly, children may not always become infected. That exposure to the small amounts of virus through faecal contamination (unlike microbes that multiply in food) would infect them, is an unrealistic expectation.

There are sufficient anomalies demanding our revision of the old paradigms. IPV is a better immunogen than OPV and is completely safe. During the interval between the cessation of wild virus transmission and the global stoppage of polio vaccination, it will be advantageous to use IPV, particularly combined with DPT vaccine, to provide individual protection, and herd effect to prevent spread in case of the introduction of wild polioviruses, whether unintentionally or otherwise, and to bolster the Expanded Programme on Immunisation.

Introduction

When all facts are not known about a scientific issue, the gaps may be filled with assumptions, and a paradigm is born. The more a paradigm is repeated in textbooks, classrooms and in health programmes, the more readily are the assumptions mistaken for facts.

Although we have been fortunate to have two excellent tools against poliomyelitis, the inactivated poliovaccine (IPV) and the live oral poliovaccine (OPV), we have not been wise enough to use them to the best advantage of children in all regions of the world. Based on limited and incomplete evidence and for reasons that are not entirely scientific, **paradigms** developed around them and policy makers have been guided more by the **paradigms** than by the **evidence** available at specific times in the history of these vaccines. **When events contrary to paradigms (anomalies) are observed, there is a tendency for adherents of the paradigms to disbelieve them, thus delaying the recognition of the meaning of such anomalies** [1]. Such delay has had serious repercussions on the control and elimination of poliomyelitis by vaccination. Eventually, when scientists observe a sufficient set of anomalous events, paradigms are modified [1]. I believe that the history of polio vaccines is going through this process, as I will describe and illustrate in this paper. As we are at the threshold of global polio eradication, it is timely and important for us to understand these issues clearly, so that the final years of the eradication era will be managed on scientific grounds rather than on paradigms. For this purpose it is necessary to re-examine paradigms and distinguish evidence from assumptions.

The OPV Paradigm

Even before OPV was developed, it was anticipated that such a vaccine would be highly desirable. As Robbins put it succinctly, "the idea of attenuated (polio) vaccine as opposed to killed vaccine appealed to many investigators, because it was presumed that an active infection most nearly reproduced the natural situation and could be expected to give longer lasting immunity and greater resistance of the bowel to re-infection" [2]. Thus, the origins of the OPV paradigm preceded its actual development, and it grew further after it gained popularity. One important quality of OPV is said to be "the known transmission pattern of the vaccine virus, which resembles that of the wild virus in being shed in large quantities and for long periods, in the stool of inoculated children" [3]. Accordingly, "by inoculating children regularly (annually or more frequently) as part of a mass vaccination programme, it is possible to spread the vaccine viruses in the environment so that children who are missed by the vaccination programme are indirectly exposed to them" [3].

In summary, OPV is considered to be almost an 'ideal' vaccine, for the following reasons [2-7]:

(i) it is given by mouth, a route which closely resembles what is believed to be the natural route of wild poliovirus infection;

(ii) it is believed to spread to unvaccinated children from the vaccinated, thus increasing immunity coverage;

(iii) it is believed to be extremely safe, as the viruses are attenuated;

(iv) being a live vaccine, it would have near 100% vaccine efficacy;

(v) it is supposed to induce not only systemic immunity for protection from disease, but also a high degree of mucosal (gut) immunity, which would lead to excellent herd effect and easy elimination of virus transmission.

When the Expanded Programme on Immunisation (EPI) was established by the World Health Organisation (WHO) in 1974, OPV was included (to the exclusion of IPV) and thereafter it became very widely used in most countries. The EPI schedule was three doses of OPV in infancy, and the goal set for vaccine coverage was 80%. It was hoped and predicted, solely based on the paradigm, that polio would be controlled when this goal was achieved. It was not to be so.

Anomalous Observations on OPV Paradigm

Two anomalous observations against the paradigm had been documented even before the establishment of EPI in1974 [8]. One was the occurrence of vaccine failure in India, with children who had been vaccinated with three doses of OPV developing paralytic polio, predominantly caused by type 3 poliovirus [8,9]. The second was the sub-optimal seroconversion rates to one, two or even three doses of OPV of proven potency, in India and Nigeria [8-10]. The explanation for the low vaccine efficacy (VE) was that the infectivity of vaccine viruses was low in these tropical developing countries [11]. The problem was geographically variable, probably determined by gastro-intestinal factors associated with an environment of poor hygiene and sanitation, and not easily overcome by enhancing 10-fold the potency (virus titre) of OPV [12]. A simple solution was actually found. A five-dose primary vaccination would induce the same effect as two doses in North America or Europe [13]. There is a mathematical relationship between the seroconversion rates of sequential doses. It would take 10 doses of OPV in India to equal the benefit of three doses in the U.S. or Europe [14].

Another anomaly was the lack of 'herd effect' of OPV against wild poliovirus infection, in countries such as India and Brazil [15,16]. Herd effect is defined as the fall in incidence in the unimmunised segment of the population as a result of immunizing a proportion of the total population; it is the consequence of retardation of the transmission of the infectious agent, indicating mucosal protection induced by the vaccine [17]. In India, the reported annual prevalence of polio did not decline for nearly 10 years after establishing EPI, in spite of achieving national three-dose OPV coverage of 80% [15]. In Brazil also, the introduction of OPV under EPI did not result in the decline of the prevalence of polio for seven years, until 1981, when additional two-dose annual immunization campaigns (national immunization days, NIDs) were started and continued for the next decade to control the disease and finally to eliminate wild virus transmission by additional mop-up campaigns [16,18].

During the 1980s, large outbreaks of polio occurred in some countries (such as Brazil, Bulgaria, The Gambia, Jordan, Israel, Kerala State in India, Namibia, Oman, Saudi Arabia and Taiwan), in which it had earlier been controlled effectively by high coverage of OPV. The experience in Taiwan is particularly educative; there was a large outbreak due to type 1 virus, in 1982 [19,20]. The official explanation for the setback was the putative pockets of population remaining unvaccinated [19]. On the other hand, polio cases were not in clusters, but widely distributed [20]. Arithmetically, the size of the unvaccinated population was too small to cluster in pockets [20]. Among the unvaccinated children, the attack rate was one in 160 children, suggesting that all unvaccinated children were infected in the epidemic [20]. The only plausible explanation was the participation of the vaccinated (and themselves protected) children in wild-virus transmission [20]. If this was true, then OPV-induced protection from disease (systemic immunity) and from infection (mucosal immunity) are dichotomous [20]. These conclusions were confirmed by direct observation in another type 1 polio outbreak in Oman [21]. In both these countries, the VE of three doses of OPV was intermediate between those in the U.S. and Europe on the one hand, and India, Nigeria and Brazil on the other [19,21]. The lack of herd effect in India and Brazil and the dichotomy of systemic and mucosal immunity found in Taiwan and Oman stood in contrast to the excellent performance of OPV in the U.S., Europe, Australia and Japan. There seem to be two factors operating. One is the VE itself, which varied geographically [14,17]. The other is the 'force of transmission' of wild polioviruses, which also varies geographically [14,17]. In countries with a high standard of living, the force of transmission is low and the VE is high. In such places, the true herd effect of OPV cannot be exposed for want of wild virus challenge. Where VE is moderate and the force of transmission is high, as in Taiwan and Oman, the herd effect was insufficient in spite of high vaccine coverage.

We have examined mucosal (gut) immunity induced by oral infection in the monkey model [22]. Four monkeys given 100 median monkey infectious doses (MID_{50}) of type 1 poliovirus (Mahoney) were found to shed virus for 18 to 20 days in the throat and faeces. The faecal virus was quantified in every sample. After cessation of virus shedding and the absence of virus in repeated samples over two weeks, all monkeys were once again fed the same dose. All monkeys became infected and shed virus for about the same duration and in the same quantities as in the first infection [22]. This is clear evidence that one infection does not induce sufficient mucosal immunity to prevent re-infection or even cause a reduction in the duration of throat and faecal virus shedding or the quantum of faecal virus shedding [22]. All monkeys were challenged again and now the duration of shedding in the throat and in faeces was reduced to less than one week and the quantum of virus reduced by about one $\log_{10}$ [22]. We did not inoculate the monkeys a fourth time, but the evidence so far shows that repeated infections are necessary to induce sufficient mucosal immunity to decrease the duration and reduce the quantum of virus shedding. It is very likely that a fourth inoculation might have failed to establish infection and virus shedding. Antibody measurement had confirmed that the first infection itself had induced excellent humoral immunity [22]. Thus, protection from disease (humoral immunity) and protection from infection (mucosal immunity) are clearly dichotomous.

There is epidemiological evidence that in polio endemic countries, mucosal immunity, herd effect or break in transmission of wild viruses requires multiple inoculations of OPV. The paradigm taught us that vaccine viruses would spread and immunize the unvaccinated children. In reality, there was no evidence for significant secondary spread contributing to herd effect. In Brazil the mean number of doses consumed by children under five was 10, and coverage virtually 100%, when transmission was interrupted [23]. In India, the mean number has exceeded 10 early in the year 2000 and a break in transmission is likely to have occurred in the vast majority of the population units. The VE of 10 doses of OPV in Brazil or India equals that of three doses in wealthy nations, as had been predicted [14]. Vaccination should achieve near 100% VE before herd effect can be expressed; for OPV about 10 doses are needed for that level of VE. For OPV the mucosal immunity is not strong; hence near 100% coverage is necessary for interrupting transmission, especially where the force of transmission is very strong, as we have witnessed in Brazil, India and many similar countries in Asia and Africa. When mucosal immunity is strong, or if the force of transmission of wild virus is low, substantially lower coverage may be sufficient to interrupt transmission.

The IPV Paradigm

The IPV was developed earlier than OPV. In a mammoth vaccine trial, involving 1,829,916 individuals, mostly in the US, and also in Canada and Finland, the safety and efficacy of IPV were established [2]. The VE of two to four doses was about 60-80%. VE correlated with the vaccine potency as measured by the antibody response in those vaccinated. With these findings, IPV was licensed in the U.S.A. in 1955 and as its use increased, the incidence of polio declined rapidly [2]. By 1963, when OPV was advocated for routine use, the incidence had fallen by about 95% [24]. In Finland, in 1960-1961, a mass vaccination programme was instituted, with two doses of IPV one month apart and a third dose 12 months later. By the time a coverage of 51% of the population was reached, the disease disappeared [25]. The circulation of wild viruses also ceased and imported viruses failed to spread. Thus, the complete safety, high VE and excellent herd effect of IPV were established in the U.S., Canada and Finland. Sweden, Norway and Holland also had adopted IPV for routine vaccination. It must be pointed out here that the immune response to IPV could be manipulated; delaying the third dose by many months is a method for improving the level of antibody response. The same approach is currently used in the case of hepatitis B vaccination. For the hepatitis A vaccine, which resembles very closely the modern IPV (see later), a second dose given six months after the first would suffice for achieving high antibody titres and long-lasting immunity. Another method is to increase the antigen content of the vaccine itself, as described later [26,27].

Once the U.S.A. shifted its policy in 1963 in favour of OPV, the OPV paradigm gained wide acceptance, and had great impact and influence on the WHO, resulting in the exclusive choice and promotion of OPV in EPI. The IPV paradigm emerged in contrast to the OPV paradigm and was articulated mostly by the OPV enthusiasts. They believed that IPV lacked all the good qualities of OPV. According to the paradigm:

(i) IPV requires more doses than OPV for satisfactory VE;

(ii) the immunity induced by it wanes and periodic boosters are needed;

(iii) it does not induce mucosal immunity in the intestines;

(iv) it does not have herd effect in developing countries where it is unsuitable for interrupting wild-virus transmission.

Every one of these assumptions has subsequently been proven unfounded. The original IPV as developed by Salk had variable antigen content and antibody response. After the D antigen of IPV was defined, the potency was standardized to 20, two and four D units of poliovirus types 1, 2 and 3 respectively, per individual dose [26]. Subsequently, the vaccine was further improved in terms of purity and potency, with the new IPV containing 40, 8 and 32 D antigen units [26]. We called it the enhanced potency IPV (eIPV), but since all currently available IPV conforms to this standard, there is no need to qualify it any more [28]. As stated earlier, the first IPV trial had predicted that the VE was determined by potency; this was confirmed after the new eIPV became available [2,26,28].

Anomalous Observations on IPV Paradigm

The excellent herd effect of the original IPV was documented in the U.S.A. and the Scandinavian countries [2,24,25]. But the paradigm predicted a lack of herd effect in countries with poor sanitation. On the contrary, in India and elsewhere, wherever IPV was introduced for field trials, excellent VE and an unexpectedly high degree of herd effect were noted [14,27,29]. From April 1980 to March 1983 a field trial of IPV was conducted in a south Indian rural community of 50,000 people [29]. Infants were given three doses of DPT-IPV (containing 20, two and four D units) combination during 19 months, followed by DPT and eIPV in the next 17 months. Among 3220 vaccinees followed up to three years of age (6911 child-years), none developed poliomyelitis. In the adjoining rural community receiving only DPT vaccination, among 3104 infants similarly followed up (6612 child-years), 17 cases of paralytic polio were recorded, for an attack rate of 2.6/1000 child-years below three years [29]. In this highly polio-endemic area, the clinical protective VE of IPV/eIPV was 100%. There was a rapid decline of incidence of polio in the non-immunised segment of children under five in the study area. In the first year the number of cases declined to about half of what was anticipated, and in the second and third years, there were no cases at all.

From 1979 to 1984, in another rural community, weekly stool shedding of polioviruses was compared sequentially between non-immunised (control) children and IPV-given (study) children below three years of age [14]. Three doses of IPV were given, along with DPT, to the study children at monthly intervals. Control children were given only DPT. Among 4527 stool samples from control children 69 strains of polioviruses were isolated, for a rate of 1.52%. Among 8159 samples from study children, only 49 strains were isolated, for a rate of 0.52% ($p<0.001$) [14]. This degree of decline in the circulation of polioviruses among vaccinated children is a reflection of mucosal immunity, which is the basis of herd effect.

Professor Renu Patel (currently Dean, CS Medical College, Thane, Maharashtra, India) had conducted an experiment during 1988 to 1991 (unpublished, but presented at the World Conference on Poliomyelitis, January 7-12, 1992, New Delhi). She was in charge of the Integrated Child Development Scheme in several slum communities in Bombay (now Mumbai). Until 1989, while the three-dose OPV coverage was over 90%, polio used to occur annually in five or more children below five years of age, per block of 100,000 population, mainly as three-dose vaccine failure cases. Then in 1988 she introduced three-dose IPV in one block, keeping all other blocks on OPV. From1989 there was no case of polio in the IPV block, while it continued to occur in the OPV blocks. In 1989 and 1990, she introduced IPV in one new block each, while maintaining one block on OPV as control. From 1990 and 1991, the two blocks on IPV had no polio, while the control block continued to have cases. The first block remained polio-free for three years, the second for two years and the third for one year, while on IPV. The control block on OPV continued with polio every year. This study was closed in 1992, when the investigator was transferred out of Mumbai.

In Kolda, a rural region of Senegal, the introduction of eIPV was followed by a dramatic decline of polio [27]. Data like these have forced us to re-examine the paradigm in a monkey model [30]. We defined mucosal immunity as the degree of resistance to intestinal infection by wild poliovirus. Sixteen monkeys without poliovirus antibodies were given three doses of IPV at monthly intervals. All developed excellent antibody levels to the three poliovirus serotypes. They were kept in quarantine and at three months' intervals four animals were brought to the experimental area and fed 100 MID_{50} of poliovirus type 1 (Mahoney). Up to 12 months, none of the challenged monkeys shed any virus either in the throat or in the stool. This experiment has unequivocally shown excellent mucosal (gut) immunity induced by IPV against intestinal infection by oral inoculation of wild poliovirus [30]. This experiment is in direct contrast to the finding of the lack of protection against re-infection, induced by one or two earlier infections, as noted earlier [22].

What is the Route of Transmission of Polioviruses in Countries Like India?

This is an important question with bearing on the paradigms of OPV and IPV. It is generally assumed that in countries with good environmental sanitation, poliovirus transmission is via the respiratory route and in countries with poor sanitation, the transmission is via the faecal-oral route [3]. It is also generally believed that in countries with respiratory transmission, IPV will be effective for control and elimination of polioviruses, whereas in countries with faecal-oral transmission, only OPV will be effective. It has been shown above that IPV and OPV are very effective in countries with good sanitation. In such places, the force of transmission of wild viruses is also low, and either vaccine has sufficient VE and mucosal immunity to interrupt transmission. Contrary to the paradigm, OPV does not perform well in countries with poor sanitation, where the force of transmission is very high and the VE of OPV is low. On the other hand, the available evidence indicates that IPV performs better in such countries. The VE of IPV is certainly high, but does it induce sufficient mucosal immunity to prevent transmission? Is transmission respiratory or faecal-oral? The vaccine viruses do not seem to spread much among children, in spite of ample opportunities for faecal-oral transmission. This anomaly, together with the herd effect of IPV in such environments, may partly be explained if wild poliovirus transmission is not faecal-oral, but respiratory. If the route of transmission is respiratory in rich countries, surely respiratory transmission must occur where there is overcrowding and close contact among young children. Poor sanitation per se cannot prevent or reduce the probability of respiratory transmission.

OPV is given by mouth and it infects. It is shed in the stool. Wild viruses are shed in the stools of infected children. Therefore it is assumed that they also infect via the oral route. Since wild virus spreads, it is assumed that vaccine viruses must also spread. Where environmental sanitation is poor, many pathogens spread by the faecal-oral route; hence it is possible that wild polioviruses may also spread by the faecal-oral route, but evidence for it is hard to obtain. Vaccine-virus-induced polio among contacts is one clear evidence, but the extent of such transmission is not clear. The respiratory route is likely to be the more important portal of virus entry; as in rich countries, so also in poor ones. Overcrowding may be the main reason for the high force of transmission in poor countries lacking sanitation. The reason for the decreased force of transmission in rich nations may be better housing and living standards and not necessarily the level of sanitation. The vaccine viruses colonise the upper respiratory tract poorly, and that may be the reason why they do not spread efficiently [31].

The median age of poliomyelitis was 12 to 18 months before the widespread use of OPV in India. Even after high vaccination coverage day the median age continues to be below two years [32]. By five years, the risk of polio is virtually eliminated. The median age of measles in the pre-vaccine era was two to three years [33]. Such early infection and rapid saturation is possible only with respiratory transmission. No faecal-oral infection has such an age profile. While faecal-oral transmission of wild polioviruses may occur, this circumstantial evidence suggests that the predominant route of infection might be respiratory. If this is the case, OPV administration by mouth does not mimic natural infection. And, IPV induces sufficient mucosal immunity to prevent respiratory spread.

Had there been substantial transmission and circulation of vaccine viruses, there would not have been the need to achieve near 100% coverage of vaccination, especially with repeated doses. The success of NIDs in rapidly reducing the incidence of polio as well as the circulation of wild viruses has been assumed to be due to the vaccine virus spread to the unvaccinated children [3]. If we take the example of Brazil, what NIDs achieved was the rapid reduction of incidence of disease [16]. There are two alternate explanations for this phenomenon, which a three-dose routine (year-round and age-specific) immunization programme could not achieve. First, with NIDs, each child gets two additional doses of OPV each year; more doses mean greater probability of seroconversion and also the increased chance of repeated infections (in the already seroconverted) leading to better mucosal immunity and herd effect. By four years of age, each child would have had the opportunity to receive three doses in the EPI schedule and 10 additional doses in NIDs. It is not easy to dissect the specific contribution by the many doses versus the process of NIDs, in the rapid reduction of incidence of infection and disease. Second, whatever gut immunity is induced, it is simultaneous in a large proportion of children, thereby reducing the probability of wild virus circulation temporarily and temporally associated with NIDs. That the effect is temporary is the reason why we have to repeat NIDs year after year.

If two doses given simultaneously achieve some success, what will be the effect of three doses given at monthly intervals? There is experimental evidence to show that one three-dose course of 'pulse vaccination' interrupted wild virus transmission in a community highly endemic for polio [34]. Our interpretation was that the herd effect of three-dose pulse is far superior to that of two-dose NIDs or three-dose routine immunisation [14,17]. In summary, there are sufficient plausible explanations for the documented success achieved by the tactical use of OPV in annual pulses, other than the belief that vaccine viruses set up circulation among unvaccinated children. Vaccine viruses do not perpetuate themselves even in communities with very poor sanitation, in spite of weeks of virus shedding in the stools of children with virus 'take'.

Mucosal Immunity and Parenteral Vaccines

The organisation of the mammalian immune system is conceptualized as being in two compartments, systemic and mucosal. The IPV paradigm is that it induces good systemic immunity (and protection from disease), but poor mucosal immunity [2-4]. The immunogen in IPV elicits excellent IgM and IgG and also some non-secretory IgA responses [3,5]. In the absence of a substantial secretory IgA response it was believed that there would be little or no mucosal protection [5,7]. The function of systemic immunity is to prevent the extension of virus infection to the spinal cord and thus to prevent disease; the role of mucosal immunity is to render the mucosa resistant to subsequent infection by the same virus, wild or vaccine. This paradigm is found in many textbooks. To cite one example, it was stated that "mucosal and gut immunity to wild virus" was "very low" for IPV and also that the "potential for circulation of wild virus in vaccinated population" would continue in spite of vaccination with IPV [6]. Thus, according to the paradigm, IPV offers little or no protection against wild-virus infection, hence it has no herd effect nor any role in the elimination of wild polioviruses [7]. However, we have already seen many anomalies to this paradigm.

Secretory IgA response is a marker of infection, and of detectable mucosal immunity, but not necessarily the sole mediator of mucosal protection. This view has clearly emerged largely due to the excellent herd effect of a new parenteral subunit antigen, the *Haemophilus influenzae* b vaccine [35]. Such herd effect (hence mucosal protection) has been shown with acellular pertussis vaccine also [36]. Historically, the earliest successes of polio vaccination were the rapid decline of poliomyelitis in the U.S.A. and in Finland while using IPV [8,9]. The decline in incidence of disease was out of proportion to the vaccination coverage, this phenomenon being attributable to herd effect, which in turn is due to mucosal protection [8,9,10]. In Finland, when 51% of population were (cumulatively) covered by vaccination, the disease disappeared; in parallel, transmission also ceased [9]. The WHO had investigated the safety and efficacy of OPV and IPV in eight countries, over a period of 10 years [37]. The clear conclusion was that both vaccines protected the vaccinated individual and had excellent herd effect also. Thus, we have always known that IPV did induce significant mucosal protection, but the paradigms had overshadowed this information.

The Relevance of the Anomalies to the Final Phase of Polio Eradication

After reasonable evidence of the absence of poliomyelitis is gathered in all countries of the world, we will be unwise to discontinue polio immunization abruptly. It is possible that undetected or silent transmission (without acute flaccid paralysis) of wild polioviruses could occur in some communities, at least for a short period. Stocks of wild virus are available in many virus laboratories and it will take time and extraordinary effort to ensure their destruction or secure containment. During this interval, it will be prudent to continue polio immunization sufficiently to keep up the immunity of new annual birth cohorts so that wild virus may not spread rapidly through a susceptible childhood population. Which vaccine is preferable in this interregnum, IPV or OPV?

Obviously, OPV is easier to give and also cheaper than IPV. One problem with OPV is the rare instance of vaccine-associated paralytic poliomyelitis (VAPP). There are at least two cases of VAPP annually in the United Kingdom [38]. Until OPV was discontinued in the U.S.A., about 10 cases of VAPP have been documented per year since its introduction in 1963. There is a geographical variation in the risk of VAPP, with some countries having many times the risk cited above [37]. While a small risk of VAPP was accepted during the intense eradication phase, the exclusive occurrence of VAPP in the face of no disease due to wild viruses will certainly pose an ethical dilemma. A second problem with OPV is the need for annual immunization campaigns, which is out of step with the EPI mode of normal routine immunization with other vaccines. Routine, schedule based, OPV inoculation alone was not able to interrupt transmission of wild viruses; hence, between routine and pulsed immunization, obviously the latter method is the logical choice if the intention is to interrupt any introduced virus from spreading, even if there has been a time lag between introduction and detection, or between introduction and immunization. Ideally both routine and pulsed immunization should be used, but there is likely to be increasing resistance from programme managers to do both even after zero disease is achieved.

Another problem with OPV is the potential for chronic infection in immunodeficient individuals [39]. The viruses are shed in their faeces, often for years together. Such viruses are OPV derived, but they show increased neurovirulence in monkeys, indicating their reversion from attenuation. These individuals may potentially trigger local spread and possible outbreaks [39,40].

The potential of IPV is that it can easily be combined with DPT; hence it will merge with the EPI schedule, while offering both individual protection and herd effect [37,41]. The main problem with IPV is its higher cost per dose than that of OPV. However, since only two or three doses of IPV are sufficient, the cost per child may indeed be less than that of OPV, but this has to be calculated, taking into account the price of IPV, if manufactured in sufficient quantities.

References

1 Kuhn TS: The structure of scientific revolutions. University of Chicago Press, Chicago. 1996;1-212.

2 Robbins FC: Polio. Historical, in Plotkin SA, Mortimer EA (eds): Vaccines. Second edition. Philadelphia, WB Saunders, 1994, Chapter 6, pp 137-154.

3 Monto AS: The epidemiology of viral infections, in Mahey BWJ, Collier L (eds): Topley and Wilson's Microbiology and Microbial Infections. Ninth Edition. London, Arnold, 1998; Vol 1, pp 235-257.

4 Robbins FC, Nightingale EO: Poliomyelitis, in Walsh JA, Warren KS (eds): Strategies for Primary Health Care. Technologies Appropriate for the Control of Diseases in the Developing World. Chicago, University of Chicago Press, 1986, pp 189-202.

5 Brooks GF, Butel JS, Ornston LN: Picornaviruses, in Jawetz, Melnick, Adelberg (eds): Medical Microbiology. London, Prentice Hall International, 1991, Chapter 36, pp 410-423.

6 Jamison DT, Torres AM, Chen LC, Melnick JL: Poliomyelitis, in Jamison DT, Mosley WH, Measham AR, Bobadilla JL (eds): Disease Control Priorities in Developing Countries. Oxford, Oxford University Press, 1993, pp 117-129.

7 Hull HF, Ward NA, Hull BP, Milstien JA: Paralytic poliomyelitis: seasoned strategies, disappearing disease. Lancet 1994;343:1331-1337.

8 John TJ: Problems with oral poliovaccine in India. Indian Pediatr 1972;9:252-256.

9 John TJ, Jayapal P: Oral polio vaccination in the tropics: 1. The poor seroconversion rates and the absence of viral interference. Amer J Epidemiol 1972;96:263-269.

10 Oduntan SO, Lucas AO, Wennen EM: The immunologic response of Nigerian infants to attenuated and inactivated poliovaccines. Annals Trop Med Parasitol 1978;72:111-115.

11 John TJ: Oral poliovaccination of children in the tropics.2. Antibody response in relation to vaccine virus infection. Amer J Epidemiol 1975;102:414-421.

12 John TJ, Devarajan LV, Balasubramanian A: Immunisation in India with trivalent and monovalent oral poliovirus vaccines of enhanced potency. Bull WHO 1976;54:115-117.

13 John TJ: Antibody response of infants in tropics to five doses of oral poliovaccine. Brit Med J 1976;1:811.

14 John TJ: Immunisation against polioviruses in developing countries. Rev Med Virol 1993:3;149-160.

15 John TJ: Did India have the world's largest outbreak of poliomyelitis associated with injections of adjuvanted DPT? Indian Pediatr 1998;35:73-75.

16 Risi JB Jr: The control of poliomyelitis in Brazil. Rev Infect Dis 1984;6(Suppl):S400-S403.

17 John TJ, Samuel R: Herd immunity and herd effect. New insights and definitions. Europ J Epidemiol 2000;16:601-606.

18 de Quadros CA, Andrus JK, Olive J-M, da Silveira CM, Guerra de Macedo C, Henderson DA: Polio eradication from the western hemisphere. Annual Rev Public Health 1992;13:239-252.

19 Kim-Farley RJ, Rutherford G, Lichfield P, Hsu ST, Orenstein WA, Schonberger LB, Bart KJ, Lui KJ, Lin CC: Outbreak of poliomyelitis in Taiwan. Lancet 1984;2:1322-1324.

20 John TJ: Poliomyelitis in Taiwan. Lessons for developing countries. Lancet 1985;1:872.

21 Sutter RW, Patrirca PA, Brogan S: Outbreak of paralytic poliomyelitis in Oman: evidence for widespread transmission among fully vaccinated children. Lancet 1991;338:715-720.

22 Selvakumar R, John TJ: Intestinal immunity to poliovirus develops only after repeated infections in monkeys. J Med Virol 1989;27:112-116.

23 de Quadros CA, Andrus JK, Olive JM, Carrasco P: Strategies for poliomyelitis eradication in developing countries. Public Health Rev 1993/94;21:65-81.

24 Kim Farley RJ, Bart KJ, Schoneberger LB, Orenstein WA, Nkowane BM, Hinman AR, Kew OM, Hatch MH, Kaplan JE: Poliomyelitis in the USA. Virtual elimination of the disease caused by wild viruses. Lancet 1984;2:1315-1321.

25 Lapinleimu K: Elimination of poliomyelitis in Finland. Rev Infect Dis. 1984;6(Suppl.2):S457-S460.

26 van Wezel AL, va Steenis G, van der Marel P, Osterhaus ADME: Inactivated poliovirus vaccine: current production methods and new developments. Rev Infect Dis 1984;6(Suppl.2).S335-S340.

27 Stoeckel P, Sclumberger M, Parent G, Maire B, van Wezel A, van Steenis A, Evans A, Salk D: Use of killed poliovirus vaccine in a routine immunization programme in West Africa. Rev Infect Dis 1984;6(Suppl.2):S463-S466.

28 Simoes EAF, Padmini B, Steinhoff MC, Jadhav M, John TJ: Antibody response of infants to two doses of inactivated poliovaccine of enhanced potency. Amer J Dis Child 1985;139:977-980.

29 John TJ, Selvakumar R, Balraj V, Rajarathinam A: Field studies using killed poliovirus vaccine, in Proceedings of the third international seminar on vaccination in Africa, Niamey, Niger, 1987. Paris, Association for the Promotion of Preventive Medicine, 1987, pp 173-181.

30 Selvakumar R, John TJ: Intestinal immunity induced by inactivated poliovirus vaccine. Vaccine 1987;5:141-144.

31 Melnick JL: Live attenuated poliovirus vaccines, in Plotkin SA, Mortimer EA (eds): Vaccines. Second edition. Philadelphia, WB Saunders, 1994, Chapter 7, pp 154-204.

32 Singh J, Khare S, Bhatia R, Jain DC, Sokhey J: Epidemiological characteristics of poliomyelitis in Delhi, 1997. Indian Pediatr 1999;36:1211-1219.

33 John TJ, Joseph A, George TI, Radhakrishnan J, Singh RPD, George K: The epidemiology and prevention of measles in rural south India. Indian J Med Res 1980;72:153-158.

34 John TJ, Pandian R, Gadomski A, Steinhoff MC, John M, Ray M: Control of poliomyelitis by pulse immunization in Vellore, India. Brit Med J 1983;286:31-32.

35 Barbour ML: Conjugate vaccines and the carriage of *Haemophilus influenzae* type b. Emer Infect Dis 1996;2:176-182.

36 Trollfors B, Taranger J, Lagergard T, Sundh V, Bryla DA, Schneerson R, Robbins JB: Immunisation of children with pertussis toxoid decreases spread of pertussis within the family. Pediatr Infect Dis J 1998;17:196-199.

37 WHO Consultative group: The relation between acute persisting spinal paralysis and poliomyelitis vaccine – results of a ten-year enquiry. Bull WHO 1982;60:231-242.

38 Finn A, Bell F: Polio vaccine: is it time for a change? Arch Dis Child 1998;78:571-574.

39 Bellmunt A, May G, Zell R, Pring A, Kerblom P, Vergagen W, Heim A: Evolution of poliovirus type 1 during 5.5 years of prolonged enteral replication in an immunodeficient patient. Virology 1999;265(2):178-184.

40 Minor P: Characteristics of poliovirus strains from long-term excretors with primary immunodeficiencies, in Brown F (ed): Progress in Polio Eradication: Vaccine Strategies for the End Game. Dev Biol. Basel, Karger, 2001, vol 105, pp 75-80.

41 Lancet (Editorial). Polio reconsidered. Lancet 1984;2:1309-1310.

Dr. J.T. John, Institute of Virology of Infectious Diseases, Kerala, 439 Civil Supplies Godown Lane, Kamalakshipuram, Vellere TN 632002, India.

Brown F (ed): Progress in Polio Eradication: Vaccine Strategies for the End Game.
Dev Biol. Basel, Karger, 2001, vol 105, p 209

Poster Session III

Brown F (ed): Progress in Polio Eradication: Vaccine Strategies for the End Game.
Dev Biol. Basel, Karger, 2001, vol 105, pp 211-217

Evaluation of the New Control Methods for Oral Poliomyelitis Vaccine

V.P. Grachev, G.G. Karganova, A.A. Rumyantsev, O.E. Ivanova, T.P. Eremeeva, S.G. Drozdov

Chumakov Institute of Poliomyelitis and Viral Encephalitides RAMS, Moscow Region, Russia

Key words: Polio vaccine, MAPREC, transgenic mice, control methods.

Abstract: In the draft recommendations for production and control of OPV the WHO proposed new control methods: (i) mutant analysis with PCR and restriction enzyme cleavage (MAPREC) assay that allows evaluation of poliovirus population heterogeneity at the molecular level; (ii) neurovirulence (NV) test using transgenic mice susceptible to polioviruses and (iii) control of the seed lots for the presence of the simian virus 40 (SV40) DNA sequence. This paper is focused on our experience in the practical implementation of the new methods at the Institute of Poliomyelitis and Viral Encephalitides (IPVE). Using methods based on PCR we have demonstrated that working seed viruses used by IPVE for OPV production are free from SV40 DNA sequences. Our experience on the conduction of the OPV type 3 control using TgPVR21 mice NV test (seven vaccine lots) and the MAPREC assay (more than 150 samples of single harvests and monovalent bulks) showed that these methods may be used instead of the monkey NV test, because they could not pass the vaccine failed monkey NV test. The necessity for single harvests control is discussed.

INTRODUCTION

Regularly increasing demands on the quality and safety of vaccines in general, especially live vaccines, requires constant improvement of production technology and vaccine control methods. Several new tests for OPV safety control have been developed during the past decade: (i) the MAPREC assay that allows evaluation of poliovirus population heterogeneity at the molecular level; (ii) the NV test using transgenic mice susceptible to polioviruses and (iii) control of the seed lots of OPV for the presence of the simian virus 40 (SV40) DNA sequences by PCR [1-3]. Successful evaluation of these methods during the WHO collaborative study allows us to reconsider the recommendations for OPV production and to propose these methods as alternative or obligatory controls [4]. This paper focuses on our experience with the practical implementation of the new control methods at the IPVE manufactory.

Materials and Methods

Molecular biological assays

MAPREC-assay for mutations at positions 472 in OPV type 3, and position 481 in OPV type 2 have been previously described [1, 5-7]. All tested OPV samples were provided by the WHO and IPVE manufactory.

Control of OPV contamination by SV40 DNA sequences was performed according to the WHO recommendations [3]. SV40 was kindly placed at our disposal by Dr. P. Minor.

TgPVR21 mice neurovirulence (NV) assay

The TgPVR21 mouse strain was developed in Dr. A. Nomoto's laboratory [2] and was provided by Dr. T. Nomura (Central Institute of Experimental Animals, Japan). Viruses were supplied by WHO and IPVE manufactory (H-67). The NV test was performed as described previously [8].

Results

Control of SV40 DNA sequence contamination

We have tested working seed viruses used for production of live OPV types 1, 2 and 3 at IPVE for SV40 DNA sequence contamination according to WHO recommendations. The DNA from mock-infected VERO cells and AGMK were used as negative controls. SV40 DNA after one passage of the virus in VERO cell was used as a positive control. The titre of infectious virus was 6,7 log PFU/ml. The WHO recommended method allowed us to demonstrate the specific amplification product in the 10^{-7} dilution; this corresponds to approximately 1 PFU/ml of virus. Our results demonstrated that working seed viruses of OPV types 1, 2 and 3 used at IPVE were free from SV40 DNA sequences (Fig. 1). The products of non-specific amplification might occur in the OPV samples and negative mock-infection cell DNA controls. This may be the reason for the false failing of the OPV seed virus.

TgPVR21 mice neurovirulence test

In the draft recommendations for production and control of OPV, WHO proposed two new methods of testing the genetic stability of virus population of OPV

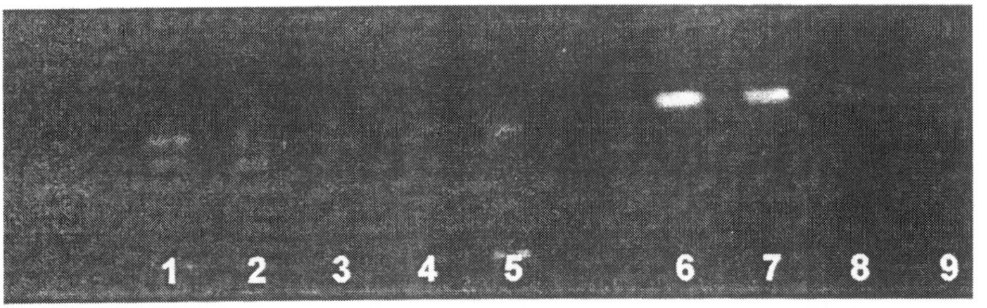

Fig. 1: Control of Simian virus 40 (SV40) DNA sequence contamination in OPV seed viruses (ethidium bromide stained agarose gel). – 1,2,3: seed viruses OPV type 1,2 and 3 respectively; 4,5: VERO and AGMK cell substrates respectively negative control; 6,7,8 and 9: 10^{-3}, 10^{-5}, 10^{-7}, 10^{-8} – SV40 DNA dilutions positive control.

type 3 vaccine strains: (i) in vivo NV test using transgenic mice carrying the PVR receptor (TgPVR21 line) as alternative to the monkey NV test, and (ii) in vitro - MAPREC as obligatory test instead of rct40-test [4].

We participated in the WHO collaborative study on evaluation of the TgPVR21 mouse NV test. Six samples of OPV type 3 obtained from different production lots were tested; three of them had failed and three had passed the monkey NV test. These were tested in five blind experiments. Samples were compared with the WHO reference in two doses. As shown in Table 1, there was a high correlation between the results of the monkey and Tg mice NV tests with one exception – sample 98/652. This OPV type 3 was not derived from WHO seed virus and requires special reference for the mice NV test. Moreover, we studied one dose of the OPV type 3 bulk (H-67) produced by the IPVE and this passed the monkey and Tg mice NV tests.

Table 1: Comparative analysis of the WHO proposed methods (MAPREC and NV in transgenic (Tg) mice) and the monkey NV test for control of OPV type 3 bulks from different manufacturers.

OPV 3 type lots	% 472-C	MAPREC	NV on Tg mice	NV on monkeys
93/568	2,02	failed	failed	failed*
93/636	3,30*	failed	failed	failed*
95/526	1,70*	failed	failed	failed*
93/650	1,14	likely to fail	passed	passed*
98/652	0,34	passed	failed	passed*
93/664	0,86	passed	passed	passed*
H-67	0,64	passed	passed#	passed

* Data from [12].
\# Tested in one dose.

Mutant analysis

In the WHO draft recommendations for the production and control of OPV the MAPREC was proposed as an obligatory in vitro test to control filtered OPV type 3 bulks and was recommended for monitoring consistency of production of single harvests (SH) [4]. MAPREC is a very sensitive method that allows to evaluate quantitatively the heterogeneity of viral population as low as 0,1%. It makes the test a powerful tool for analysis of the genetic stability of the OPV type 3 [1]. We studied over 150 different samples of OPV type 3 to evaluate the proportion of viruses with reversion to the neurovirulent genotype characterized by UÆC replacement in the 472 nucleotide position of the 5’ untranslated region. Standard operating procedure (SOP) for the OPV type 3 MAPREC test recommends the use of the set of standards 95/542 and 94/790- cDNA standards, 96/572 and 96/578 – that should respectively pass and fail the MAPREC test [6]. The results of the MAPREC test of these standards (Table 2) were similar to the results obtained in other laboratories during collaborative study and demonstrate a high reproducibility of this method [9]. According to the SOP, OPV type 3 that contains 472-C in

Table 2: Analysis of MAPREC OPV type 3 standards.

Standard (number of experiments)	472-C	Minimum	Maximum
96/572 (23)	0,95±0,06	0,47	1,57
96/578 (23)	1,70±0,07	0,56	2,02
95/542 (26)	1,15±0,07	0,72	2,33
94/790 (28)	91,46±0,57	87,11	94,87

excess of that in the standard vaccine 95/542 (1,0%) fails MAPREC. We have tested 55 bulks of OPV type 3 produced by IPVE over several years. The mean content of 472-C mutants among all bulks was 0,38%±0,02 and the upper limit level for the manufactory was calculated as 0,65%. All bulks of the OPV type 3 studied passed the MAPREC test. Four of the tested bulks had 472-C concentration above the upper limit.

Ninety-eight unfiltered SH which were combined into 12 bulks of OPV were studied to assess the consistency of OPV production. The mean content of 472-C revertants was 0,66%±0,05. Eleven SH failed the MAPREC test.

We explored the possible influence of some slight technology breaches during OPV propagation on the accumulation of 472-C revertants in the vaccine population. We possessed samples of OPV type 3 SH which had been failed at different stages of OPV production: (i) 10 SH cultivated at elevated temperature (upper limit 35°C); (ii) four SH propagated on poor substrate cell monolayers due to non-specific cell pathogenic effect resulting from contamination by an unknown agent; (iii) two SH propagated on subconfluent cell monolayer. All samples passed the MAPREC test.

We have analysed the influence of storage condition on the consistency of the poliovirus population at 472 position of seed viruses OPV type 3 and bulks derived from them. Long-term storage of seed-working viruses at –20°C did not influence the accumulation of 472 mutants in bulks of OPV derived from them. Storage study results of OPV type 3 bulks derived from SO and RSO seed viruses are shown in Table 3.

Table 3: The influence of different storage conditions on the amount of 472-C in SO and RSO derived OPV type 3.

Incubation temperature	Incubation period	472-C			
		RSO-a	RSO-b	RSO-c	SO
42°C	12 hours	0,32±0,15	0,50±0,06	0,62±0,09	0,60±0,05
	1 day	0,48±0,22	0,63±0,19	0,84±0,12	0,35±0,11
	2 days	0,71±0,12	0,68±0,15	**2,89**±0,23	0,30±0,03
37°C	5 days	0,44±0,18	**1,19±0,05**	0,66±0,07	**0,96±0,57**
	10 days	**1,52±0,11**	0,76±0,13	**1,07**±0,08	0,44±0,04
25°C	7 days	0,34±0,09	0,46±0,02	n.d.*	0,36±0,02
	14 days	0,34±0,03	0,48±0,05	n.d.	0,41±0,06
4°C	4 months	0,41±0,07	0,63±0,03	0,83±0,08	0,66±0,09
Freezing-thawing (eight times)		0,40±0,04	0,36±0,02	n.d.	0,32±0,06
Control		0,24±0,08	0,58±0,08	0,61±0,06	0,27±0,11

* Not determined.

The MAPREC assay for OPV type 2 as the method for monitoring production consistency is based on the determination of the proportion of 481-G revertants [7]. Commercially produced monovalent bulks of Sabin type 2 were found to contain between 0.4 and 1.1% 481-G mutants. Using MAPREC we have analysed nine bulks of OPV type 2 by MAPREC (Table 4) and have discovered one bulk that later failed the monkey NV test.

Table 4: Results of OPV type 2 control by MAPREC assay.

Code	% 481-G	Prediction	MNVT
F-59*	0,48±0,09	will pass	passed
F-60	0,52±0,07	will pass	passed
H-81	0,53±0,01	will pass	passed
E-15	0,54±0,02	will pass	passed
H-25	0,55±0,02	will pass	passed
H-33	0,58±0,09	will pass	passed
H-79	0,60±0,05	will pass	passed
H-80	0,64±0,09	will pass	passed
H-27	0,67±0,11	will pass	passed
H-31	0,68±0,11	will pass	passed
H-32	5,49±0,67	will fail	failed

* All bulks were prepared at IPVE manufactory.

Discussion

Modern molecular biological methods provide manufacturers with new ways for the safety control of live vaccines. Several articles on the discovery of SV40 DNA sequences in some human tumours were published during the past few years. However, no epidemiological relationship between the development of these tumours and contamination of the earlier poliovaccines by this virus was found [3,10]. To avoid the introduction of SV40 into the human population during vaccination, a new method based on PCR diagnostic technique that permits identification of SV40 DNA sequences in OPV was developed [10]. Using this approach we demonstrated that working seed viruses used by IPVE for OPV production are free from SV40 DNA sequences.

Our experiments with the OPV controls using the TgPVR21 mice NV test and MAPREC assay demonstrated that these methods may be used instead of the monkey NV test. They are less labour-consuming, faster, and easy to standardize. Results of all three methods used to control several OPV type 3 bulks are shown in Table 1.

The vaccines which failed the monkey NV test were not found to pass using the new methods. MAPREC appeared to be the more discriminating approach. Sometimes the OPV type 3 bulks that passed the monkey NV test failed the MAPREC, for example lot 98/650 (Table 1). The standard vaccine 96/572 with elevated 472-C (but less than 1%) nevertheless have failed MAPREC four times out of 23 experiments. The 96/578 vaccine standard that had 472-C mutants above 1% have passed the MAPREC assay seven times out of 23 experiments. Moreover, OPV type 3 bulk H-66 (Table 5), one of 55 IPVE bulks studied, has failed MAPREC once but passed it upon re-test. However, it contained 472-C mutants above the calculated upper limit level (0,65%) for the IPVE bulks. Thus, the OPV type 3 with approximately 1% 472-C may or may not fail the MAPREC test. Nonetheless, all this vaccines that contained 472-C above the upper limit for bulks produced at IPVE passed the monkey NV test. We consider that MAPREC can be used as an alternative test to the monkey NV test. We consider that the strategy of OPV type 3 control should be as follows: (i) if 472-C content is less than the upper limit calculated, it is allowed to pass; (ii) if it is higher, the decision will be obtained by the in vivo test. For example, among analysed IPVE type 3 bulks, four samples contained 472-C above the upper limit but all of them passed the monkey NV test. One of them, H-67, which was tested in TgPVR21 mice in one dose (Table 1), also passed this test.

Table 5: Characteristics of OPV type 3 containing single harvests (SH) which failed the MAPREC assay.

OPV type 3 bulks	% 472-C in the bulk	Number of SH forming the bulk	Number of analyzed SH	Failed MAPREC	Additional information
H-66	0,83	12	11	5	Not used for vaccination
H-67	0,66	11	8	2	2 VAPP*
H-95	0,38	13	10	3	1 VAPP*
H-96	0,35	13	13	1	2 VAPP*

* VAPP: vaccine associated paralytic poliomyelitis.

To determine the possible role of elevated 472-C content in bulks we studied 12 OPV type 3 bulks included in 14 lots of polyvalent OPV connected with 12 cases of vaccine associated paralytic poliomyelitis (VAPP) and two cases compatible with VAPP among OPV recipients registered in Russia from 1998 (Table 5). The H-67 bulk with elevated 472-C content was associated with two VAPP cases but all other bulks contain 472-C mutants close to the mean level for IPVE products (0,38%). Thus we revealed no correlation between VAPP cases and content of 472-C mutants in vaccines. We have revealed 11 type 3 SH which failed MAPREC. Five of them were included in the H-66 bulk not used for vaccination (Table 5). Another six SH have been included in bulks associated with VAPP. The reason for developing VAPP is not yet clear. Possibly, in the first place it is associated with the health of the recipient. It is impossible however to eliminate completely the possibility that some vaccine characteristics could promote a manifestation of immunity defects in the recipient. Evidently the content of 472-C revertants is the marker of accumulation of other poliovirus mutants that promoted VAPP development. We suppose that elimination of SH with high 472-C content could increase OPV safety even for persons with immune disorders.

To identify factors in the manufacturing process that may influence the accumulation of viruses with 472-C reversion we have analysed SH produced under slightly faulty conditions at different stages of production (elevated temperature (upper limit 35°C) of cultivation, non-specific cell pathogenic effect and poor quality of cell monolayers) and revealed no correlation. Obviously vaccine quality depends mostly on the individual nature of the animal donor used for cell substrate preparation. The results of genetic structure changes in the virus population kept at different conditions are given in Table 3. In the experiments vaccine samples have been used without any stabilizers. Commercial vaccines that are more stable during storage at an elevated temperature could result in different MAPREC data [11]. However, it must be taken into consideration that any decrease of OPV infectious titres may result in changes in genetic consistency of the population and increase in neurovirulence.

References

1 Chumakov KM, Powers LB, Noonan KE, Roninson IB, Levenbook IS: Correlation between amount of virus the altered nucleotide sequence and the monkey test for acceptability of oral poliovirus vaccine. Proc Natl Acad Sci USA 1991;88(1):199-203.

2 Kioke S, Taya C, Kurata T, Abe S, Ise I, Yonekawa H, Nomoto A: Transgenic mice susceptible to poliovirus. Proc Natl Acad Sci USA1991;88:951-955.

3 Sangar D, Pipkin PA, Wood DJ, Minor PD: Examination of poliovirus vaccine preparations for SV40 sequences. Biologicals 1999;27:1-10.

4 Draft recommendations for poliomyelitis vaccine (oral). Expert committee on biological standardization. WHO 1999.

5 Chumakov KM, Dragunsky EM, Norwood LP, Douthitt MP, Ran Y, Taffs RE, Ridge J, Levenbook IS: Consistent selection of mutations in the 5-'untranslated region of oral poliovirus vaccine upon passaging in vitro. J Med Virology 1994;42:79-85.

6 Chumakov KM: Mutant Analysis by PCR and Restriction Enzyme Cleavage (MAPREC) for Oral Poliovirus (Sabin) Vaccine. Standard Operating Procedure for the WHO Collaborative study on MAPREC. 1999.

7 Taffs RE, Chumakov KM, Rezapkin GV, Lu Z, Douthitt M, Dragunsky EM, Levenbook IS: Genetic stability and mutant selection in Sabin 2 strain of oral poliovirus vaccine grown under different cell culture conditions. Virology 1995;209:366-373.

8 Dragunsky E, Taffs R, Chernokhvostova Y, Nomura T, Hioki K, Gardner D, Norwood L, Levenbook I: A poliovirus-susceptible transgenic mouse model as a possible replacement for the monkey neurovirulence test of oral poliovirus vaccine. Biologicals 1996;24:77-86.

9 Matherials of Working group on the use of the MAPREC assay in the quality control of oral polio vaccine. WHO 1999.

10 Lewis AM Jr, Egan W: Workshop on simian virus 40 (SV40): a possible human polyomavirus. Meeting report. Biologicals 1997;25:355-358.

11 Pipkin PA, Minor PD: Studies on the loss of infectivity of live type 3 poliovaccine on storage. Biologicals 1998;26:17-23.

12 Materials of Working group on transgenic mice as animal model for neurovirulence test of OPV. WHO 1999.

Dr. G.G. Karganova, Institute of Poliomyelitis, Moscow Region, 142782, Russia.

Brown F (ed): Progress in Polio Eradication: Vaccine Strategies for the End Game.
Dev Biol. Basel, Karger, 2001, vol 105, pp 219-223

Poliomyelitis in Russia in 1998-1999

O.E. Ivanova[1], *T.P. Eremeeva*[1], *G.G. Karganova*[1], *A.A. Rumyantsev*[1], *E.V. Leshinskaya*[1], *G.Y. Lipskaya*[2], *E.A. Cherkasova*[2], *E.A. Korotkova*[2], *V.P. Grachev*[1], *S.G. Drozdov*[1]

[1] M.P. Chumakov Institute of Poliomyelitis and Viral Encephalitides of Russian Academy of Medical Science, Moscow Region, Russia

[2] A.N. Belozersky Institute of Physical-Chemical Biology, Moscow State University, Moscow, Russia

Key words: Acute flaccid paralysis, vaccine-associated paralytic poliomyelitis, oral poliovaccine, polioviruses.

Abstract: After introducing surveillance for poliomyelitis and AFP cases in the Russian Federation in 1998, 740 AFP cases have been registered in 1998-1999, and 18 of that number were considered as vaccine-associated paralytic poliomyelitis (VAPP). Of 18 cases 11 were classified as VAPP of vaccine recipients and confirmed by virus isolation; from two of the vaccine recipients virus was not isolated, and five were poliomyelitis cases in contact non-vaccinated children. In all the cases the disease was characterised with the typical clinical picture with residual pareses and paralyses. One case was fatal. Vaccine virus type 3 has been isolated from all the vaccine recipients. The MAPREC test has shown that the quality of monovaccine type 3 bulks used for vaccinating these children did not differ from the quality of other bulk vaccines produced by the Chumakov Institute of Poliomyelitis. Patients surveyed for gammaglobulin were positive. Polioviruses type 1 isolated from two of the contact cases had changed antigenic properties and were recombinants of types 1 and 2.

Introduction

The last isolation of wild poliovirus in the Russian Federation (RF) was registered in 1995 during an outbreak of paralytic poliomyelitis in the Chechen Republic. To raise the level of individual and collective immunity and to banish the circulation of wild poliovirus, National Days of Immunization (NDI) have been conducted in 1996-99 in the RF. During these NDIs, 99,3% of children less than three years old have been vaccinated [1]. Since 1998, a precise system of registration of acute flaccid paralysis (AFP) has been introduced in Russia. This system raised the efficacy of epidemiological surveillance for poliomyelitis and AFP and virological investigation of each case. In 1998-1999 740 AFP cases were registered in Russia, and 18 of that number were considered as poliomyelitis. This communication analyses these cases.

Materials and Methods

Stool samples were prepared as described [2]. Virus isolation was performed using RD, Hep-2 and/or L20B cells [2]. Identification of isolated cytopathogenic agents with type-specific antisera to polioviruses (RIVM, Bilthoven, The Netherlands) were carried out by microneutralization in RD cells [2]. Intratypic differentiation has been done using ELISA with cross-absorbed rabbit antisera [3] and polymerase chain reaction (PCR) with primer pairs specific for Sabin strains [4].

Genetic analysis was performed by:

1) Restriction fragment length polymorphism (RFLP) assay [5];
2) Nucleotide sequencing. DNA copies of selected genomic portions were amplified by PCR with appropriate primers (the sequences are available upon request). PCR products were purified in the QIAquick system (Quiagen) and directly sequenced by using the Sequenase version 2.0 kit (US Biochemical).

Genetic stability of the virus population of oral poliovaccine (OPV) types 2 and 3 was determined by the MAPREC test (Mutant Analysis with PCR and Restriction Enzyme Cleavage) [6].

Results

Of 18 poliomyelitis cases 11 were classified as vaccine-associated paralytic poliomyelitis (VAPP) of vaccine recipients, one as a case compatible with poliomyelitis, possible vaccine recipient, one as poliomyelitis of unknown aetiology, possible vaccine recipient (virus has not been isolated during adequate investigation of the case), five as poliomyelitis cases in contact non-vaccinated children. The cases have been classified according to [7].

In all the cases diseases were characterised with the typical clinical picture: spinal (16 cases) and bulbo-spinal (one case) localisation of the process with residual pareses and paralyses. One case was fatal.

The VAPP cases were noted in 10 vaccine recipients aged four to five months and in one eighteen-month old child. In nine cases paralysis was noted after the first dose of trivalent OPV 11-32 days post vaccination. Two children (age of four and five months) had paralysis after the second dose of OPV (on the 7th and 16th day, respectively).

In all the VAPP cases only vaccine viruses have been isolated. The spectrum of isolated viruses is presented in Table 1.

The cases compatible with VAPP and poliomyelitis of unknown aetiology were registered in children aged of three and four months after the first dose of OPV 22 and 17 days before paralytic manifestation respectively.

For vaccination, 12 lots of trivalent OPV (Manufactory of Chumakov Institute of Polio) including 14 bulks of monovaccine type 3, five bulks of monovaccine type 2 and 18 bulks of monovaccine type 1 have been used.

Analysis of OPV (11 bulks of type 3 and three bulks of type 2) used for vaccination of these children was accomplished. All the tested bulks of monovaccines successfully passed the MAPREC test. The mean number of reversions in position 472 of monovaccine type 3 associated with VAPP was the same as in all the tested bulks (more than 50) of monovaccines type 3 produced by the Chumakov Institute of Poliomyelitis.

VAPP contact cases have been observed in children aged three to nine months. The spectrum of isolated viruses is presented in Table 1. Polioviruses of type 3 have been characterised as vaccine-related. Poliovirus type 1 isolated from one child was also vaccine-related. Polioviruses type 1 isolated from two other chil-

Table 1: Spectrum of polioviruses isolated from VAPP cases.

Classification of the cases	Type of isolated polioviruses				
	1	3	1+2+3	1+3	2+3
Recipients of vaccine	–	6	2	1	2
Non-vaccinated contacts	3	2	–	–	–

dren had changed antigenic properties and were detected in ELISA as wild but in PCR they were shown to be vaccine-related. Restriction analysis showed that the two strains were recombinants of types 1 and 2. Partial sequencing of genomic fragments of these strains proved the recombinant nature of the isolates and allowed us to determine precisely the regions of recombination. One isolate had a point of crossing over in the genomic region encoding protein 2A and another isolate had that point on the 3'- end of the genomic fragment encoding protein VP1. Comparison of partially sequenced poliovirus genomic fragments encoding capsid protein VP1 and non-structural proteins 2A and 2B with the corresponding genomic fragments of vaccine strains 1 and 2 types showed nucleotide and aminoacid replacements randomly distributed within these fragments.

Of 11 children with illness after vaccination, four were investigated for serum proteins. All those investigated had hypogammaglobulinaemia from 6 to 8.7%. Two of the patients (one of them with hypogammaglobulinaemia) had recurrent purulent paraproctitis.

Discussion

Risk of VAPP after vaccination with live OPV is very low and according to different authors varies from one case per 1.4 million vaccine doses [8] to one case per 2.5 million vaccine doses [9]. According to Andrus et al, in 1989-1991 in Latin America, the frequency of VAPP cases after the first dose of OPV was one case per 1.2 million doses, and after subsequent vaccinations was one case per 3.6 million doses. Contacts had a much lower risk: one case per 5.6 million doses [10].

Between 1988 and 1999 in Russia, 48 million doses of trivalent OPV (Chumakov Institute of Poliomyelitis) were distributed. This means one VAPP case after the first dose of OPV per 5.3 million doses or, if two possible VAPP cases, one case per 4.4 million doses. After the second vaccination, there would be one case per 24 million doses, and for contact VAPP, one case per 9.6 million doses. The mean index of VAPP in RF was one case per 2.6 million doses of trivalent vaccine for two years.

Mostly, VAPP cases in vaccine recipients are associated with poliovirus type 3 [11]. In this investigation, vaccine virus type 3 has been isolated from all the registered cases in vaccine recipients (Table 1). We tried to connect the quality of monovaccine type 3 used for vaccination with VAPP. Using the MAPREC test, we analysed 11 out of 14 OPV type 3 bulks (78.6%) and, retrospectively, five bulks included in four trivalent lots associated with four cases of post-vaccinal complications during 1995-1998. This analysis did not reveal a rise in the level of neurovirulent revertant polioviruses in the OPV population compared with the mean level of such revertants in the vaccine series produced by the Chumakov Institute of

Poliomyelitis. This means that the quality of the vaccine did not play a significant role in VAPP cases in recipients.

We do not possess complete information concerning the immune status of all the patients. However there is one notable fact: four out of 11 patients (vaccine recipients) had immunological insufficiency in the form of hypogammaglobulinaemia, and one of these cases was fatal and two cases had purulent paraproctitis. The question about the correlation of immunological damage in children and VAPP requires further study.

From five VAPP cases (vaccine recipients) we isolated mixtures of different poliovirus types while from contact children we isolated one poliovirus type only. It is possible that non-vaccinated contacts excrete only the virus that caused illness.

Contact cases in non-vaccinated children are frequently associated with type 2 and, to a lesser degree, 3 type virus [11]. In our investigation, virus of type 2 in contact patients has not been detected but two recombinant strains of types 1 and 2 have been isolated. In the region encoding the structural proteins which in both cases is derived from Sabin strain type 1, about 1% of nucleotide replacements with regard to vaccine ancestor has been registered. Approximately the same number of replacements as compared with Sabin strain type 2 have been accumulated in the regions encoding proteins 2A and 2B. Based on the information on the speed of accumulation of replacements (about 1-2% per genome per year), it is possible to consider that the revealed number of replacements was not possible to have been accumulated in the patients during the period of illness. Approximately equal numbers of replacements in the genome regions derived from different serotype ancestors suggests that this recombinant event took place before invasion of the organism (in both cases). Amino-acid replacements in the VP1 protein do not explain their antigenic changes; we plan to carry out an analysis of other capsid proteins.

Acknowledgements

We thank Mrs. M.S. Trofimchik, M.P. Chumakov Institute of Poliomyelitis and Viral Encephalitides of Russian AMS, for technical assistance, and Dr. V.N Sadovnykova from Federal Centre of Sanitary and Epidemiological Surveillance of Russian Ministry of Health for access to epidemiological data.

References

1 Monisov AA, Ivanov SI, Mikchailova LG: Epidemiological control for poliomyelitis and acute flaccid paralyses. Ministry of Health, Federal Center of sanitary and epidemiological surveillance. Health of population and environment quarterly rep 1998;3-4:6-9.

2 World Health Organization: Manual for the virological investigation of poliomyelitis.WHO/EPI/CDS/90.1, Geneva, 1990, pp 29-66.

3 van Loon AM, Ras A, Poelstra P, Mulders MN, van der Avoort HGAM: Intratypic differentiation of polioviruses, in Kurstak E (ed): Measles and Poliomyelitis. Vienna, Springer Verlag, 1993, pp 359-369.

4 Yang C, De L, Holloway BP, Pallansch MA, Kew OM: Detection and identification of vaccine-related polioviruses by the polymerase chain reaction. Virus Research 1991;20:159-179.

5 Balanant J, Guillot S, Candrea A, Delpeyroux F, Crainic R: The natural genomic variability of poliovirus analyzed by a restriction fragment length polymorphism assay. Virology 1991;184:645-654.

6 Chumakov KM: Mutant Analysis by PCR and Restriction Enzyme Cleavage (MAPREC) for Oral Poliovirus (Sabin) Vaccine. Standard Operating Procedure for the WHO Collaborative study on MAPREC. 1999.

7 Leshinskaya EV, Laticheva IN: Clinic, diagnostic and treatment of acute poliomyelitis. Methodical recommendations. Moscow, 1998, pp 3-48 (in Russian).

8 Joce R, Wood D, Brown D, Begg NT: Paralytic poliomyelitis in England and Wales. Brit Med J 1992;304:79-82.

9 Strebel PM, Sutter RM, Cochi SL, et al: Epidemiology of poliomyelitis in the United States one decade after the last reported case of indigenous wild virus - associated disease. Clin Infect Dis 1992;14:668-679.

10 Andrus JK, Strebel PM, de Quadros CA, Olive JM: Risk of vaccine-associated poliomyelitis in Latin America. Bull WHO 1995;73:33-40.

11 Assaard F, Cockburn WC: The relation between acute persisting spinal paralysis and poliomyelitis vaccine - results ten year enquiry. Bull WHO 1982;60:231-242.

Dr. O.E. Ivanova, M.P. Chumakov Institute of Poliomyelitis and Viral Encephalitides of Russian AMS, 142782, Moscow, Russia.

Brown F (ed): Progress in Polio Eradication: Vaccine Strategies for the End Game.
Dev Biol. Basel, Karger, 2001, vol 105, pp 225-230

Inhibition of Poliovirus RNA Synthesis as a Molecular Mechanism Contributing to Viral Persistence in the Mouse Central Nervous System

T. Couderc[1], *S. Girard*[1], *I. Pelletier*[1], *A.S. Gosselin*[1], *J. Destombes*[2], *D. Thiesson*[2], *F. Colbère-Garapin*[1], *B. Blondel*[1]

[1] Unité de Neurovirologie et Régénération du Système Nerveux, Institut Pasteur, Paris, France

[2] UMR 7000, Faculté de Médecine Pitié-Salpétrière, Paris, France

Key words: Poliovirus, poliomyelitis, persistence, RNA synthesis, central nervous system, nerve cells.

Abstract: Many survivors of poliomyelitis, several decades after the acute phase of the disease, develop a set of new muscle symptoms called post-polio syndrome. The persistence of poliovirus (PV) in the central nervous system (CNS) may be involved in the aetiology of this syndrome. By using a mouse model, we have shown that PV persists in the CNS of paralysed mice for over a year after the acute disease. Detection of PV plus- and minus-strand RNAs in the spinal cord of paralysed mice suggested continuous PV RNA replication in the CNS. However, infectious PV particles could not be recovered from homogenates of CNS from paralysed mice beyond 20 days post-paralysis, indicating that PV replication was restricted. In an attempt to identify the molecular mechanism by which PV replication was limited, PV plus- and minus-strand RNA levels were estimated in the CNS of persistently infected mice by a semi-quantitative RT-nested PCR method. Results revealed that RNA replication was inhibited at the level of plus-strand RNA synthesis during persistent infection. Similar results were obtained in neuroblastoma IMR-32 cell cultures persistently infected with PV. Restriction of PV RNA synthesis could be involved in persistence by limiting PV replication.

INTRODUCTION

After decades of clinical stability, many poliomyelitic patients develop a disease called post-polio syndrome (PPS). This syndrome involves a variable set of symptoms ranging from muscle and joint pain to slowly progressive muscle weakness [1]. The persistence of poliovirus (PV) in the central nervous system (CNS) may be involved in the aetiology of this syndrome. Although the link between PV persistence and PPS remains controversial, several studies suggest that PV is present in the human CNS a long time after the acute paralytic poliomyelitis. Analyses of the spinal fluid from PPS patients have revealed the presence of anti-PV IgM antibodies [2] and of fragmentary genetic sequences of PV RNA or PV-related RNA [3-5]. In vitro, it has been shown that PV can establish persistent infection in human cell cultures of neural origin such as neuroblastoma cells IMR-32 [6].

Experimentally, poliomyelitis can be transmitted to monkeys with all three serotypes of PV and to mice with mouse-adapted PV strains by inoculation into the CNS. We have previously isolated and characterized a PV mutant pathogenic for mice, PV-1/Mah-T1022I, derived from the PV-1/Mahoney strain [7, 8]. This mouse-adapted mutant causes paralytic poliomyelitis in Swiss mice which is not always lethal. We have taken advantage of this mouse model to study the ability of PV to persist in the CNS after the acute phase of the disease.

Materials and Method

Animal infections

Twenty-one day old female OF1 (Iffa-Credo) mice were inoculated intraventrically with 3 x 10^6 plaque forming units of the mouse-adapted strain PV-1/Mah-T1022I. Surviving paralysed mice were sacrified at various times after inoculation.

Histological analysis and immunofluorescence

Mice were killed under deep anaesthesia with Sagatal and perfused with Bodian fixative as described [9]. Longitudinal sections (10 µm thick) of the spinal cord were cut and deparaffinized, and one section was stained with cresyl violet. On one adjacent section, PV antigen was detected by immunofluorescence with monoclonal antibody C3, directed against the structural polypeptide VP1 of PV-1 [10] and with the biotin-avidin complex conjugated to fluorescein isothiocyanate [9].

Ultrastructural immunodetection

Mice were killed as described above and perfused with a fixative solution of 4% paraformaldehyde and 0.1% glutaraldehyde in 0.1M phosphate buffer, pH7.4. Following post fixation, longitudinal sections (50µm) were cut with a vibratome and immunoperoxidase staining was performed with monoclonal antibody C3, then with the biotin-avidin complex conjugated to horseradish peroxidase (Vectastain Elite ABC kit; Vector Labs) to label PV particles [9]. Sections were then treated as described [9] before performing ultrathin sections. Electron microscope, Jeol CX 100, was used for observation.

Reverse transcription-nested polymerase chain reaction (RT-nested PCR) of CNS RNA

Total RNA was extracted from mice spinal cords with the RNA Plus reagent (Bioprobe Systems). PV plus- and minus-strand RNA molecules were detected independently by RT-nested PCR [9]. To estimate the ratio of plus-strand RNA to minus-strand RNA, serial dilutions were performed on total RNA extracted from the mouse spinal cord and each dilution was submitted to eight independent RT-nested PCR for plus-strand RNA and for minus-strand RNA detection, respectively. PCR products were visualized after electrophoresis on agarose gels. The dilution for which 50% RT-nested PCR are positive (D-PCR50) was calculated by the Reed and Muench end point method [11]; the plus-strand RNA to minus-strand RNA ratio corresponds to the D-PCR50 for plus-strand RNA to the D-PCR50 for minus-strand RNA.

Results

Poliovirus persistence in the mouse spinal cord after the onset of paralysis.

To investigate the ability of PV to persist in the spinal cord after the acute phase of poliomyelitis, Swiss mice were inoculated intracerebrally with the mouse-adapted mutant PV-1/Mah-T1022I and surviving paralysed mice were studied at 10 days and at three, six, nine, and 12 months after the onset of symptoms [9]. Histological examination of the spinal cord sections stained with cresyl violet revealed neuronal damage in a limited area of the ventral horn which corresponds to the distribution of clinical paralysis (data not shown). In this area, neuronal chromatolysis could be observed at each time point. Inflammatory cell infiltration was pronounced at 10 days and at 3 months after the onset of paralysis, and then decreased but did not disappear entirely, at later time points.

Viral antigens were detected by immunofluorescence in motor-neurons of the affected ventral horn at each time studied (data not shown). Moreover, PV particles were observed in the cytoplasm of motor-neurons by ultrastructural immunodetection until 12 months post paralysis (Fig. 1). These results showed that PV persists in the CNS of paralysed mice for over a year after the acute disease. More-

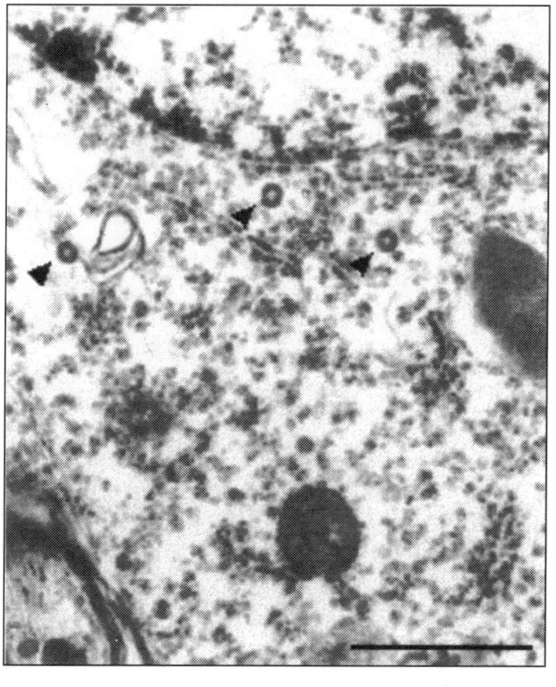

Fig. 1: Ultrastructural immunodetection of PV particles (arrowheads) in the cytoplasm of motor neurons of the mouse spinal cord at 6 months after the onset of paralysis (the appearance and the size of these viral particles are identical to those detected by the same procedure in the PV-infected epithelial cell cultures) [9]. Bar, 1μm.

over, detection of PV plus- and minus-strand RNAs, by RT-nested PCR, in the spinal cord of paralysed mice suggested continuous PV RNA replication in the CNS (Fig. 2). However, infectious PV particles could not be recovered from homogenates of CNS from paralysed mice beyond 20 days post-paralysis, indicating that PV replication was restricted. Limited replication has been shown with other neurotropic viruses such as the measles virus and mouse hepatitis virus, for which viral antigens and genome were detected although infectious virus could rarely, if ever, be isolated during persistent infection of the CNS [12, 13].

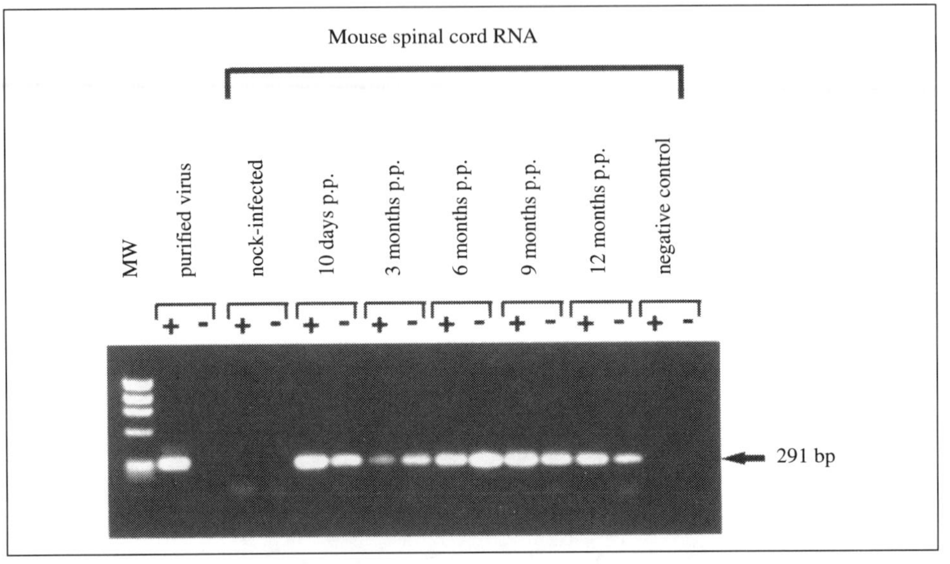

Fig. 2: Nested PCR products following RT of RNA extracted from the mouse spinal cord at the indicated time points post paralysis (p.p.). Positive (+) and negative (-) RNA strands were specifically amplified using appropriate primers [9]. Purified infectious PV particles devoid of minus-strand RNA were used as a negative control for minus-strand RNA. A mock-inoculated mouse was used as a negative control for the mouse spinal cord. A negative control for RT/PCR, which contained water instead of RNA, was also included. DNA molecular weight marker (MW): phiX174/*Hae*III.

Restriction of poliovirus RNA synthesis during persistent infection in nerve cells

We were interested in the molecular mechanism of PV persistence in the mouse CNS. One of the main mechanisms by which non-retroviral RNA viruses, and picornaviruses in particular, persist in vivo is an abnormal regulation of RNA production at the level of plus-strand RNA as observed for Coxsackievirus B or at the level of minus-strand as observed for Theiler's virus [14,15]. To investigate whether such a mechanism was involved in PV persistence in the mouse CNS, the PV plus- and minus-strand RNA ratio in the spinal cord of mice was estimated at the time of the onset of paralysis and at later times after paralysis (one, three and 12 months) by using an end point method of RT-nested PCR detection. Our results showed that this ratio decreased during persistent infection (Fig. 3) indicating that PV RNA replication is restricted at the level of plus-strand RNA synthesis during persistent infection.

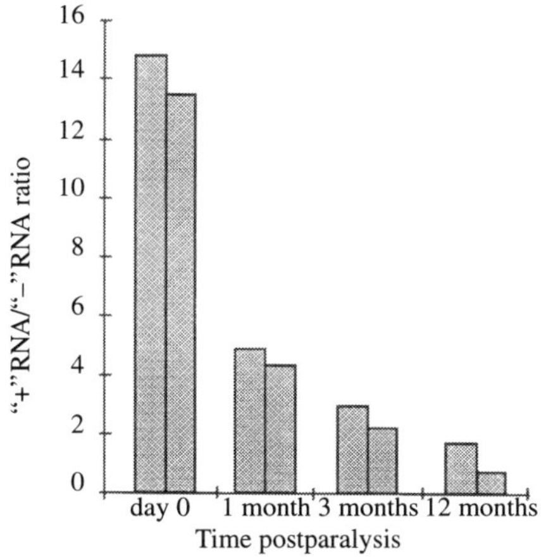

Fig. 3: Evolution of PV plus-strand RNA to minus-strand RNA ratio during persistent infection of the mouse spinal cord. Each bar represents one PV-infected mouse.

To investigate whether PV RNA replication is inhibited during PV persistence in vitro, we analysed PV RNA synthesis in human neuroblastoma IMR-32 cells persistently infected with PV-1/Mah-T1022I. The ratio of PV plus-strand RNA to minus-strand RNA was estimated in these cells until six months post infection. The results revealed that the plus-strand RNA to minus-strand RNA ratio decreased during persistent infection (data not shown), indicating that, as observed in the mouse CNS, RNA replication in persistently infected IMR32 cells was inhibited at the level of plus-strand RNA synthesis.

Discussion

Altogether our results show that PV is able to persist in the spinal cord of paralysed mice for a long period of time after the acute phase of poliomyelitis. Furthermore, PV plus-strand RNA synthesis is restricted during the persistent infection in the mouse spinal cord as well as in human neuroblastoma IMR-32 cells. This restriction could be involved in persistence by limiting PV replication. The IMR-32 cell model will allow us to characterize the molecular mechanisms involved in the inhibition of PV RNA synthesis; in particular we will study the respective contribution of cellular and viral factors in this inhibition.

Conclusion

Studies on PV persistence in human spinal fluid and in human neuroblastoma cells, as well as those in the mouse spinal cord raise the question of the ability of PV to persist in the CNS of poliomyelitis survivors. This issue is particularly important in the context of the poliomyelitis eradication programme.

Acknowledgements

This work was supported by grants from the Association Française contre les Myopathies (contracts 3720, 5082, 5740, 6495 and 6932 and by the Direction des Recherches sur l'Environnement (Recherche Environnement 6724).

References

1 Dalakas MC, Bartfeld H, Kurland LT: The post-polio syndrome, The New York Academy of Sciences, New York, 1995.

2 Sharief MK, Hentges MR, Ciardi M: Intrathecal immune response in patients with the post-polio syndrome. N Engl J Med 1991;325:749-755.

3 Leparc-Goffart I, Julien J, Fuchs F, Janatova I, Aymard M, Kopecka H: Evidence of presence of poliovirus genomic sequences in cerebrospinal fluid from patients with postpolio syndrome. J Clin Microbiol 1996;34:2023-2026.

4 Muir P, Nicholson F, Sharief MK, Thompson EJ, Cairns NJ, Lantos P, Spencer GT, Kaminski HJ, Banatvala JE: Evidence for persistent enterovirus infection of the central nervous system in patients with previous paralytic poliomyelitis, in Dalakas MC, Bartfeld H, Kurland LT (eds): The Post-Polio Syndrome. New York, The New York Academy of Sciences, 1995, vol 753, pp 219-232.

5 Leon-Monzon ME, Dalakas MC: Detection of poliovirus antibodies and poliovirus genome in patients with post-polio syndrome (PPS), in Dalakas MC, Bartfeld H, Kurland LT (eds): The Post-Polio Syndrome. New York, The New York Academy of Sciences, 1995, vol 753, pp 208-218.

6 Colbère-Garapin F, Christodoulou C, Crainic R, Pelletier I: Persistent poliovirus infection of human neuroblastoma cells. Proc Natl Acad Sci USA 1989;86:7590-7594.

7 Couderc T, Hogle J, Le Blay H, Horaud F, Blondel B: Molecular characterization of mouse-virulent poliovirus type 1 Mahoney mutants: involvement of residues of polypeptides VP1 and VP2 located on the inner surface of the capsid protein shell. J Virol 1993;67:3808-3817.

8 Couderc T, Delpeyroux J, Le Blay H, Blondel B: Mouse adaptation determinants of poliovirus type 1 enhance viral uncoating. J Virol 1996;70:305-312.

9 Destombes J, Couderc T, Thiesson D, Girard S, Wilt SG, Blondel B: Persistent poliovirus infection in mouse motoneurons. J Virol 1997;71:1621-1628.

10 Blondel B, Akacem O, Crainic R, Couillin P, Horodniceanu F: Detection by monoclonal antibodies of an antigenic determinant critical for poliovirus neutralization present on VP1 and on heat inactivated virions. Virology 1983;126:707-710.

11 Reed LJ, Muench M: A simple method for estimating fifty percent endpoints. Amer J Hyg 1938;27:493-497.

12 Schneider-Schaulies S, ter Meulen V: Molecular aspects of measles virus induced central nervous system disease, in Roos RP (ed): Molecular Neurovirology. Totowa, NJ, Human Press Inc, 1992, vol pp 419-449.

13 Kyuwa S, Stohlman SA: Pathogenesis of a neurotropic murine coronavirus, strain JHM in the central nervous system of mice. Sem Virol 1990;1:273-280.

14 Cash E, Chamorro M, Brahic M: Minus-strand RNA synthesis in the spinal cords of mice persistently infected with Theiler's virus. J Virol 1988;62:1824-1826.

15 Cunningham L, Bowles NE, Lane RJM, Dubowitz V: Persistence of enteroviral RNA in chronic fatigue syndrome is associated with the abnormal production of equal amounts of positive and negative strands of enteroviral RNA. J Gen Virol 1990;71:1399-1402.

Dr. B. Blondel, Unité de Neurovirologie et Régénération du Système Nerveux, Institut Pasteur,
28 rue du Docteur Roux, F-75724 Paris Cedex 15, France.

Brown F (ed): Progress in Polio Eradication: Vaccine Strategies for the End Game.
Dev Biol. Basel, Karger, 2001, vol 105, pp 231-237

Outbreak of Paralytic Poliomyelitis in the Chechen Republic in 1995

O.E. Ivanova[1], T.P. Eremeeva[1], G.Y. Lipskaya[2], E.A. Cherkasova[2], E.V. Gavrilin[2], S.G. Drozdov[1]

[1] M.P. Chumakov Institute of Poliomyelitis and Viral Encephalitides, Russian Academy of Medical Science, Moscow Region, Russia

[2] A.N. Belozersky Institute of Physical-Chemical Biology, Moscow State University, Moscow, Russia

Key words: Poliomyelitis, outbreak, wild poliovirus type 1.

Abstract: An outbreak of poliomyelitis with 146 cases among children of whom six died occurred in the Chechen Republic in 1995. Sporadic cases of poliomyelitis have been reported in the neighbouring Ingush Republic. The outbreak lasted for five months (from May to September) and the maximum number of cases was registered in July. The age of the patients did not exceed 11 years, and more than 90% of the patients were children aged from one month to four years. The overwhelming majority of the patients had not been vaccinated in the routine OPV immunization programme. The outbreak was due to wild poliovirus type 1 belonging to genotype T previously known to circulate in the territory of the former Soviet Union (FSU). Chechen and Ingush isolates were very closely related to each other and to isolates from Central Asia, Tajikistan, 1994. Only a very distant relatedness of the Chechen and Ingush isolates was found with the strains isolated at about the same time outside the FSU (China 1994, Pakistan 1995). The presence of high numbers of non-vaccinated/poorly vaccinated persons and the poor sanitary and hygienic conditions for civilians due to the military conflict were factors that had a role in the outbreak.

Introduction

In the Soviet Union systematic mass vaccination against poliomyelitis, introduced in 1959, reduced the number of cases from 13,492 in 1958 to 17 in 1991 [1]. The collapse of the Soviet Union (1991) resulted in the destruction of the union system of vaccine prophylaxis and surveillance, and outbreaks have been noted in some regions [2].

In 1995, sanitary and hygienic conditions for civilians and health services in the Chechen Republic worsened. Migration of large groups of the population increased sharply. An outbreak of paralytic poliomyelitis occurred with 146 cases among children (six of them lethal). Due to cross-border movement of refugees, sporadic cases of poliomyelitis have been reported in the neighbouring Ingush Republic.

THE OUTBREAK

Background

The Chechen and Ingush republics are situated in the southern part of Russia – northern Caucasus. They have an area of 19,000 km^2 with a population of 1.29 million. Endemic focus of poliomyelitis with sporadic cases has been existing in this territory for several years and poliovirus vaccination of children was carried out with difficulty. Thus, in 1993 in the Chechen Republic only 53,6% of children aged one year had complete vaccination, and 17,4% were not vaccinated at all. In 1994 poliovirus vaccination was not carried out.

The first child became ill in March 1995 (retrospective clinical data). The majority of the cases took place in June-July (Fig. 1). The last cases were noted in November. The cases in the Ingush Republic were noted in September and October, and the last case was registered in December 1995. Patients were admitted to hospital in Grozny; 26 children with mothers were admitted to the First Infections Hospital in Moscow. All the admitted children had typical development of the disease. Various degrees of residual symptoms after two months of onset of the disease were observed for all the patients. The outbreak covered a large area (Fig. 2). The majority of the cases were registered in regions with the most intensive shift of the population. The age of the patients (Fig. 3) did not exceed 11 years. The highest morbidity rates in the Chechen Republic were in children younger than one year.

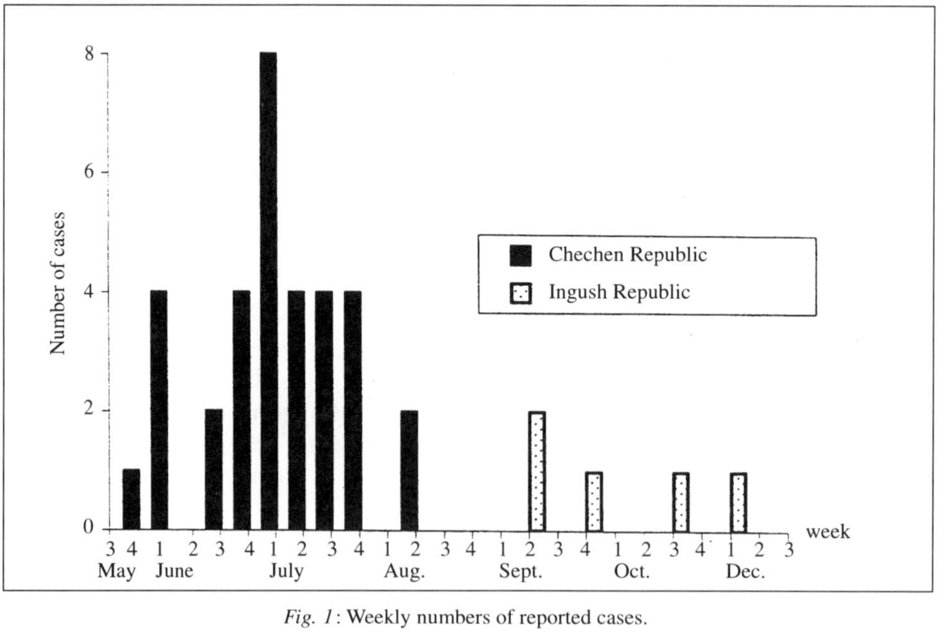

Fig. 1: Weekly numbers of reported cases.

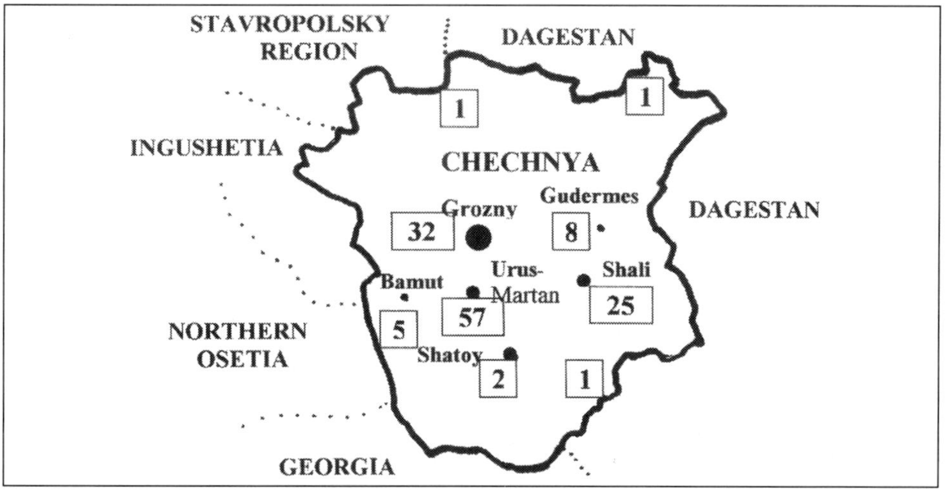

Fig. 2: Geographical distribution of cases. In squares – number of documented cases.

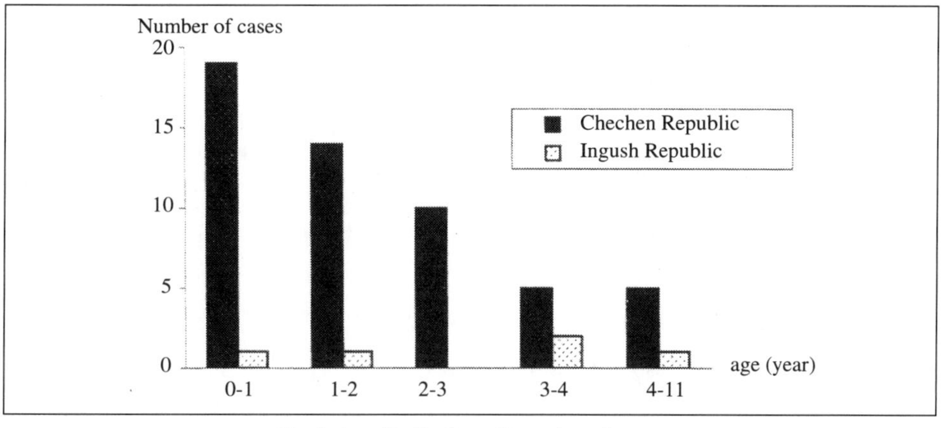

Fig. 3: Age distribution of investigated cases.

Materials and Methods

Chechen Republic

Faeces (155 samples) from 53 patients and sera (55 samples) from 29, and faeces (61 samples) and sera (23 samples) from 25 adult contacts (mothers of children hospitalized in the Moscow clinic) were investigated. None of the patients had been vaccinated in the routine OPV immunization programme with the exception of three children who had a history of having received one or two doses of trivalent OPV.

Ingush Republic

Six stool samples from five patients were obtained. Two of the patients had not been vaccinated in the routine OPV immunization programme; the three others had received one, two and eight doses of trivalent OPV. Materials (91 stool samples and three serum samples) from 64 contact children (two-13 years) and from seven contact adults have also been investigated. From contact children 33 (51%) had received one to three doses of OPV, 26 (41%) – six to 12 doses of OPV and five (8%) had no information about vaccination.

Stool samples have been prepared according to procedure [3]. The viruses have been isolated in RD cells [3]. Identification of cytopathogenic agents with type-specific antisera to polioviruses (RIVM, Bilthoven, The Netherlands). have been carried out by micro-neutralization in RD cells [3].

Intratypic differentiation of isolated strains has been carried out using ELISA with cross-absorbed rabbit antisera [4] and PCR with primer pairs specific for Sabin strains [5]. For determination of the virus genotype, specific primers have been used [6]. Partial sequencing has been carried out according to the method in Ref. [7]. The dendrogram was generated using the PUZZLE program version [8].

Virus-neutralizing titres of antibodies to Sabin vaccine polioviruses types 1-3 were determined by microneutralization in Hep-2 cells (Cincinnati) [3].

RESULTS

Chechen Republic

As shown in Table 1, 72% of the patients (despite rather late sampling of stool samples) and 7% of contact cases were positive for wild poliovirus type 1. Wild poliovirus type 1 has been isolated from 51% of stool samples of patients and from 3,2% of stool samples of contacts. No polioviruses of type 2 and 3 have been isolated.

Stool samples of 22 patients admitted to the Moscow hospital were taken several times to observe the duration of excretion of the virus. Eleven patients (50%) showed excretion of the virus for one month after onset, nine patients (41%) within two months, and two patients (9%) excreted the virus for more than two months.

Sera from 29 patients were investigated: using eight single and 21 paired sera (two to four samples). The late sampling of samples did not allow us to observe seroconversion. Table 2 shows that all the samples had neutralizing antibodies to poliovirus type 1. The majority of the patients had no antibodies ($<3 \log_2$) to poliovirus types 2 and 3. The rather high titre of antibodies to all three types was detected in the sera of adult contacts.

Ingush Republic

Table 1 shows that 60% of the patients and 21% of the contacts (12 children and three adults) excreted wild poliovirus type 1. From one to 10 days before collection of stool samples all the contact children had been vaccinated with OPV. So the spectrum of isolated viruses was manifold: 13 contacts excreted wild poliovirus type 1, eight, vaccine virus type 1, two contacts excreted wild and vaccine

Table 1: Results of virological investigations of patients and contacts.

Groups	Number of investigated persons		Number of faecal samples	
	Total	With wild polio 1	Total	With wild polio 1
	Chechen Republic			
Patients	53	38	155	79
Contacts	27	2	61	2
	Ingush Republic			
Patients	5	3	6	3
Contacts	71	15	91	17

Table 2: Results of serological investigations of patients and contacts.

Poliovirus type	Total	Number of investigated persons										
		With antibody titres (log_2) to polioviruses										
		<3	3	4	5	6	7	8	9	10	11	>11
		Patients										
1	29					1	3	1	12	4	4	4
2	29	28								1		
3	29	27		1						1		
		Contacts										
1	22					1		2		3		16
2	20			1		2		5	4	3		5
3	20		4	1	3	2	4	4	2			

viruses type 1 simultaneously, one contact, vaccine virus type 2, and one contact, a mixture of vaccine polioviruses types 1 and 3.

Only three serum samples from three contact children taken three weeks after contact with the patient were available. The children had a history of administration of six to seven doses of OPV. The children had antibody titres to poliovirus type 1 of 9,10 and >> 11 log_2; to poliovirus type 2-<3, >11 and >>11 log_2; to poliovirus type 3 - < 3,6 and <3 log_2, respectively. Wild strains of poliovirus have been isolated from stool samples of these children.

Genetic analysis of the virus

The analysis by PCR of some randomly selected isolates of wild poliovirus type 1 from the Chechen and Ingush Republics with genotype-specific primers showed that they belonged to genotype-T previously known to circulate in the territory of the former Soviet Union [1]. Partial genomic sequencing of the VP1/2A junction region [3] of some of the isolates was carried out to determine the possible genetic relatedness of the strains to other representatives of the T genotype (Fig. 4). The Chechen and Ingush isolates (6490CHE95 and 6405ING95, 6427ING95) are very closely

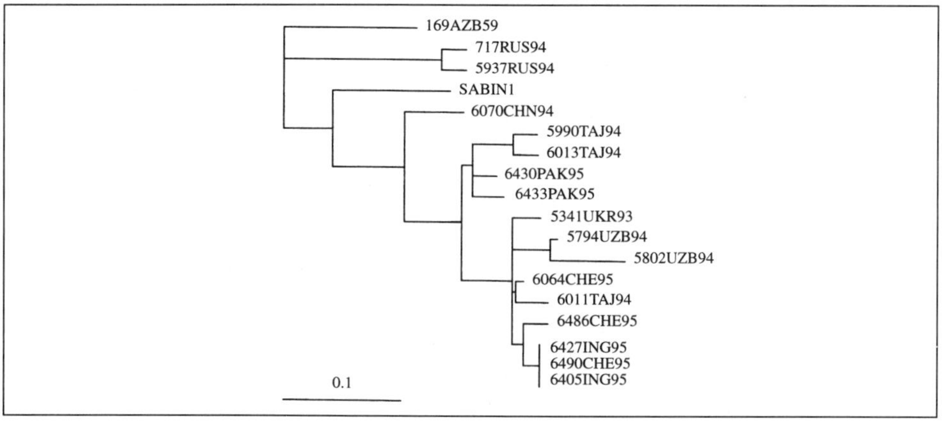

Fig. 4: The VP1/2A maximum likelihood tree (PUZZLE 4.0) rooted on 169AZB59 showing the relationships of polio type 1 wild strains. The scale corresponds to 10% of the nucleotide divergence.

related to each other (1.3-3.4%%). The close relatedness of the Chechen strains with the isolate from Central Asia, Tajikistan (6011TAJ94) was shown (Fig.4). Only a relatively distant relatedness (exceeding 10%) of the Chechen and Ingush isolates was found with the strains isolated at about the same time outside the FSU (6070CHN94, 6430PAK95, 6433PAK95).

Discussion

The epidemiological picture of the outbreak, and the clinical manifestations were similar to those of classical outbreaks of poliomyelitis in developing countries in the pre-vaccine era; as with the majority of outbreaks of that period it was caused by wild poliovirus type 1 [9].

The outbreak was characterized by wide circulation of the virus among the population. Many contact persons were involved in the epidemic. Of 98 investigated contacts (totally or partially vaccinated with OPV), 17% excreted wild virus. The contacts comprised two groups: (i) adult contacts from the Chechen and Ingush republics and (ii) mainly children aged two to 12 years from the Ingush Republic. The frequency of wild virus isolation among adults was 15%, and 19% among children. In the sera of adult contacts, high-titered antibodies were detected both to type 1 and to types 2 and 3. The ability of the virus to multiply in the intestines of the people with a high level of humoral immunity may be explained by a decrease in local immunity in the intestines and/or by massive invasion of the virus that exceeds the protective level of secretory antibodies (IgA). Unfortunately we had only three serum samples from Ingush contact children; this does not allow us to judge the status of humoral immunity in the group and to explain the fact that the majority of the contacts excreted wild virus. It is possible to suggest only that besides the mentioned causes, there were various violations during vaccination. For example, a child after seven vaccinations had high level antibodies to poliovirus type 1 and no antibodies to types 2 and 3 which demonstrates low efficacy of vaccination. Similar causes of widespread epidemic poliovirus among the partially or totally vaccinated population had been observed during many recent outbreaks in developing countries [9]. The presence of healthy excretors of the virus in the population provided virus circulation during the rise of morbidity and long-term conservation of the virus, at least to December 1995.

Transmission of the wild-type virus to the population was also supported by patients with long-term excretion of the virus (for two and more months). Long-term excretion of the virus in the background of adequate immune response to infection (high level of antibody titres) is probably connected with non-mature intestinal immunity of children. At the same time there was no circulation of wild poliovirus in Russia outside the borders of the Chechen and Ingush Republics. None of the isolations of wild viruses from AFP cases and the environment were from contacts moving into Moscow by municipal transport. Evidently the level of collective immunity was sufficient to prevent virus expansion.

In spite of the steps being taken to stop the circulation of wild virus (NID-s in Spring 1996), three cases of poliomyelitis (only clinically confirmed) were registered in the summer of 1996 in the Chechen Republic. In the following years, AFP surveillance programme in this region has not been carried out. The coverage of trivalent OPV in one-year-old children was 32,5% in 1997 and 43,4% in 1998 (data from the MOH of the RF). Resumption of military activity in 1999 aggravated the situation again. The Ministry of Health of the RF ensured that more than 90% of the children in the northern Caucasus were vaccinated during NIDs in April 2000. But only the institution of active AFP surveillance in the Chechen and Ingush republics can confirm the absence of wild poliovirus circulation.

Acknowledgements

We thank the virologists from the M.P. Chumakov Institute of Poliomyelitis and Viral Encephalitides of Russian AMS: Dr. V.B. Kontorovitch, Mrs M.S.Trofimchik for technical assistance, Dr. V.B.Seibil, Mrs L.P. Malyshkina, and Ms. V.F.Yefimova) for their contribution of some virus isolates, and Professor E.V.Leshinskaya and Dr I.N.Martynenko for access to clinical data.

References

1 Infectious diseases in Russia. Statistical guide. State Committee of Sanitary and Epidemiological Surveillance. Moscow, 1992, pp 26-27 (in Russian).

2 Centers for Disease Control and Prevention. Status of poliomyelitis eradication – Europe and the Central Asian Republics, 1993. MMWR Morb Mortal Wkly Rep 1994;43:518-521.

3 World Health Organization: Manual for the virological investigation of poliomyelitis.WHO/EPI/CDS/90.1, Geneva, 1990, pp 29-66.

4 van Loon AM, Ras A, Poelstra P, Mulders MN, van der Avoort HGAM: Intratypic differentiation of polioviruses, in Kurstak E (ed): Measles and Poliomyelitis. Vienna, Springer Verlag, 1993, pp 359-369.

5 Yang C, De L, Holloway BP, Pallansch MA, Kew OM: Detection and identification of vaccine-related polioviruses by the polymerase chain reaction. Virus Research 1991;20:159-179.

6 Lipskaya GY, Chervonskaya EA, Belova GI, Maslova SV, Kutateladze TN, Drozdov SG, Mulders M, Pallansch MA, Kew OM & Agol VI: Geographical genotypes (genotypes) of poliovirus case isolates from the former Soviet Union: relatedness to other known poliovirus genotypes. J Jen Virol 1995;2:1687-1699.

7 Rico-Nesse R, Pallansch M, Nottay B, Kew OM: Geografic distribution of wild poliovirus type 1 genotypes. Virology 1987;160:311-322.

8 Strimmer K, von Haeseler A: Quartet puzzling: a quartet maximum likelihood method for reconstructing tree topologies. Mol Biol Evol 1996;13:964-969.

9 Patriarca PA, Sutter RW, Oostvogel PM: Outbreaks of paralytic poliomyelitis, 1976-1995. J of Infect Dis 1997;175:S165-172.

Dr. O.E. Ivanova, M.P. Chumakov Institute of Poliomyelitis and Viral Encephalitides of Russian AMS, 142782, Moscow, Russia.

List of Participants

AGOL Vadim, Institute of Poliomyelitis, Russia Academy Medical Science, 142842 Moscow, Russia.
ALMOND Jeffrey, Aventis Pasteur, Campus Merieux, 1541 av. Marcel Mérieux, F-69280 Marcy-l'Etoile.
ANDRE Francis E., SmithKline Beecham Biologicals, 89, rue de l'Institut, B-1330 Rixensart.
ARITA Isao, Agency for Cooperation in International Health, 4-11-1 Higashi-machi, Kumamoto City, Kumamoto 862-0901, Japan.
ARMAND Jacques, Aventis Pasteur, Campus Mérieux, 1541 av. Marcel Mérieux, F-69280 Marcy l'Etoile.

BARRETO Luis, Aventis Pasteur Limited, 1755 Steeles Ave. West, Willowdale, Ontario M2R 3T4, Canada.
BERGER Jacques, Aventis Pasteur, 2, avenue Pont Pasteur, F-69007 Lyon.
BLONDEL Jacques, Aventis Pasteur, 2, avenue du Pont Pasteur, F-69007 Lyon.
BOGAERTS Hugues, Smithkline Beecham, 89, rue de l'Institut, B-1330 Rixensart.
BOTTIGER Margareta, WHO Europe Commission, Gransäter, S-13236 Saltsjö-Boo.
BRO-JORGENSEN Klaus, Statens Serum Institut, Artillerivej 5, DK-2300 Denmark.
BROWN Fred, Plum Island Disease Center, P.O. Box 848, Greenport, NY 119 44, USA.

CACERES Victor M., Centers for. Disease Control, 1600 Clifton Rd, Mailstop E-05, Atlanta, GA 30340, USA.
CARO Valérie, Institut Pasteur, Epidémiologie des Entérovirus, 25, rue du Dr Roux, F-75724 Paris Cedex 15.
CHALUMEAU Hervé, Aventis Pasteur, Campus Mérieux, 1541, av. Marcel Mérieux, F-69280 Marcy l'Etoile.
CHINO Fumitoshi, Tokyo Vaccination Clinic, 1-8-2 Marunouchi, Chiyoda-ku, Tokyo 100-0005, Japan.
CHUMAKOV Konstantin, FDA/CBER, 1401 Rockville Pike, HFM-255, Rockville, MD 20852, USA.
COCHI Stephen, CDC / National Immunization Program, Mailstop E-05, Atlanta, GA 30333, USA.
COLBERE-GARAPIN Florence, Institut Pasteur, Génétique Virale – NRSN, 25, rue du Dr Roux, F-75724 Paris Cedex 15.
CRAINIC Radu, Institut Pasteur, Epidémiologie des Entérovirus, 25, rue du Dr Roux, F-75724 Paris Cedex 15.
CUERVO Nancy, Institut Pasteur, Epidémiologie des Entérovirus, 25, rue du Dr Roux, F-75724 Paris Cedex 15.

DA SILVA Edsom, Institut Oswald Cry, Av. Brasil 4365, 21045-900 Rio de Janeiro, Brazil.
DELPEYROUX Francis, Institut Pasteur, Epidémiologie des Entérovirus, 25, rue du Dr Roux, F-75724 Paris Cedex 15.
DESMYTER J., Katholieke Universiteit Leuven, Rega Instituut, Minderbroedersstraat 10, B-3000 Leuven.
DIDELEZ Jean, Smithkline Beecham Biologicals, 89, rue de l'Institut, B-1330 Rixensart.
DOI Yutaka, Japan Poliomyelitis Research Inst., 5-34-4 Kumegawa-cho, Higashimurayama, Tokyo 189-000 Japan.
DREJER Dik, European Committee Certification Eradication of Polio, Leeuwerikenlaan 100, NL-2215 NT Voorhoub.
DROZDOV Sergei, Inst. of Poliomyelitis, 142782 Moscow Region, Russia.
DUCHENE Michel, SmithKline Beecham Biologicals, 89, rue de l'Institut, B-1330 Rixensart.

EGAN William M., FDA/CBER/OVVR, 1401 Rockville Pike, Bethesda, MD 20892, USA.

FEDSON David, Aventis Pasteur MSD, 8, rue Jonas Salk, F-69367 Lyon Cedex 07.
FLETCHER Mark Andrew, Aventis Pasteur, Medical Affairs, 2, av. du Pont Pasteur, F-69367 Lyon 07.
FRIEDERICH Klaus, Chiron Behring GmbH & Co., P.O. Box 1630, D-35006 Marburg.
FUCHS Florence, Agence du Médicament/Direction des Laboratoires et Contrôles, 321, av. Jean Jaurès, F-69007 Lyon
FURESZ John, 1805 Apt, 20 The Driveway, Ottawa, Ontario K2P 1C8, Canada.

GARY Howard, Centers for Diseases Control & Prevention, NIP (E05), CDC, Atlanta, GA 30333, USA.
GEMMIL Ian, Canadian Public Health Assoc., 221 Portsmouth Avenue, Kingston, Ontario M2R 3T4, Canada.
GILCHRIST Shawn, Aventis Pasteur, 1755 Steeles Av. West, Bldg 83, Toronto, Ontario M2R 3T4, Canada.
GRACHEV Victor, P.O. Inst. of Poliomyelitis, Russian Academy of Med. Science, 142782 Moscow Region, Russia.
GRAF Hughes, Aventis Pasteur, Production Virologie V8-V6, Campus Mérieux, 1541, av. Marcel Mérieux, F-69280 Marcy l'Etoile.
GRECO Michel, Aventis Pasteur SA, Le Confluent 1, 2, av. Pont Pasteur, F-69367 Lyon Cedex 07.

HALKJAER-KNUDSEN Vibeke, Staten Serum Institut, Artillerivej 5, NL-2300 Copenhagen S.
HALSEY Neil, John Hopkins University, 615 N. Wolfe Street, Baltimore, MD 21205, USA.
HERREMANS Tineke, Lab. Of Infectious Diseases, RIVM, P.O. Box 1, NL-3720 BA Bilthoven.
HO Mei-Shang, Inst. of Biomedical Sciences, IBMS, Academia Sinica, Taipei 11529, Taiwan.
HOVI Tanapi, National Public Health Inst., Mannerheimintie 166, FIN-00300 Helsinki.
HULL Harry, WHO, Avenue Appia, CH-1211 Geneva 27.

JALBY Jean-Marc, Aventis Pasteur, Campus Mérieux, 1541, avenue Marcel Mérieux, F-69280 Marcy l'Etoile.
JOHN Jacob T., Inst. of Virology & Infectious. Diseases, Kerala, 439 Civil Supplies Godown Lane, Kamalakshipuram, Vellere TN 63, India.

KADO-BOLL Gustavo, Inst. Nacional de Virologia Birmex, Prolongacion de Carpio 492, DF 11340 Mexico, Mexico.
KAUFHOLD Achim, Smithkline Beecham Biologicals, 89, rue de l'Institut, B-1330 Rixensart
KIM Kyung Ho, Green Cross Vaccine Corp. 303 Bojung-Ri, Koosung-Myun, Yongin City 449-910, South Korea.
KIMMAN Tjeerd, National Inst. of Public Health, P.O. Box 1, NL-3720 BA Bilthoven.
KNUDSEN Birgitte W., Statens Serum Institut, 5, Artillerivej, DK-2300 Copenhagen S.
KOURILSKY Philippe, Institut Pasteur, 28 Rue du Docteur Roux, F-75724 Paris Cedex 15.

LEVY-BRUHL Daniel, Institut de veille sanitaire, 12 rue du Val d'Osnes, F-94415 St-Maurice Cedex.
LINA Bruno, Centre national de référence pour les Entérovirus, Domaine Rockfeller, F-69373 Lyon Cedex 08.
LIPSKAYA Galina, W.H.O., Sherfigsvej 8, DK-2100 Copenhagen.

MACADAM Andrew, N.I.B.S.C., Blanche Lane, South Mimms, Potters Bar, Herts EN6 3QG, U.K.
MALLET Laurent, Aventis Pasteur, campus Mérieux, 1541, av. Marcel Mérieux, F-69280 Marcy l'Etoile.
MARTIN Javier, N.I.B.S.C., Blanche Lane, South Mimms, Potters Bar, Herts EN6 3QG, U.K.
MENDELSON Ella, Central Veterinary Lab., Public Health Laboratories MOH, Chaim Sheba Medical Center, Tel-Hashomer 52621, Israel.
MILSTIEN Julie, W.H.O., 20, av. Appia, CH-1211 Geneva 27.
MINOR Philip, N.I.B.S.C., Blanche Lane, South Mimms, Potters Bar, Herts. EN6 3QG, U.K.
MONTAGNON Bernard J., 5, rue des Ecoles - Le Bourg, F-69210 Lentilly.
MORER Isabelle, Agence française de Sécurité Sanitaire des Produits de Santé, 143-147 Bld Anatole France, F-92385 Saint-Denis Cedex.
MORGEAUX Sylvie, AFSSAPS, 321 avenue Jean Jaurès, F-69007 Lyon.
MORGON Pierre, Aventis Pasteur, 2, avenue Pont Pasteur, F-69367 Lyon.

NOMOTO Akio, University of Tokyo, Dept. of Microbiology, 7-3-1 Hongo, Bunkyo-ku, Tokyo 113-0033, Japan.

ORENSTEIN Walter, CDC, National Immunization Program, 1600, Clifton Road NE, Mail Stop E-05, Atlanta GA 30333, USA.

PALLANSCH Mark, Center for Disease Control & Prevention, 1600 Clifton Road, Mail Stop G17, Atlanta, GA 30333, USA.

PELLEGRINI Vittoria, Chiron SpA, Via Fiorentina 1,I-53100 Siena.

PELLETIER Isabelle, Institut Pasteur, 25, rue du Dr Roux, F-75724 Paris Cedex 15.

PEREZ BERCOFF Raul, University of Roma - La Sapienza, Dept of Cellular & Dev. Biology, Viale di Porta Tuburtina 28, I-00185 Roma.

PETRICCIANI John C., P. O. Box 1925, Palm Springs, CA 92263-1925, USA.

PLESNER Anne-Marie, National Board of Hearth, Amaliegade 13, DK-1012 Copenhagen.

POELOENGAN Thamrin, Bio Farma, J.I. Pasteur, 40161 Bandung-West Java, Indonesia.

ROUMIANTZEFF Micha, 1, rue Dangon, F-69004 Lyon.

SALISBURY David, Wellington House, Room 707, 133-155 Waterloo Road, London SE1 8UG, U.K.

SALUZZO Jean-François, Aventis Pasteur, Campus Mérieux, 1541 avenue Marcel Mérieux, F-69280 Marcy l'Etoile.

SANDERS Ray, W.H.O., 20, av. Appia, CH-1211 Geneva 27.

SCHILD Geoffrey C., N.I.B.S.C., Blanche Lane, South Mimms, Potters Bar, Herts. EN6 3QG, U.K.

SCHOUB Barry, National Institute for Virology, Private Bag X, Sandringham 2131, South Africa.

SCHUERMAN Lode, Smithkline Beecham Biologicals, 89, rue de l'Institut, B-1330 Rixensart.

SETYANINGSIH Harry, Bio Farma, JL Pasteur 28, 40161 Bandung, West Java, Indonesia.

SEVER John, Children's National Medical Center, Potomac, MD 20854, USA.

SHULMAN Lester, Central Virology Laboratory, Sheba Medical Center, 52621 Tel Hashomer, Israel.

SILBER Jeffrey, Merck & Co, Inc., P.O. Box 4, UNC-141, West Point, PA 19486-0004, USA.

SMITH Joseph, 95 Lofting Road, London N1 1JF, U.K.

SO Hashizume, Japan Polyomyelitis Research Institute, Hagashimurayama, 5-34-4 Kumegawa-cho, Tokyo 189-0003, Japan.

SOAVE Marie-Christine, Aventis Pasteur, Bâtiment F4 Nord, Campus Mérieux, 1541, av. Marcel Mérieux, F-69280 Marcy l'Etoile.

STOECKEL Philippe, AMP/Fondation Mérieux, 28, rue du Dr Roux, F-75015 Paris Cedex 15.

SUTTER Roland, Center for Diseases Control & Prevention, NIP (E05), CDC, Atlanta, GA 30333, USA.

SVETNER Michael, Statens Serum Institut, Artillerivej 5, DK-2300 Copenhagen S.

SWARTZ Tiberio Alex, Tel-Aviv University, Dept. of Epidemiology & Preventive Medicine, Scaekler School of Medicine, P.O. Box 39040, Ramat-aviv, 61390 Tel-Aviv, Israel.

TEUWEN Dirk, Aventis Pasteur MSD, 8, rue Jonas Salk, F-69367 Lyon.

THOELEN Stefan, Smithkline Beecham Biologicals, 89, rue de l'Institut, B-1330 Rixensart.

THYSMAN Pierre, Smithkline Beecham Biologicals, 89, rue de l'Institut, B-1330 Rixensart.

TRALLERO Gloria, Centro Nacional de Microbiologia, Instituto de Salud Carlos III, Crta Majadahonda-Pozuelo Km 102, E-28220 Madrid.

VAN DER AVOORT Harrie, RIVM/LIS, P.O. Box 1, NL-3723 WY Bilthoven.

WAETERLOOS Geneviève, Scientific Inst. of Public Health, 14, rue J. Wytsman, B-1050 Bruxelles.

WIMMER Eckard, School of Medicine, State University of New York, Dept. Molecular Genetics & Microbiology, .Stony Brook, NY 1794-5222, USA.

WOOD David J., N.I.B.S.C., Blanche Lane, South Mimms, Potters Bar, Herts EN6 3QG, U.K.

YONEYAMA Tetsuo, National Inst. of Infectious Diseases, 4-7-1 Gakuen, Musashimurayama, Tokyo 208-0011, Japan.

ZIMMERMANN Hanspeter, Swiss Federal Office of Public Health, Sägestrasse 65, CH-3098 Köniz/Berne.

Index of Authors

Symposia Series in Immunobiological Standardization

Vol. 1: Talloires 1965	Rabies
Vol. 2: Munich 1965	Neurovirulence of viral vaccines
Vol. 3: Stockholm 1965	Biotechnical developments in bacterial vaccine production
Vol. 4: Royaumont 1965	Immunological methods of biological standardization
Vol. 5: London 1966	Laboratory animals
Vol. 6: Utrecht 1966	Adjuvants of immunity
Vol. 7: Marburg/L. 1967	Assay of combined antigens
Vol. 8: Lyon 1967	Foot-and-Mouth Disease: Variants and immunity
Vol. 9: Paris 1967	Pseudotuberculosis
Vol. 10: London 1967	Biological assay methods of vaccine and sera
22nd Symp., London 1968	Standardization of immunofluorescence. Ed. Blackwell
Vol. 11: London 1968	Rubella vaccines
Vol. 12: Tunis 1968	Brucellosis. Standardization and control of vaccines and reagents
Vol. 13: Utrecht 1969	Pertussis vaccine
Vol. 14: London 1969	Standardization of interferon and interferon inducers
Vol. 15: Berne 1969	Enterobacterial vaccines
Vol. 16: Versailles 1970	Anti-lymphocytic serum
29th Symp., Brighton 1969	Hazards of handling simians. Ed. Lab. Animals Ltd. (4)
Vol. 17: Frankfurt 1970	BCG vaccine
Vol. 18: Copenhagen 1972	HL-A reagents
Vol. 19: Utrecht 1972	Smallpox vaccines
Vol. 20: London 1972	Influenza
Vol. 21: Lyon 1972	Rabies II
Vol. 22: Monaco 1973	The use of vaccines

Developments in Biological Standardization

Vol. 23: Madrid 1973	Sterilization and sterility testing of biological substances
Vol. 24: San Francisco 1973	Preservatives in biological products
Vol. 25: Lyon 1973	Requirements for poultry virus vaccines
Vol. 26: Budapest 1973	Selected veterinary vaccines
Vol. 27: Budapest 1973	Purity of human plasma proteins
Vol. 28: London 1974	Immunity to infections of the respiratory system in man and animals
46th Symp., London 1974	Breeding of simians and their uses in developmental biology. Ed. Lab. Animals Ltd. (6)

Vol. 29: Geneva 1974 (WHO/IABS)	Standardization and control of allergens administered to man
Vol. 30: Milan 1974	Viral hepatitis
Vol. 31: Rabat 1975	Brucellosis (II)
Vol. 32: Paris 1975 (OIE/IABS)	Colstridial sera and vaccines for veterinary use
Vol. 33: Douglas 1975	Vaccination by the non-parenteral route
Vol. 34: Budapest 1976	Pyrogenicity, innocuity and toxicity test systems for biological products
Vol. 35: Lyon 1976	Foot-and-mouth disease vaccines
Vol. 36: Lyon Washington D.C. 1976	Freeze-drying of biological products
Vol. 37: Geneva 1976	Standardization of cell substrates for the production of virus vaccines
Vol. 38: London 1977	Biological preparations in the treatment of cancer
Vol. 39: Geneva 1977	Influenza immunization (II)
Vol. 40: Marburg 1977	Standardization of rabies vaccines (III) (WHO/IABS)
Vol. 41: Guadeloupe 1978	Vaccinations in the developing countries
Vol. 42: Paris 1978	Second General Meeting of European Society of Animal Cell Technology
Vol. 43: Brussels 1978	Immunization: Benefit versus risk factors
Vol. 44: Villars 1979	Test methods for the quality control of plasma proteins
Vol. 45: San Antonio 1979	The Standardization of animals to improve biomedical research, production and control
Vol. 46: Oxford 1979	Third General Meeting of European Society of Animal Cell Technology
Vol. 47: Bilthoven 1980	Reassessment of inactivated poliomyelitis vaccine
Vol. 48: Geneva 1980	Standardization of albumin, plasma substitutes and plasmapheresis
Vol. 49: Leetown 1981	Fish biologics: Serodiagnostics and vaccines
Vol. 50: Heidelberg 1981	Joint ESACT-IABS Meeting on the use of heteroploid and other cell substrates for the production of biologicals
Vol. 51: Lyon 1981	Immunization of adult birds with inactivated oil adjuvant vaccines
Vol. 52: Lyon 1981	Herpes virus of man and animal: Standardization of immunological procedures
Vol. 53: Dublin 1982	Enteric infections in man and animals: Standardization of immunological procedures
Vol. 54: Athens 1982	Viral hepatitis: Standardization in immunoprophylaxis of infections by hepatitis viruses
Vol. 55: Copenhagen 1982	Fifth General Meeting of European Society of Animal Cell Technology
Vol. 56: Algeria 1983	IIIrd International Symposium on Brucellosis
Vol. 57: Paris 1983	Monoclonal antibodies: Standardization of their characterization and use
Vol. 58: Budapest 1983	BCG vaccines and tuberculins
Vol. 59: Geneva 1983	Standardization and control of biologicals produced by recombinant DNA technology
Vol. 60: Gardone Riviera 1983	Production and exploitation of existing and new animal cell substrates
Vol. 61: Geneva 1984	Proceedings of the Fourth International Symposium on pertussis
Vol. 62: Stockholm 1985	Diagnostics and vaccines for parasitic diseases
Vol. 63: San Francisco 1985	Use and standardization of chemically defined antigens
Vol. 64: London 1985	Reduction of animal usage in the development and control of biological products
Vol. 65: Amsterdam 1985	Use and standardization of combined vaccines
Vol. 66: Baden 1985	Advances in animal cell technology: cell engineering, evaluation and exploitation
Vol. 67: Melbourne 1986	Standardization in blood fractionation including coagulation factors
Vol. 68: Geneva 1986	Cells – Products – Safety
Vol. 69: London 1987	Cytokines: Laboratory and clinical evaluation

Developments in Biologicals

IMPRIMERIE MEDECINE m+h HYGIENE
octobre-2001